RADICAL
MEDICINE

D1117121

ARP Books (Arbeiter Ring Publishing)
205-70 Arthur Street
Winnipeg, Manitoba
Treaty 1 Territory and Historic Métis Nation Homeland Canada R3B 1G7
arpbooks.org

Design and layout by Relish New Brand Experience
Printed and bound in Canada by Friesens on paper made from 100% recycled
post-consumer waste.

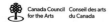 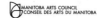

Canada Council   Conseil des arts
for the Arts   du Canada

MANITOBA ARTS COUNCIL
CONSEIL DES ARTS DU MANITOBA

Canada   Manitoba

ARP Books acknowledges the generous support of the Manitoba Arts Council
and the Canada Council for the Arts for our publishing program. We acknowledge
the financial support of the Government of Canada through the Canada Book
Fund and the Province of Manitoba through the Book Publishing Tax Credit
and the Book Publisher Marketing Assistance Program of Manitoba Culture,
Heritage, and Tourism.

LIBRARY AND ARCHIVES CANADA CATALOGUING IN PUBLICATION

Title: Radical medicine : the international origins of socialized health care in
    Canada / Esyllt W. Jones.
Names: Jones, Esyllt W., 1964- author.
Identifiers: Canadiana (print) 20190071044 | Canadiana (ebook) 20190071052 |
    ISBN 9781927886168 (softcover) | ISBN 9781927886175 (EPUB)
Subjects: LCSH: National health insurance—Canada—History—20th century. |
    LCSH: Health insurance—Saskatchewan—History—20th century. | LCSH:
    Medical policy—Canada—History—20th century. | LCSH: Medical policy—
    Saskatchewan—History—20th century. | LCSH: National health insurance—
    History—20th century. | LCSH: National health services—History—20th
    century. | CSH: Saskatchewan—Politics and government—1944-1964.
Classification: LCC RA412.5.C3 J66 2019 | DDC 368.4/200971—dc23

RADICAL MEDICINE

THE INTERNATIONAL ORIGINS OF
SOCIALIZED HEALTH CARE IN CANADA

ESYLLT W. JONES

ARP BOOKS   WINNIPEG, MB

For my family, whom I love.

And for those who made this history,
believing in the dream of health equality.

CONTENTS

ACKNOWLEDGMENTS

In December 2018, I was making final revisions to this book when Harry Leslie Smith died. Author of *Harry's Last Stand: How the World My Generation Built is Falling Down*, the octogenarian Smith's recollections about his childhood in England before the creation of the National Health Service made him a media sensation. This dignified elderly man's speech to the 2014 British Labour Party convention in Manchester brought his audience to tears. It has been watched tens of thousands of times on YouTube. What moved me most about it was how familiar it felt to me. Born in 1923, he was about the same age as my parents. Like them, he emigrated in the 1960s from Britain to Canada to find a better life for his family, and yet remained psychologically, culturally, and socially tied to the country of his birth. Having lost a sister to tuberculosis during his childhood, Smith's commitment to universal public health care arose out of his experiences of dire poverty and unequal access to medical care. Despite the adversity he faced as a young person, the history he lived through generated his belief that government could help people. Smith's story, a transnational tale of strength and hope, also embodied an obvious connection—that between lived experience and political belief.

Unlike my first book, this one is not about the lives of working families, or the bodily experience of ill health, as much as it is a history of ideas, policies, and movements. Neither is it a local story. I move across continents to follow the threads of socialized medicine. For a long time, I was motivated to track down every strand of political connection in the transnational world of health advocacy. I met the most extraordinary people in these archival meanderings, who during their lifetimes became collaborators, instigators, and then people in power. It's a long way from writing about single working class mothers and fathers, to writing about civil servants and key political advisors. And yet this journey will, I hope, make sense to my readers.

Eventually I had to come to my senses, and finish the job. The years had passed, and I had drawn on the help and advice of a lot of friends, students, colleagues, and archivists. I am going to forget to name some of those people here, probably only to recall them the minute the book is printed. My apologies in advance for these oversights.

The project began with post-doctoral funding from SSHRC, and a home at the Centre for Contemporary British History, then at the Institute for Historical Research in London, England. My supervisor there was Pat Thane. Virginia Berridge, of the London School of Hygiene and Tropical Medicine has also shown interest in this work over the years, and answered many questions, as has Martin Gorsky. While researching in Britain, I used a number of local archives and local studies libraries. Associated Medical Services funded a year of further post-doctoral study under James Hanley at the University of Winnipeg, during which the more local elements of this study began to take shape.

I took up a faculty position at University of Manitoba, and SSHRC again funded my research, which allowed me to visit archives in Regina, Montreal, Toronto, New Haven, Chapel Hill, North Carolina, and Oxford. Archivists and staff at all of the archives I consulted were wonderful. The amazing social medicine collection at Yale University held endless treasures for me. The Section for the History of Medicine at Yale gave me research space for part of a sabbatical term, where I worked on book chapters and tried not to allow myself too much time in the seductive archives. Naomi Rogers and I had many conversations about this project, and health activism in general, and her family welcomed me into their home.

Several of my former students contributed valuable research for this book, including Leah Morton, Heather Graham, and Chris

Thomas. Chris and I still frequently talk about health politics, and I like to take some credit for his career path in public health. Leah also helped me rein in my unruly citation habits to get the book ready to submit. Katrina Ackerman in Regina and Michael Chiarello in Ottawa tracked down some late stage details. James Naylor helped me with primary sources on the CCF's history; an archival tip of his allowed me to unravel what happened to Mindel and Cecil Sheps.

In Winnipeg there is a small but mighty history of medicine community, and I cannot say enough about what this has meant to me over the years. As friends and colleagues, they are an exceptional group of people. Delia Gavrus, James Hanley, Marion McKay, Chris Dooley and the late Dr. Peter Warren have all been there through some part of this project. James Hanley has been especially supportive. Any embarrassing errors about the British health system are my fault, not his. My friend and fellow historian of health Geoffrey Hudson in Thunder Bay early on encouraged me, inviting me to present my research on London health centres at the Northern Ontario School of Medicine. I have presented papers on this research at too many conferences to list here, but I thank all of my audiences for their comments and suggestions.

Adele Perry, Karen Dubinsky and Henry Yu were kind enough to invite me to contribute to their book on transnationalism and nation. Sarah Carter and Nanci Langford asked me to submit work to their forthcoming collection, *Active Women*, despite my last-minute conference bailout. It turned out that instead of presenting my research, I went on strike with my UMFA colleagues that eventful fall of 2016.

I also want to thank the family of Mindel Cherniack Sheps for their help in researching her life. Her brother Saul Cherniack, who died just last year aged 101, gave me essential information about her as I was starting out. In 2016, I delivered the Switzer-Cooperstock

Prize lecture in Western Canadian Jewish History, with Mindel's son, Sam, and his family, Saul, and other members of the extended Cherniack clan in attendance. It was a special honour to discuss Mindel's life and contribution to medicare with them. She has loomed so very large in this work, as one of the only powerful women in a book filled with men. She was brilliant and fierce and I quite fell in love with her.

The manuscript had two readers, and I've done my best to incorporate their suggested changes. When you've been with a project as long as I have been with this one, letting anyone see it can become a daunting prospect. Their generous, enthusiastic responses and useful interventions did a lot to keep me going during the end stages of preparing the manuscript.

My appreciation also goes to the scholarly community at St. John's College, University of Manitoba, where I am currently Dean of Studies. The College has been a sheltering space for me, among other things keeping me cheerful with endless light flowing through its large, prairie modernist windows, and providing me with a lot of good coffee. All of my colleagues and the staff there have a special place in my heart.

My publisher, ARP Books, has been an important part of my life for many years. It is an honour to have them take this project out into the world. Years ago, I walked through Clerkenwell with our dear friend John Samson, ARP's co-founder, to see the Finsbury Health Centre. John understood why I wanted this to be an ARP book, and supported it from the start. Todd Besant and Irene Bindi are fabulous to work with, not to mention incredibly patient with my fussiness, footnote anxieties, and delays. Thank you as well to Terry Corrigan of Relish for designing the book's interior, Jessica Antony for copy editing, and Paula Butler for indexing.

This project began its life with my younger son, Owen. I cherish a photo, taken during my first post-doctoral fellowship, of a four-month-old baby perched on my lap in front of a computer in our rented flat in Highgate. My son Dylan celebrated his four-teenth birthday with a barbeque on the roof of our neighbour's flat in London; now he is a father himself, and partner to Sarah. Our grandson Sebastian's acrobatic joy brightens our lives. I have to thank my family for their tolerance when the demands of academic life were overwhelming, and made me cranky. Which I think Owen would say was a lot of the time.

To my partner of over twenty years, Todd Scarth, I owe every-thing. Todd is an outstanding editor, and a perfectionist in the best way. His passion for this project gave me the stamina to polish the book when I was out of gas. The list of things I could not do, or ever want to do without him is long. Writing books is just one of them.

INTRODUCTION

A TRANSNATIONAL IDEA

Health Centres and the History of
Socialized Medicine in Canada

Universal health insurance, or medicare, is Canada's most cherished social program. Even more than that, it has become a touchstone of Canadian national identity. Medicare is said to embody Canada's humanitarian values and politics, especially in comparison to health policy in the United States. These associations are often mobilized today to defend the program at a time when its very survival appears constantly challenged by austerity measures, or the ideologically based claim that only private medicine can solve medicare's flaws. At the same time, the popular story of medicare has given its existence an air of historical inevitability, its inexorable emergence in the post-World War II years a natural outgrowth of Canadians' political and social identity. This is what historians call the whiggish narrative of liberal progress, one that is partly sustained by what historian Ian Mackay calls the "charismatic aura" surrounding T.C. "Tommy" Douglas, known as the father of medicare.[1] Every national myth needs a hero. Although investigated and surveilled by the RCMP during his lifetime for his leftist beliefs, a politically pacified version of Douglas's persona is now incorporated into our national story.

The other major element in that story is the birthplace of medicare: the province of Saskatchewan. Here, too, social and political complexities typically are flattened out in the service of a mythology in which pragmatic prairie people supported medicare as one of the various co-operative institutions they used to survive rural isolation and resist exploitation from heartless eastern bankers. In other words, medicare was endogenous to Saskatchewan, based fundamentally in local values and traditions, with little if any international influence. Stories such as these reconcile a belief that medicare defines us and therefore will always be with us, with a limited understanding of its history and the movement out of which it was born.

Radical Medicine tells a more complex, and less well-known story about medicare's origins in Canada. Rather than focusing solely on the national emergence of medicare in the post-war era, it moves between the local and the transnational. Douglas's Co-operative Commonwealth Federation (CCF) government in Saskatchewan created the first universal public hospitalization program in North America in 1944. *Radical Medicine* argues that the ideas and people that came together in Saskatchewan in the 1940s and early '50s to build the CCF health program were part of a transnational, and on occasion explicitly internationalist, movement for greater health equality that percolated in the context of war, pandemic, and the October Revolution, then moved across the Atlantic world, reaching its apex at the close of World War II. Admittedly, I am far from the first scholar to suggest that the "national" and the "transnational" are not completely separate and distinct spheres, but this argument is one that historians of medicare have neglected.

I first began to conceive of this research project while writing my book, *Influenza 1918: Disease, Death and Struggle in Winnipeg* (University of Toronto Press, 2007). One of the unexpected sub-themes of that book, which combined medical, labour, and social history into an examination of the differential effects of the global influenza pandemic in Winnipeg, was the struggle against medical care inequality. Researching and writing that book drew my attention to the early recognition by ordinary people that health care was a key site in the struggle for a more equal society. While it was apparent that working people had long organized themselves politically around health care, this raised another question: what was their ultimate goal? What health care system did working people want? This is not an abstract question, but rather one that mandates close attention to the ways in which institutions reflect political power.

Although *Radical Medicine* is not primarily an intellectual history, there is an idea, or an ideal, at the heart of this story. Naming it, however, is not easy. It may be helpful to begin with what it is *not*. This is not a book about liberal health politics, with an attendant emphasis on the rights and responsibilities of the individual or debates around health insurance. Rather, it is a book about collective health politics that might be labeled socialist, left wing, social democratic, communist, radical, or grassroots. While these categories apply in different ways to my subject, none on its own fully captures or adequately explains the nature of the movement I am centrally concerned with, and so I have chosen not to pick one and use it throughout. This is a history of how people engaged with the problem of health inequality that was rooted in social relations more generally, but in the problem of limited access to health care decision-making and institutional power more specifically. For some, including the radical physicians who make their way into this story, medicine itself was the target of reform: an elite institution that needed to be changed. When the CCF ran for office in 1944, one of its promises was to increase opportunities for those from all backgrounds to go to medical school and become doctors, without financial barriers. It was these young men and women trained in a socialized health care system who would lead the way to a more progressive model of care, the party believed. The CCF government's first health advisors were physicians who were actively engaged in transforming the politics of their own profession: Henry Sigerist, the Swiss historian of medicine whose book, *Socialized Medicine in the Soviet Union*, inspired a generation of young physicians to challenge

their own profession; and Mindel Cherniack Sheps, a Jewish socialist who overcame gender and anti-Semitic quotas at the University
of Manitoba School of Medicine to emerge as a brilliant political
advocate for socialized medicine.

This book focuses on the period bracketed by the Russian
Revolution and the dawn of the Cold War. These years of global
crises were also a time when "access to health care became the defining issue in the controversies surrounding the relationship between
state and society."[2] Out of these debates and controversies came a
template for health equality through socialized medicine referred to
here as the health centre model. Elements of this model were shared
among radical health advocates across the Atlantic world, who bor-
rowed and learned from each other. Strands can be found in the
health politics of the Soviet October Revolution, British Labour,
the United States during the New Deal, and beyond. The health
centre model challenged social inequality, professional hierarchy,
and elite control over health care—it was about a new way of defining the obligations of the state to guarantee health and collective
well-being. Examining this health centre model brings us closer to
understanding what advocates meant when they talked about "socialized" or "state" medicine in Canada, and how they thought it could
be achieved.

When elected in 1944, Saskatchewan's first CCF government
embraced the health centre model with considerable fanfare, but
ultimately failed to achieve its implementation. The tension between
radical aspirations and the cold realities of economic and political
power curtailed Canada's pioneering medicare programs. Rather
than a radical re-organization of health and fully socialized provision, Douglas created government health insurance for hospital (and
later physician) care. So it is in part a story that ends in failure. It is
nonetheless a powerful story with resonance for us today, as existing
government health programs face perhaps the most serious challenge
in their post-war history. Some government health programs, such

as the Affordable Care Act in the US and Britain's National Health Service, have become the focus of fierce political struggles engaging thousands of ordinary people, as well as health care professionals and policy commentators. The history of grassroots involvement in health care movements is rich ground for research.

Yet despite a high level of public interest in medicare, historians in recent decades have had relatively little to say about its political development. The most recent scholarly monograph on the history of Canadian medicare was David Naylor's *Private Practice, Public Payment: Canadian Medicine and the Politics of Health Insurance, 1911–1966*, published in 1986. It was followed in the 1990s by several important studies in related disciplines that took a comparative approach, such as Antonia Maioni's *Parting at the Crossroads: The Emergence of Health Insurance in the United States and Canada*, and Carloyn Hughes Tuohy's *Accidental Logics: The Dynamics of Change in the Health Care Arena in the United States, Britain, and Canada*. In 2012, public policy analyst Gregory Marchildon edited the volume *Making Medicare: New Perspectives on the History of Medicare in Canada*. The collection has proven a valuable resource for *Radical Medicine*, especially the contributions by health historians Heather MacDougall and Gordon Lawson.

Radical Medicine has been influenced to a greater extent than were these earlier works by a desire to interrogate the meanings of nation and nation-state development, and to explore how health advocacy slipped beyond and across national borders. Editors Karen Dubinsky, Adele Perry, and Henry Yu observe in *Within and Without the Nation: Canadian History as Transnational History*: "even the most iconic Canadian moments are forged by, and continue to be read through, a global context."[3] In a contribution to that volume, "Health and Nation Through a Transnational Lens: Radical Doctors and the History of Medicare in Saskatchewan," (an early draft of parts of chapter 4 of this book) I suggested some ways to write a history of medicare that is not simultaneously a history in service of the nation.

The book also incorporates the pertinent critiques of the welfare state that have emerged from multiple political directions over the past several decades, without rejecting the value people have ascribed to public programs.[4] Patients, providers, and advocates all have agency in any health care system, as social historians of medicine have often demonstrated. Working-class or immigrant mothers in the first half of the twentieth century, for example, accepted what was useful for their families, and attempted to ignore or reject the more normative aspects of state or quasi-public programs.[5]

Nevertheless, health care, like all state institutions, rests upon social hierarchy and inequality.[6] For the contemporary reader, it is impossible to read a history of Canadian health care without acknowledging exclusion, segregation, and experimentation upon Indigenous bodies in the name of medicine. As several historians have proven, health care programs in Canada are integral to colonialism, despite a long history of resistance.[7] Such critiques are not merely valid; they are essential. I draw from them in my evaluation of the political beliefs and actions of health care activists, because the movement for socialized medicine was not without its oversights, silences, mistakes, and bigotry. The women and men in this book wanted to change health care, through a movement to create health programs intended to help regular people exert greater control over their bodies and live better, healthier lives. It is no surprise that theirs was only a partial success. I've struggled with how to represent historical actors who were simultaneously fierce advocates for a more equitable health system, and capable of callous disregard toward, and exclusion of, Indigenous peoples. Or, how to depict socialists who expressed open anxiety about Jews in their government. In these instances, I must let my subjects speak for themselves. I have not tried to silence them, but rather to understand the intricacies and entanglements of the movement they helped to build, and to assess its record in a balanced way.

Programs such as universal medical care insurance were the

outcome of historical struggle, motivated by a belief that government could do good in the lives of ordinary people. Social and political movements in the mid-twentieth century were not naïve about the powers of the state, even a democratic state. The people in this book were survivors of and witnesses to the Depression, the struggle against fascism, a "total" war, and state-sanctioned anti-Semitism. And yet they believed in the possibility of social equality and health equity, and in their own capacity to create and run democratic state institutions. I attempt to approach the political commitment that made medicare possible on its own terms, and to probe the complex meanings of socialized medicine to a generation of activists, including physicians.

Recent histories from the US, such as Jennifer Klein's *For All These Rights*, Alan Derickson's *Health Security for All*, or Beatrix Hoffman's *Health Care for Some*, demonstrate the need to historicize health movements.[8] Especially relevant for this study, their work challenges the view that physicians and public health elites were inherently conservative (or at best moderately reformist), and that physicians predominantly opposed state health care provision. In Saskatchewan, organized medicine had a powerful oppositional voice, but so too did the health centre model of socialized medicine, whose advocates reached the highest echelons of government. The health professionals and policy experts who shaped health programs at the elite level in Saskatchewan can and should be viewed as activists. Their lifelong careers in support of movements for health equality in multiple countries illustrate this point.

Radical Medicine tells a large story, transnational in scope and taking place over several decades. Giving shape to a story this complex is definitely a challenge. The book's narrative follows a specific thread, the influence of a key idea—the health centre model of socialized medicine—and through it traces the growth of a movement across space and time. An idea is an abstract and sometimes elusive thing to pursue through history, especially if cut off from human agency and action. I have used a number of linked biographies to help me clarify and enrich this history. As sociologist James Jasper argues in *The Art of Moral Protest: Culture, Biography and Creativity in Social Movements*, individual lives matter because individuals are what movements for social change are made of.[9] Individual biographies, relationships, and encounters have proven essential, not just for the discovery of facts, but as tools through which I can convey the extraordinary nature of the connections that I, at first, read as almost chance meetings of minds and bodies, but which grew into a history of ideas shared in common across vast distances, lifelong bonds created out of shared values and experiences, a web of human debate, learning, and advocacy.

My subjects had commonalities. They were often raised in cosmopolitan households, and some of them were greatly influenced by the progressive politics of their parents (or affected by their conservatism). A significant number came from Jewish backgrounds and were enmeshed in a leftist and, for the women, feminist Jewish medical culture, again transnational in nature. They were highly educated and were swimming in the socially progressive art of the era—visual art, literature, and theatre. They were not afraid to be politically non-conformist, and perhaps drew pleasure from it. Their careers took them across nation-state boundaries, and they developed relationships shaped by their professional backgrounds, but just as importantly by their shared political commitments.

The focus of *Radical Medicine's* analysis is the Douglas government in Saskatchewan, especially its first two mandates from 1944–1952. This is where the strands of the story come together. Canada has a federalist system of government, and health care is constitutionally a provincial responsibility. The national government, beginning in the post-World War II era, contributed to and shaped health care provisions in important ways. However, it was the Saskatchewan government led by the CCF that enacted Canada's first universal government hospital coverage in 1946 and medical care insurance in 1962, after a bitter physicians' strike. The CCF, a social democratic party founded in 1932 in Canada, viewed the availability of medical care, alongside economic security, as necessary for individual self-development and self-expression.[10] The policies of the Saskatchewan CCF set the mold for federal legislation introduced in 1966, which subsequently saw universal public medical care provision introduced in all the Canadian provinces by 1972.

Premier Douglas appointed a Health Services Survey Commission almost immediately after the CCF was elected to government in Saskatchewan in June 1944. The Chair and Secretary of the 1944 Health Services Survey Commission were Henry Sigerist of Johns Hopkins University, a well-known physician, academic, and political advocate for state medicine in the US during this era, and Mindel Cherniack Sheps, an up-and-coming CCF politician and physician from Winnipeg, Manitoba. The Sigerist Commission developed the CCF's blueprint for a regionally organized health centre model. Between 1944 and 1952, the CCF embraced and then stepped away from a health centre model for socialized medicine. The Sigerist Commission's report led to the passage of the CCF's first health legislation, the Health Services Act (1945), which provided comprehensive health care for pensioners and widows, and created the Saskatchewan Health Services Planning Commission. However, implementing the Sigerist recommendations proved politically and practically challenging, encountering physician opposition and floundering in a highly decentralized framework of regional authority. In 1945, Douglas turned his focus to hospitalization insurance. The Saskatchewan Hospitalization Act was passed in 1946 and instituted universal state coverage for the cost of hospitalization, the first government program in North America to do so. The Sigerist health centre model, however, languished.

Seeking to understand this trajectory, I begin by asking: how did the health centre model come to be the gold standard for health advocates on the political left? Although the historical roots of the

health centre model are too numerous to fully identify here, the
notion that health centres could form the backbone of a socialized
system was in the air internationally beginning in the 1920s. Soviet
health care was an especially powerful source of inspiration to health
reformers. Widely read studies such as *Red Medicine: Socialized
Health in Soviet Russia*, published in 1933 by Sir Arthur Newsholme
(former Medical Officer of Health of the Local Government Board
of England and Wales) and John Adams Kingsbury (Secretary of the
Milbank Memorial Fund in New York) spoke positively of developments such as the Soviet "polyclinics," which were large health
centres, often located in industrial and factory districts, close to
workers and their families.[11] Other iterations of the health centre
model emerged in Germany, Sweden, and Britain.[12]

Chapter 1 explores western understandings of Soviet socialized
medicine, and the movement of the Soviet model into Canadian discourse. The 1920s and '30s saw thousands of western reformers and
radicals visit the Soviet Union to witness the socialist experiment,
including its health system. The most obvious connection between
the ideals of Soviet health care and Saskatchewan's vision for socialized medicine was via Henry Sigerist, who had published *Socialized
Medicine in the Soviet Union* in 1937 after his visits to the country.[13]
However, Sigerist was not the only conduit for Soviet ideals in
Canada. In 1935, prominent Canadian physicians Frederick Banting
and Norman Bethune traveled to the Soviet Union to attend the 15th
International Physiological Congress in Moscow and Leningrad, and
to witness firsthand the accomplishments of the Soviet health care
system, its embrace of science, its integration of preventive and primary care, and its progress in medical training. Like many others,
the two men were compelled by the Soviet Union's vision for health
care; both became avowed supporters of Soviet medicine and "socialized health" more generally. This chapter is based upon research in
their archival records, and offers a new interpretation of their Soviet
travels, informed by recent literature on the interaction between the

Soviet Union and the West in the inter-war period, and of the Soviet influence on the emergence of the health centre model.[14]

Historians of health in Britain have similarly argued that the Soviet Union was significant to health debates in that country. The British Labour Party's Advisory Committee on Public Health issued a report endorsing health centres in 1919. In 1920, Lord Bernard Dawson, Chair of the national government's Medical Consultative Council, proposed that health centres form the nucleus of primary care delivery in a state health system.[15] According to historian of public health, Virginia Berridge, Dawson was "in part inspired by the revolutionary changes in health care in the Soviet Union … after the October Revolution."[16] The leader of the Socialist Medical Association (SMA), Somerville Hastings, also visited the Soviet Union, and published his impressions as *Medicine in Soviet Russia*, in 1931. By the early 1930s, health centres operated by local councils featured prominently in the health policy proposals coming out of the SMA, the Medical Practitioners' Union, and the Labour Party at national and local levels. A handful of municipal health centres were built during the 1930s and early 1940s in Britain, including those constructed by four Labour-controlled borough councils in the city of London, the most famous being the landmark modernist Finsbury Health Centre, designed by Soviet émigré Berthold Lubetkin. These centres are examined in Chapter 2.

A version of the health centre model appeared again in the 1942 Interim Report of the British Medical Planning Commission, which had been established by the British Medical Association in 1940. The Medical Planning Commission's vision for model health centres appears in the archival records of Saskatchewan's Sigerist Commission, highlighting a point of connection between British and Canadian policy debates. According to historian Charles Webster, the Interim Report was "the first important planning document since the ill-fated Dawson report of 1920 to devote detailed attention to health centres as the basis for primary care."[17] The Medical

Planning Commission, although it supported health centres, did not support municipal government control. It was this relatively de-politicized version of the health centre, without local democratic control, that made its way into the Beveridge Report and ultimately influenced the Labour framework for the National Health Service (NHS). Some of the same compromises that characterized the formation of the NHS can be seen in the health policy of the Douglas government.

Chapter 3 follows this transnational dialogue into Saskatchewan's movement for socialized medicine. A.W. Johnson, in *Dream No Little Dreams*, and Bill Waiser and Stuart Houston, in *Tommy's Team*, have demonstrated that the Douglas Government brought men (mostly) from Britain, the US, and across Canada to work on policy in areas such as economic development and planning, health, and education. As he moved to establish new state-run health services, Douglas recruited to Saskatchewan "the best advisors he could find … from among people with very broad experience."[18] To a significant extent, Douglas turned to the talents of outsiders with international reputations in fields like health and economic planning. Henry Sigerist, Mindel Cherniack Sheps, her husband Cecil Sheps, Frederick Mott, Leonard Rosenfeld, Milton Roemer (the latter three all from the US, two of whom had worked in New Deal rural health programs), and later J. Wendell Macleod, the first Dean of the University of Saskatchewan College of Medicine, were among those "carpetbaggers" who brought an outside perspective to Douglas's signature early forays into health care. Their presence and ideas reflect how Saskatchewan's experience fits into a larger radical conversation about equality of the body.[19]

The movement of ideas such as the health centre model was also evident in the work of the State Hospital and Medical League, the most important grassroots health advocacy organization in the province. The League frequently articulated a transnational perspective on health care reform and, like advocates elsewhere, held

Soviet health care organization in high regard. Chapter 3 discusses
the League's development and draws together its detailed program
for socialized medicine, a program that was quite influential on the
CCF before the party came to power. By the early 1940s, the League
had an expansive publication program, supported largely by the farm
movement. In its pamphlets and booklets, the League shared knowledge with its supporters, but also advocated for a model of health
reform very similar to those proposed by advocates of socialized
medicine elsewhere in the Atlantic world. The League's history demonstrates the remarkable reach of this movement, and the power of
the health centre model of reform. It also adds a new element to our
understanding of the political base that brought the CCF to power.

Grassroots views can also be glimpsed in the proceedings of
the Sigerist Commission. The Commission received briefs from
dozens of groups and individuals advocating public health care for
Saskatchewan, from trade unions to women's organizations and
farmer groups. These briefs have never been examined by historians
to any significant extent. They are remarkable for their sophistica-
tion and their commitment to mobilizing knowledge for the good of
ordinary people. Judging from these briefs, and the publicity work of
the League, health advocacy in Saskatchewan had generated a high
level of public engagement from people who believed in their own
right and capacity to influence not just the overall direction of CCF
health policy, but its thorny, politicized details.

Chapter 3 concludes with an evaluation of the Sigerist Report
and its immediate aftermath. Henry Sigerist's role in Saskatchewan
has long been of interest to historians of medicine in Canada. In the
1990s, medical historian Jacalyn Duffin co-authored two pioneering articles about Sigerist's influence and the international attention
his involvement in the Commission brought to this small Canadian
province. *Radical Medicine* situates Sigerist's time in Saskatchewan
within his long career of health advocacy, including his calls for
health reform in the United States, and his embrace of the Soviet

health care system. Sigerist's views had an extremely long reach in the transnational movement for socialized medicine. His extensive professional networks crossed Europe and North America, and he was, as Duffin has put it, a "guru" to many physicians on the medical left.[20] Among those who revered Sigerist was the Secretary of the Sigerist Commission, the Winnipeg physician and CCF politician Mindel Cherniack Sheps. This book discusses for the first time her experience as an influential Jewish woman in the earliest days of the CCF government.

The first two years of Douglas's health policy development were shaped, then, by local politics, and by the views of Henry Sigerist and Mindel and Cecil Sheps. Mindel Cherniack Sheps worked with Sigerist on the commission itself, played an important role in planning Saskatchewan's first health care programs, and mobilized public support for a regional health centre model in rural communities. Their time together touring Saskatchewan in fall of 1944 as part of the commission had a lasting impact on both of their lives. Cecil Sheps became the first Acting Chair of the Health Services Commission in 1945, after being demobilized from venereal disease control work in the Canadian Army. Mindel and Cecil became close friends and political allies with Henry Sigerist, corresponding with him into the 1950s. Sigerist was a key point of professional and political contact between the Sheps and a broader transnational medical left in this period.

Their relationship reveals the hopeful early days of the Douglas health department, and also the emerging political realities that generated frustration and conflict, as Mindel struggled to see the Sigerist recommendations come to fruition. Mindel's brief experience in government is worth reflecting upon because she was female and Jewish and had direct access to the Premier. Mindel broke several glass ceilings. Yet her experience in Saskatchewan was ultimately a great disappointment to her personally and politically. Chapter 4 focuses on how gender and ethnic identity, along with her radicalism, shaped Mindel's political career, up to and including her time in Regina. Mindel's ideas about health and inequality emerged out of health policy research for the Manitoba and national branches of the CCF in the early 1940s. In Saskatchewan, these ideas were put to the test and Mindel, if anything, was radicalized. Her views moved closer to the health centre model of socialized medicine. Her identity and her politics, however, put her on a collision course with the Saskatchewan CCF and the Saskatchewan Medical Association. This conflict was resolved in an unfortunate way for Mindel and Cecil, who left Saskatchewan for the US in 1946, where Cecil earned his Masters degree in Public Health from Yale University. The couple's role as key health advisors was taken over by Frederick Mott, a former US Assistant Surgeon General, who had spent a decade building health programs for the rural poor through the Roosevelt Government's Farm Security Administration (FSA). Mindel and Cecil had expected to return to Saskatchewan when Cecil finished his degree, but in 1947 they were told there were no positions for them. Their time in Saskatchewan was over.

For the next several years, Fred Mott would be the single most influential health planner in Saskatchewan. A figure in the background of so many histories of this period, his contributions to Saskatchewan's health programs are under-appreciated. Perhaps this has been because he was an American and, as such, does not fit our nationalist narrative about medicare's history. Chapter 5 examines what Mott and his American colleagues learned from their experiences in the US about rural health, health care organization, and the value of a health centre model. Mott, his New Deal colleague Milton Roemer, and Leonard Rosenfeld, a former student of Henry Sigerist's, all served as senior health department staff and advisors in the first decade of the CCF government. When Mott arrived in Saskatchewan in 1946, he had been at the head of the FSA rural health programs for four years. At its peak, the FSA provided health care to as many as 200,000 of the US's most impoverished migrant farm workers, and supported the operation of health care co-operatives.[21] In their influential book *Rural Health in America*, based on their years of experience with rural health in the US, Mott and his co-author, Milton Roemer, attempted to re-define health politics in keeping with a critique of rural economies that linked the failures of capitalism, rural poverty, and inadequate access to medical services for rural populations as key to shaping the experience of rural workers—from sharecroppers, to agricultural labourers, to family farmers and Indigenous peoples.[22] A technical expert operating at an elite level of policy influence and program development, Mott was a member of what Richard Couto refers to as the "heroic bureaucracy"—a cohort of civil servants who had a "predilection for experiment over precedent and the creation and utilization of new forms of citizen-client participation in their programs" during the US's New Deal era.[23] The New Deal experiment in health care provision collapsed after the end of World War II. Mott, Roemer, and others who had supported failed national health insurance legislation while they were employees of the federal public health service, were driven out of the US government by intensifying Cold War politics.[24] Saskatchewan thus became a haven, and an opportunity.

During his tenure in Saskatchewan, Mott was responsible for an ambitious planning agenda, including the introduction of regional health boards to take over from municipal medical plans, organizing financing and administrative mechanisms for hospital care, and designing health services for widows and the impoverished (Milton Roemer was brought as a consultant on the latter). Chapter 6 follows Mott's years in Saskatchewan, when he oversaw the development of the CCF's key health care policies, including North America's first universal hospitalization scheme, introduced in 1947. In 1946, at Sigerist's recommendation, Leonard Rosenfeld joined Mott in Regina as the first Director of the Saskatchewan Hospital Services Plan. After studying with Sigerist at Johns Hopkins University from

1942–46, Rosenfeld started a public health program in Nicaragua. This public health work was part of Roosevelt's "good neighbour" policy and sponsored by the Institute of Inter-American Affairs.[25] Rosenfeld worked closely with Mott, particularly on regional boards and the framework for hospital care. Both men continued to have ongoing connections with friends, colleagues, and fellow members of the medical left in the US. These relationships were especially valuable as Mott and Rosenfeld did the intense work of building the hospitalization plan.

As Martin Lipset observed decades ago, an idea more recently re-iterated by Gordon Lawson, "the universal medical services plan introduced in Saskatchewan in 1962 was not what the CCF had intended when it first came to power in 1944."[26] While Lawson focuses on the question of physician remuneration and the debate between salaried and fee-for-service payment, my analysis in the concluding chapter of the book integrates the political struggle over physician remuneration into a bigger story about the variance between the health centre model of socialized medicine, and the actual services built by the Saskatchewan government. The health centre model, so central to the vision of progressive health advocates, was never realized and has been largely forgotten. Consequently the overwhelming focus in Canadian public policy history has been on "insurance" for hospital care and physician services. Over the course of the CCF's first two mandates, Saskatchewan's health care policies moved further and further away from the early health centre model envisioned in the Sigerist Report, and in early efforts at a regionally based rural system. Historians Joan Feather and Gordon Lawson have focused on two specific ways in which Saskatchewan diverted from its early intentions: the erosion of the role of lay governance in a regionalized system of health care; and the apparent capitulation to organized medicine through a fee-for-service model of physician payment with unlimited fee billings. Both of these lines of argument are essential to understanding the realities of CCF health policy, and indeed the two issues are tightly intertwined, though largely unsynthesized in the literature. Both scholars are addressing issues that were shaped by professional power and resistance to the health centre model.

When Fred Mott, the Health Services Planning Commission's first permanent head, took over from Cecil Sheps in 1946, decisions were made on health policy that would have longstanding repercussions for Canadian health care, particularly the introduction of the Saskatchewan Hospitalization Act. However Mott continued to hope for broader transformations through the creation of regional health units, in which treatment and preventive services would be melded. Regional boards were to be elected by district health councils, themselves made up of municipal representatives. In 1947, Mott referred to this as a network of health care, built upon district hospitals and regional centres where specialist care and recent technologies would be accessible to local practitioners and their patients. This network would rely upon the principles of co-operative group physician practice, with a cap on the overall costs of physician care in each region, to ensure affordability in a public system.

Telling the story of the regional health centre model shifts long-standing interpretations of medicare's development. Malcolm Taylor's classic 1987 study of Canadian health care, *Health Insurance and Canadian Public Policy*, referred to Saskatchewan's decision in 1946 to create a system of compulsory hospital care insurance as the "first decisive action in the long chain of events leading to our present system."[27] Yet this reading, in its presentism, should be revisited. While the decision to provide universal hospital coverage through a combination of personal and family premiums and government revenues was a hallmark accomplishment in the CCF's first mandate, hospitalization was at the time intended to be one part of an integrated system of care. Only by virtue of the fact that other elements of the health centre model failed to materialize can we place pre-paid hospital care on its own as one of the "seven decisions that created the Canadian health insurance system," as the sub-title of Malcolm Taylor's book argues.

Moreover, the political, financial, and organizational energy taken up by the early implementation of universal, compulsory public hospital care insurance is key to understanding the government's successes and its failures. The "major health reform initiated in the early years of the CCF government," it tilted health services heavily towards the institutional, tertiary end of the care spectrum.[28] As the CCF's lynchpin policy, hospitalization had to be made a success. The CCF's re-election depended upon it. The effort it took to establish accessible, universal hospitalization crowded out other elements of the CCF's original health planning framework—an opportunity that has also been lost to history.

Radical Medicine concludes in the mid-1950s, just as the first universal federal health care funding programs were being introduced in Canada (the Hospital Insurance and Diagnostic Services Act was passed in 1957). Full medicare inclusive of physician services would not be introduced until 1966, after Saskatchewan had again played a historic role by insuring physician care, despite a bitter physicians' strike in opposition to medicare in 1962. The periodization of my study is chosen to correspond to a span of political openness, during which the ideals of the medical left remained influential. By the mid-1950s the Cold War had altered the landscape of health politics in North America. Henry Sigerist was driven out of the US in the late 1940s as a communist sympathizer. Milton Roemer, hired by the World Health Organization, was investigated by the US government and the FBI, and had his passport withdrawn in Geneva in 1951. Mott and Rosenfeld both returned to the US, where they would never again hold positions in government. In 1951 Mott departed Saskatchewan for Washington, where he worked to establish a series of hospitals for the radical United Mine Workers of America, led by John L. Lewis. He would later work with Walter Reuther and the

United Automobile Workers to establish a network of community health centres in Detroit. Late in his life, he would return to Canada as a professor of public health at the University of Toronto. Like the Sheps's, his was a life lived across borders.

In 2001, Harvard historian and writer for *The New Yorker,* Jill Lepore, published an influential essay called "Historians Who Love Too Much: Reflections on Micro-History and Biography." As Lepore notes, writing about people, living or dead, is "tricky work," asking the historian to balance intimacy with distance.[29] Falling in love with one's subject is the biographer's pitfall, and yet it is also our opportunity for insight. The feelings that come with even a modest amount of intimacy—reading letters, looking at photographs, talking to family members, following the contours of a life—can make objective assessment more difficult. Yet, without that connection to our subjects, our work can become lifeless and without empathy. A historian who writes biography must convince her audience that her evaluation of a life is fair and balanced, but also that her examination of subjectivity and life history lends greater insight. By attending to the emotions and mental life of both author and subject, biography can humanize intellectual and policy history.

My subjects frequently experienced emotional connections with one another, something often neglected in political histories of medicare. Jeff Goodwin points to the reciprocal emotions present in social movements, the close affective ties of friendship, love, and loyalty generated by the practice of politics.[30] All social movements involve emotions and emotional work, Goodwin argues, "even the most professional and bureaucratic movements."[31] This is an important point, because many of the central actors in this story are not typical social activists. They are elite professionals, who have direct access to state power. At the same time, advocates of socialized medicine were passionate people. Their relationships to each other, and to the shared goal of health equality, shaped their lives and careers.

Sometimes these relationships were formalized (within political parties or activist groups, for example), sometimes they were informal (hearing an inspirational speech or reading a key author). Linkages could be direct, when historical actors related to each other in personal relationships, and they happened in varied types of connection: from kinship, friendship, or romantic love; to the exchange of information; to joint participation in specific social movement activities. Ties making up a social movement network need not mean face-to-face interaction in a specific organization or group. "Linkages may also consist of more ideational, cognitive and emotional exchanges."[32] They can be constituted purely through ideas and knowledge. Social movement networks can therefore be shaped indirectly, reflecting common participation in a broader movement in which individuals may never meet or correspond.

The history covered by this book was characterized by optimism that the welfare state could generate a more equal society. This belief engendered passion, formed the basis for relationships, and helped to create a health care movement that crossed the borders of nation states. In 1971, Barbara Cadbury (wife of George Cadbury, a key economic advisor to the Douglas Government), an English immigrant, socialist, and one of the future founders of Planned Parenthood Canada, spoke at the memorial service for her friend and comrade Mindel Cherniack Sheps. Cadbury's reflections suggest the emotional power of the friendship between two "carpetbagger" families who had been recruited to Saskatchewan, and the ways that the first Douglas government evoked memories of political idealism and personal loyalty:

My family first met the Sheps, Mindel and Cecil, right after the last war. We were helping to build the first democratic socialist government in North America, in the province of Saskatchewan, on the Canadian prairies, and the air was lively with meaning and hope. There was a great gathering of social democratic comrades from this continent, and my husband from England, all qualified in their different fields to be the finest of public servants, all inspired to be more than that. ... That prairie town was never lonely for me, a Londoner, with Mindel a block away.[33]

In this moment of mourning, Barbara Cadbury recalled the power of the political beliefs that had brought the two families together, and their sense of being present, alongside each other, as history was being made. She admitted that there came a time when "inspiration diminished... In youth you do not realise that the dawn cannot last all day." But this realization was also a part of their shared history.

Ideas, however powerful, are not on their own sufficient to help us understand the past. Neither are political parties, policies, or institutions. *Radical Medicine* is the story of all these things, but it is also, perhaps more fundamentally, the story of people who acted together to make socialized medicine a movement, to give it life.

ENDNOTES

1 Ian McKay, "For A New Kind of History: A Reconnaissance of 100 Years of Canadian Socialism," *Labour / Le Travail* 46 (Fall 2000), 96.

2 Antonia Maioni, *Parting at the Crossroads: The Development of Health Insurance in Canada and the United States* (Princeton, NJ: Princeton University Press, 1998), 5.

3 Karen Dubinsky, Adele Perry, and Henry Yu, *Within and Without the Nation: Canadian History as Transnational History* (Toronto: University of Toronto Press, 2015), 4.

4 For a US example see Sheila D. Collins and Gertrude Schaffner Goldberg, eds., *When Government Helped: Learning from the Successes and Failures of the New Deal* (New York: Oxford University Press, 2014).

5 Denyse Baillargeon, *Babies for the Nation: The Medicalization of Motherhood in Quebec, 1910-1970* (Waterloo: Wilfred Laurier University Press, 2009).

6 Cynthia R. Comacchio, *Nations Are Built of Babies: Saving Ontario's Mothers and Children, 1900-1940* (Montreal and Kingston: McGill-Queen's University Press, 1998); Mona Gleason, *Small Matters: Canadian Children in Sickness and Health* (Montreal and Kingston: McGill-Queen's University Press, 2013); Nancy Christie, *Engendering the State: Family, Work and Welfare in Canada* (Toronto: University of Toronto Press, 2000).

7 Mary-Ellen Kelm, *Colonizing Bodies: Aboriginal Health and Healing in British Columbia, 1900-1950* (UBC Press, 1999); Maureen K. Lux, *Separate Beds: A History of Indian Hospitals in Canada, 1920s-1980s* (Toronto: University of Toronto Press, 2016); Mary Jane Logan McCallum, *Indigenous Women, Work, and History: 1940-1980* (Winnipeg: University of Manitoba Press, 2000).

8 Jennifer Klein, *For All These Rights: Business, Labor, and the Shaping of America's Public-Private Welfare State* (Princeton NJ: Princeton University Press, 2004); Alan Derickson, *Health Security for All: Dreams of Universal Health Care in America* (Baltimore: Johns Hopkins University Press, 2005); Beatrix Hoffmann, *Health Care for Some* (Chicago: University Of Chicago Press, 2012).

9 James M. Jasper, *The Art of Moral Protest: Culture, Biography, and Creativity in Social Movements* (Chicago; Chicago: University Of Chicago Press, 1999), 215.

10 A.W. Johnson, *Dream No Little Dreams: A Biography of the Douglas Government in Saskatchewan, 1944-1961* (Toronto: University of Toronto Press, 2004).

11 Arthur Newsholme and John Adams Kingsbury, *Red Medicine: Socialized Health in Soviet Russia* (Garden City, New York: Doubleday, 1933).

12 Paul Weindling, "Public Health in Germany," in *The History of Public Health and the Modern State*, ed. Dorothy Porter (Amsterdam: Rodopi, 1994), 125; K. Johannisson, "The People's Health: Public Health Policies in Sweden," in *The History of Public Health and the Modern State*, ed. Dorothy Porter (Amsterdam: Rodopi, 1994), 179.

13 Henry E. Sigerist, *Socialised Medicine in the Soviet Union* (London: Victor Gollancz, 1937).

14 Michael Bliss, *Banting: A Biography* (Toronto: McClelland and Stewart, 1984); Roderick Stewart and Sharon Stewart, *Phoenix: The Life of Norman Bethune* (Montreal and Kingston: McGill-Queen's University Press, 2011).

15 Frank Honigsbaum, *The Division in British Medicine: A History of the Separation of General Practice From Hospital Care, 1911-1968* (London: Kogan Page, 1979), 64–68; Abigail Beach, "Potential for Participation: Health Centres and the Idea of Citizenship 1920-1940," in *Regenerating England: Science, Medicine and Culture in Interwar Britain*, ed. C. Lawrence and A.K. Mayer (Amsterdam: Rodopi, 2000), 208; Virginia Berridge, "Health and Medicine," in *The Cambridge Social History of Britain, 1750-1950*, ed. F.M. L. Thompson (Cambridge, UK: Cambridge University Press, 1990), 227.

16 Virginia Berridge, "Polyclinics: Haven't We Been There Before?," *British Medical Journal* 336 (2008), 1161.

17 Charles Webster, "Beveridge after 50 Years," *British Medical Journal* 305, 6859 (October 17, 1992), 901.

18 A.W. Johnson, *Dream No Little Dreams*, 77.

19 J. Wendell Macleod was significantly influenced, as were the Sheps, by the internationalism of Norman Bethune. Macleod had worked with Bethune in the Montreal Group for the Security of the People's Health. See Louis Horlick, *J. Wendell Macleod: Saskatchewan's Red Dean* (Montreal and Kingston: McGill-Queen's University Press, 2007), 20-24; Wendell MacLeod, Libbie Park, and Stanley B. Ryerson, *Bethune: The Montreal Years* (Toronto: James Lorimer & Company, 1978); Libbie Park, "The Bethune Health Group," in David A.E. Shepard and Andrée Lévesque, eds., *Norman Bethune: His Times and His Legacy* (Ottawa: The Canadian Public Health Association, 1982), 138-144.

20 Jacalyn Duffin and Lesley Falk, "Sigerist in Saskatchewan: The Quest for Balance in Social and Technical Medicine," *Bulletin of the History of Medicine* 70, 4 (1996), 658–83; Jacalyn Duffin, "The Guru and the Godfather: Henry Sigerist, Hugh MacLean, and the Politics of Health Care Reform in 1940s Canada," *Canadian Bulletin of Medical History* 9 (1992), 191–218.

21 Michael R. Grey, *New Deal Medicine: The Rural Health Programs of the Farm Security Administration* (Baltimore and London: Johns Hopkins University Press, 1999).

22 Frederick Dodge Mott and Milton I. Roemer, *Rural Health and Medical Care* (New York: McGraw-Hill, 1948).

23 Robert Couto, "Heroic Bureaucracies," *Administration and Society* 23, (1991), 123–47.

24 Alan Derickson, "The House of Falk: The Paranoid Style in American Health Politics," *American Journal of Public Health* 87, 11 (November 1997), 1836–43.

25 Rosenfeld and his wife Irene were lifelong friends of the Sheps, and both men were associated from the 1970s on with what became known as the Cecil G. Sheps Center for Health Services Research at University of North Carolina Chapel Hill, still open today.

26 Seymour Martin Lipset, *Agrarian Socialism: The Cooperative Commonwealth in Saskatchewan* (Berkeley: University of Chicago Press, 1950); Gordon S. Lawson, "The Road Not Taken: The 1945 Health Services Planning Commission Proposals and Physician Remuneration in Saskatchewan," in *Making Medicare: New Perspectives on the History of Medicare in Canada*, ed. Gregory P. Marchildon (Toronto: University of Toronto Press, 2012), 395.

27 Malcolm Taylor, *Health Insurance and Canadian Public Policy: The Seven Decisions That Created the Health Insurance System and Their Outcomes* (McGill-Queen's Press, 1987), 69.

28 Aleck Ostry, "Prelude to Medicare: Institutional Change and Continuity in Saskatchewan, 1944-1962," *Prairie Forum* 20, 1 (1995), 88.

29 Jill Lepore, "Historians Who Love Too Much: Reflections on Microhistory and Biography," *The Journal of American History* 88, 1 (June 2001), 129.

30 Jeff Goodwin, James M. Jasper, and Francesca Polletta, *Passionate Politics: Emotions and Social Movements* (Chicago: University of Chicago Press, 2001).

31 Goodwin, Jasper, and Polletta, *Passionate Politics*, 15.

32 Mario Diani, "Network Analysis," in *Methods of Social Movement Research*, ed. Bert Klandermans and Suzanne Staggenborg (Minneapolis: University of Minnesota Press, 2002), 178.

33 Transcript of "Memorial Service for Mindel Cherniack Sheps, January 18, 1973, University of North Carolina, Chapel Hill," courtesy of Saul Cherniack.

CHAPTER 1

FROM MOSCOW WITH LOVE

Soviet Medicine and Interwar Medical Advocacy for Socialized Medicine

The year 1935 saw a peak in foreign visitors arriving in the Soviet Union to witness firsthand the great socialist experiment. From the early 1920s on, Soviet agencies were actively promoting abroad the achievement of their state in areas such as education and health, as well as the advancement of science and industry. In 1935, prominent Canadian physicians Frederick Banting and Norman Bethune became two of those over 100,000 foreigners who travelled to the USSR in the 1920s and 1930s—intellectuals and writers, activists, journalists, artists, as well as economists, social scientists, physicians, and scientists. British Fabians and Labour Party activists Beatrice and Sydney Webb published *Soviet Communism: A New Civilization* in 1935, after their visit.[1] Canadian visitors included Frank Scott, Graham Spry, J.S. Woodsworth, Eugene Forsey, Hugh MacLennan, and Rose Henderson,[2] as well as former Lieutenant Governor of Manitoba Roland Fairburn McWilliams and his wife Margaret McWilliams, who visited in 1926 and published *Russia in 1926* the following year.[3] "These interwar visits marked a period of intensive Soviet-western cultural and intellectual interactions."[4]

Historians have differed in their assessments of visitors to the Soviet Union. Paul Hollander's 1981 book, *Political Pilgrims: Travels of Western Intellectuals to the Soviet Union, China and Cuba, 1928–1978*,

characterized westerners visiting the Soviet Union as "pilgrims"—
those already committed in advance to seeing the Soviet experience
in a positive light, and whose understanding of what they saw in
the USSR was both highly mediated (if not actively manipulated)
by Soviet authorities and fundamentally politically naïve. This
position has more recently been restated in the work of Ludmilla
Stern.[5] Michael David-Fox, author of the compelling and sophis-
ticated study of Soviet-western engagement during the 1920s and
1930s, *Showcasing the Great Experiment*, has observed that much of
the literature about travellers has been polemical in nature and takes
a particularly dim view of western intellectuals as willfully blind and
utopian. David-Fox's response is that such a perspective forecloses
serious study of one of the most important cultural, intellectual,
and political exchanges in twentieth century history, which shaped
Soviet culture, ideology, and politics much as it shaped Europe and
North America.[6] The same might also be said of the interconnec-
tions between Soviet health and movements for socialized medicine
elsewhere, which has yet to be fully studied.

Admittedly, Soviet visitation from the West is a complex historical problem. Why were visitors apparently so impressed, focusing on
the best and ignoring the worst? What drew them by the thousands
to witness firsthand the Soviet experiment? David-Fox notes a deep
irony in the fact that the peak of foreign admiration for the Soviets
corresponded with the height of Stalinism, with all its attendant
horrors. The question of what people knew and when they knew
it has long underpinned debates about western leftists and Soviet
communism. The most obvious way to address this issue might be to
argue that travellers had leftist commitments and let ideology blind
them. Yet, this is not a satisfying or necessarily accurate assessment.
In her study of Australian "political travellers," eminent Soviet historian Sheila Fitzpatrick notes that many were not communists or
political radicals. There was a range of opinion among them about
the so-called Soviet miracle, some of it quite critical.[7] David-Fox has

made the most nuanced evaluation of the Soviet-western exchange. He refers to the Soviet Union, with its status as neither fully western nor non-western, as the "proximate 'Other'"—an alternate modernity that "combined appealing familiarity with radical novelty."[8] David-Fox makes an observation that is quite pertinent to the appeal of Soviet medicine: aspects of Soviet development that most appealed to westerners, such as social welfare provision, were not *sui generis*, but rather had been adapted from a long-standing circulation of ideas and practices within a broader European context. Health care in the Soviet Union had acknowledged connections with German social medicine, for example. In other words, it was not that Soviet health care was entirely novel to foreigners, but rather that it combined elements of social medicine in intellectual circulation in Europe and North America with the particular capacities of the Soviet state to generate radical reform.

The response to Soviet medicine *was* utopian in the sense that, for those from elsewhere, it represented unfulfilled hopes and aspirations for better health and medical care. It helped, of course, that the Soviets, especially in the 1920s and early 1930s, valued physicians and medical researchers. Foreign physicians and medical researchers witnessed their Soviet counterparts as key actors in the Soviet experiment—a role they might desire for themselves in their own societies—hence the appeal to westerners of I.P. Pavlov (idolized up to and during the Stalinist era), or even Nikolai Semashko (the first head of the Commissariat for the People's Health, who lost his position in 1930). As David-Fox notes, during the 1920s Semashko was a star outside of the Soviet Union: "all of intellectual Berlin showed up," when he spoke publicly.[9]

In health care, the 1930s were a period of innovation, but also of extremely frustrating setbacks for advocates of social medicine, and even more so for individuals like Henry Sigerist who believed in *socialist* medicine. In an atmosphere of vocal critique of the status quo, the Soviet experiment was not only a potential source of inspiration, it was also a signal of western liberal inferiority vis-à-vis a socialist state, and a foil against which the status quo might be exposed.

Part of the goal of this project is to bring insights from the literature on Soviet travellers into the history of health policy and politics in Canada. Any attempt to do so must necessarily confront lacunae in several areas. First, Canadian travel to witness the Soviet project has not been examined in any sustained way, with the exception of work by Kirk Niegarth. A full picture of Canadian political travellers has yet to emerge. Second, those Canadians who visited specifically to view Soviet socialized medicine are largely forgotten, which really requires a project of recovery too large for this study. Finally, no full-length work exists that explores the circulation of Soviet ideas about health, science, and medicine in the West during these years, whether through direct visitation or indirectly, through books and pamphlets, political affiliations, intellectual circles, or friendships. Little of the literature on Soviet travellers discusses visits from medical experts.[10]

Useful insights into the role of Soviet health politics do exist. Peter J. Kuznick's 1987 study *Beyond the Laboratory: Scientists as Political Activists in 1930s America* devotes two chapters to the relevance of the Soviet model to American scientists and physicians.[11] Susan Gross Solomon's work focuses upon the interaction between the Soviet Union and Germany. Since the 1990s, Henry Sigerist's Soviet travels have been extensively studied (and will be discussed shortly). The literature, such as it exists, does tend to be rooted in particular nation-states, however, and has not yet tackled the question of how the Soviet model circulated across multiple borders, through wide-reaching networks of knowledge and advocacy, and itself became a conduit for the transnational interaction and movement of ideas. This gap makes the broader transnational context for Canadian discussions of Soviet medicine a challenge to establish.

Western historical interest in both Russian and post-revolutionary

Soviet medicine is long-standing, and has shifted toward social medicine, or "social hygiene," a previously neglected aspect of Soviet health care history.[12] This interest in Soviet social hygiene has itself served to reveal accounts of Soviet health care written by foreign travellers who visited Russia during the 1920s and 1930s. For the most part, these accounts were virtually forgotten, "dismissed by many as ideology," as Susan Gross Solomon has observed, until the scholarship of the past twenty years retrieved them. In the Canadian case, any assessment of Soviet traveller accounts comes from biographers. Predictably, evaluation of Banting's and Bethune's Soviet encounters has been over-determined by the political sympathies of their respective biographers, if not their subjects themselves. Michael Bliss argues that Banting was essentially duped into his positive assessment of the Soviet Union.[13] Bethune's biographers, by contrast, credit his Soviet visit as important to his conversion to communism, and do not critically evaluate his Soviet experience or set it in the broader context of mutual Soviet-western interactions, especially on the subject of health.

Nevertheless, Soviet socialized medicine circulates widely in debates germane to interwar health politics, and not only on the political left. As Kuznick has noted, "articles on Soviet socialized medicine overflowed the bounds of the medical journals, appearing with regularity in the scientific press and the popular media."[14] American material, whether for a professional or a popular audience, would have been read by Canadians. Canadian visitors like Banting and Bethune played their own role in public persuasion, taking interviews, giving speeches, organizing advocacy groups, and writing for a broad public readership. The network formed by those intrigued by Soviet medicine was fascinatingly complex and diverse. This chapter will follow several traces of Soviet influence, from direct observation, assessment, and public commentary, to points of discussion and borrowing that were less direct. The most direct link between Soviet socialized medicine and developments in Saskatchewan was

Henry Sigerist. But, as we shall see, Sigerist was only one of several participants in the conversation.

Immediately after the revolution, public health and medical care were seen by Soviet leaders as the key to the development of the new state's stability and productivity, and as fundamental to the political and social identity of a socialist society. As Tricia Starks has noted in a largely critical study, "revolutionaries characterized health programs as necessary for more than mere survival ... revolutionaries pledged to provide the people with better living quarters, improved working conditions, and universal medical care."[15] Drawing from earlier traditions in Russian health care, such as *zemstvo* and community medicine, and building upon workers' insurance medicine in the years leading up to 1917, early Soviet medicine—what came to be known as social hygiene—was nonetheless a distinct set of ideas and practices that sought to approach health as a fundamentally social issue, and to prioritize the medical needs of the proletariat *as a class*, rather than those of the patient as individual.[16] The People's Commissariat of Public Health (known as Narkomzdrav) was created in 1918. Its first leader was the physician Nikolai Semashko, who described Soviet medicine as "the offspring of October," and the "hygiene of the underprivileged."[17] In June 1918, Semashko articulated the main goals of the new Soviet medicine: unification of health care administration; universally available medical care; and preventive medicine through improved sanitation and social measures.[18]

Historians have pointed to the desire among Bolsheviks and radical health experts to create the Soviet Union's "own medicine," encompassing not only medical administration and practice, but also medical education and scientific research.[19] Any attempt to define the precise nature of Soviet medicine is, however, confronted with the tension between ideals and realities. For the purpose of this study, which looks at western perceptions of Soviet health care and the adoption of the Soviet model as an ideal type to which western medicine might aspire, ideals are, of course, important. In order to evaluate the degree to which westerners were sold an ideology that fell short in its implementation, we must also of course pay attention to the failings of early Soviet medicine, particularly the impact of the Cultural Revolution, and the Stalinist era.

While the full intricacies of Russian medical care before the revolution are beyond the scope of this study, it should be noted that the Bolsheviks did inherit a system of tsarist health care provision in which centralization and state power had long been evident. "The doctor [was] a public servant" in the tsarist tradition, as historian Neil Weissman has noted. Although private medicine existed, physicians were educated at state institutions, and were obligated to perform certain functions in service of the state and public health.[20] Toward the end of the tsarist period, the health system faced increasing demands for reform, including pressures for greater local control and self-government, and a higher degree of physician autonomy, consistent with overall moves towards medical professionalization occurring simultaneously in the West. There were also demands for improved access to medical care for the working class. In 1912, the Social Democrats led a workers' health insurance movement for medical coverage, sickness and disability benefits, and worker administration of their own hospitals and medical centres. Such attempts at reform largely failed.

In the pre-revolutionary period, the Bolsheviks promised universally available free medical care to the working class, but the specifics of their health program and how it was to be organized were not especially clear. When the dust settled after 1917, Narkomzdrav and the Soviet leadership pursued centralization. Decentralized worker control of health care, advocated earlier by the workers' movement, was set aside.[21]

Although controversial and resisted by many physicians, Narkomzdrav's leadership believed that further unification and centralized control of health care services was the only way to guarantee a genuinely Soviet system of health care and to maximize the use of

scarce resources. Central organization very quickly became important in the battle against infectious disease, which raged during the
civil war (1918–1921). Between the beginning of 1918 and mid-1920, the
Soviets recorded five million cases of typhoid alone.[22]

The Soviet leadership (including Lenin) had a very high regard
for scientific and technical expertise, held largely in this period by
social elites with access to advanced education, including physicians
and medical researchers. Thus, as Weissmann has argued, the Soviet
leadership moved to mollify physicians, and smooth over opposition to Bolshevism, sometimes through the firm suppression of
dissent and sometimes by offering physicians input and influence.
Narkomzdrav also supported occupational hierarchy in health care,
privileging the position of physicians over that of *feldshers* (physician
assistants), for example. Soviet policy wished to cultivate the growth
of specialized knowledge in medicine and saw physicians as valued
experts. A defining characteristic of Soviet medicine was to be the
universal provision of expert physician care—provision by providers
such as *feldshers* or midwives was at times viewed as second best.[23]

During the 1920s, Narkomzdrav worked to forge a new discipline of Soviet medical science, labeled social hygiene, defined by
one of its prominent supporters as "the study of the influence of economic and social factors on the health of the population and on the
ways to improve that health." A.V. Mol'kov went further to describe
the centrality of social factors and the necessity to re-orient medicine
accordingly: medicine "while not tearing itself away from its biological grounding and its natural science basis, is by its nature and
its goals a sociological problem."[24] Soviet social hygiene's new vision
for the physician of the future is worth quoting at length. Medical
education should provide:

1. a serious natural science preparation, as familiar with physico-
    chemical and biological sciences as with the laws underlying the
    biological processes;

2. enough social science background to comprehend the social environment;
3. materialist thinking without which it is impossible to understand the relationship of an organism to its environment;
4. the ability to examine the patient in relation to his work life and lifestyle;
5. the ability to study the occupational and social conditions which give rise to illness and not only to cure the illness, but to suggest ways to prevent it.[25]

Social hygiene was to provide "its own type of political literacy in the medical schools," Semashko claimed.[26] All medical instruction was to proceed according to the "synthesis of curative and preventive medicine." Universalism in Soviet medical education during the 1920s meant that all general physicians were to receive this training in a "socio-biological" approach to medicine. Soloviev, the Deputy Commissar, called for the inclusion of prevention in clinical training itself, or full integration of the care and cure concepts.

Proponents of Soviet social hygiene also had an active agenda for medical research, which was to provide knowledge of and evidence for the social underpinning of health. Solomon has pointed to the intellectual transaction between Soviet hygiene and early twentieth-century German social medicine, which Semashko openly acknowledged. Interested mostly in diseases that had a demonstrable social aspect (or one that could be documented through scientific research), the Soviet research agenda in the 1920s included studies of population (birth, death, migration), consumption and nutrition, social diseases (alcoholism, narcotic use, venereal disease), sex life, workplace health, housing, education, and leisure. Research topics in these areas were approached through emerging methodologies such as demography, social surveys and questionnaires, and analyzing patients' views of their medical histories.[27]

The height of Soviet social hygiene was reached by 1926-1927.

With the rise of Stalin and the beginning of the cultural revolution in 1928, Soviet medicine took a different course, and the ideals of social hygiene were increasingly sacrificed to the goals of rapid indus-trialization and collectivization. While the rhetoric of social hygiene remained, much of its intellectual and political underpinning, par-ticularly Semashko's notion of *zhalo* ("social sting"), a critique of social factors, had become a liability. Ironically, in this regard, the Soviet leadership became as hostile to social hygiene as were many in the West, who opposed its implicit indictment of capitalism and capitalist medicine.

Christopher Williams has documented the health impact of the revolution from above during the First Five Year Plan (FYP), from 1928–1932. The Soviet leadership began to attack those med-ical specialists it had worked so diligently to cultivate during the revolutionary and New Economic Policy (NEP) period. The NEP, brought in by Lenin to return growth to a Soviet economy dev-astated by the Civil War (1918-1922), mixed elements of a market economy and central planning. It thus represented a temporary relaxation of state control over the economy. This interval of rela-tive openness had parallels in Soviet health policy, but there, too, it was short-lived. During the first FYP, physicians and researchers were increasingly disparaged as bourgeois specialists; those not in line with Stalinist policies, including Semashko, the key architect of Narkomzdrav, were purged. The first FYP also reversed many of the health care advances made in the early 1920s. With the revolu-tion and civil war behind them, Soviet citizens had begun to enjoy improved per-capita food consumption, better sanitation, hygiene, and education, and reduced morbidity and mortality from infec-tious disease. Together, these meant a rise in life expectancy. From 1928–1932, by contrast, the industrial working class saw a decline in its overall standard of living. In Leningrad, daily caloric intake fell to levels not seen since 1921. Food rationing was introduced after 1928. Housing space and quality were declining. Labour productivity drives in the factories were causing higher rates of workplace accidents and "damaging workers' health."[28] Available data suggest that the 1920s saw improvements in overall morbidity rates from infectious diseases in urban areas, although compared with pre-World War I rates, these were relatively modest. In Leningrad, for example, Williams tracked morbidity from eight infectious diseases over time. Rates for these illnesses ranged from 244.5/10,000 in 1913, to a peak of 615.0 in 1919, to 185.5 in 1927, the year before the revolution from above was implemented. Disease rates continued to fall through the late 1920s, but then appeared to rise again in 1930. The more damning situation, however, arose in other regions of the Soviet Union. In Kiev, disease mortality more than doubled between 1930 and 1933, as it did in the Kharkov region; Odessa was not far behind.[29]

Although the improvement of labour and living conditions remained a stated goal, the main focus of health care shifted away from the principles of social hygiene towards increasing the level of medical care provision. Above all, the health care system had to prove its pragmatic utility in serving the needs of economic development. In this sense, social hygiene research and medical teaching curricula that devoted time to prevention might not have met the mark.[30] Curative, not preventive care became the main priority in a context of declining health spending and inadequate resources. Susan Gross Solomon has argued that after 1930, the principles of social hygiene survived mostly in the work of the polyclinics. Polyclinics and dispensaries were seen by western observers as particularly innovative elements of the Soviet health care system, and they would inform the health centre model.

Mark G. Field noted over forty years ago that Soviet health care, like other aspects of Soviet socialist "progress," was used to convey to people all over the world that a Soviet model of government was the best at providing health care, superior to capitalist medicine. Field argued, "Socialized medicine has, thus, an important political and ideological appeal, and becomes a part of the struggle for the minds and loyalties of men the world over." Furthermore, claims to a high-quality, universal health care system that provided for the needs of all citizens held a particular value, beyond ideology. "For the existence, or lack, of medical services has an intense emotional significance to all people: their life, their health, their well-being and the welfare of those who are most dear to them."[31]

Soviet innovation in health provision was closely watched on the European continent, in Britain, and in North America, and not only by communists or fellow travellers. Visits to the Soviet Union by physicians and public health experts were common, especially after the late 1920s. Several western visitors released high-profile studies of Soviet health. In 1933 came the release of *Red Medicine: Socialized Health in Soviet Russia*, written by Sir Arthur Newsholme (former Medical Officer of Health of the Local Government Board of England and Wales) and John Adams Kingsbury (Secretary of the Milbank Memorial Fund in New York).[32] *Red Medicine* was itself a transnational collaboration, between men in two countries with different histories and philosophies of state involvement in health and social welfare. Despite their differences of opinion over aspects of Soviet society (particularly civil rights and liberties, the suppression of religion, and Soviet attitudes towards divorce, birth control, and abortion), the authors enthused about Soviet achievements "in developing a comprehensive health system that united preventive and curative functions."[33]

Red Medicine, like the travelogues of other westerners, begins with the journey itself:

> Our journey together began on August 2, 1932, in Southampton Water on board the *S.S. Bremen*, en route from New York to Bremerhaven. We had already prepared ourselves by much reading about Russia and by conferences with others who had

recently visited that country. Summaries of information, as well as the questions we intended to ask, had been set down on paper. On board the *Bremen* was an American newspaper correspondent, long experienced in Moscow, with whom one of us had frequently conferred on the way from New York. Both of us now shared the discussion of Russia as viewed by this experienced interpreter of daily events in the Soviet Union.[34]

Newsholme and Kingsbury argued that significant overall progress had been made in the health status of the Soviet population, and in the expansion of health care provision. They were particularly interested in the mechanics of health care, including financing and administration. Their study provided knowledge to westerners about how health care was organized. Although not extremely detailed or systematic, which is unsurprising given the Soviet control over access to information, their account did clarify the mechanisms of health care delivery in the period. According to Newsholme and Kingsbury, primary health care of a non-acute nature was delivered almost entirely by public physicians in dispensaries and polyclinics, in factory or workplace clinics, or when necessary in the patient's home. For more serious illness, patients were hospitalized or treated in residential facilities or sanatoria of various types:

> In this unified medical organization the next link after the home doctor and the factory doctor is constituted by dispensaries and polyclinics. There is no sharp line of demarcation between these, but usually each dispensary serves the population of a particular district. It is claimed that, by the partial and almost complete "dispensarization" of medical practice, supervision is being exercised over the healthy as well as the sick persons in a district, including not only workers and their families, but the entire population; and that thus the integration of preventive and curative medicine for the community is being reached.[35]

Thus, Kingsbury and Newsholme's account seems to support Solomon's view that the polyclinics were the practical embodiment of Soviet social hygiene.

The other major English-language study of Soviet health was Henry Sigerist's *Socialized Medicine in the Soviet Union* (1937). The book was more overtly pro-Soviet than that of Newsholme and Kingsbury, and has long been interpreted by historians as overly enthusiastic and insufficiently critical.[36] Indicative of the range of debate even among prominent health reformers who admired the Soviet Union's health policies, Newsholme criticized Sigerist after the book's publication for its "missionary spirit."[37] Yet in the context of the global political and economic crises of the 1930s, *Socialized Medicine in the Soviet Union* was the more influential text. Sigerist had a critical impact upon a generation of radical physicians and public health experts in the US and Canada. Sigerist's personal role in shaping the Saskatchewan CCF's approach to health care is discussed in chapter 3. His broader influence in North America, and his embrace of the Soviet model and socialized medicine, helps to illustrate the significance of Douglas's choice in bringing Sigerist to Saskatchewan.

Born in Paris in 1891 to wealthy Swiss parents, Henry Sigerist was educated in France, Switzerland, Germany, and England. After studying philology and languages, he took degrees in medicine and science in Zurich and Munich. As a young man, he enjoyed the financial freedom to study whatever he chose without pursuing a career or supporting himself. Sigerist was a cosmopolitan and something of a polymath; according to his biographers, he chose to become a historian of medicine because "he could essentially avoid specialization and combine his varied interests in languages, the humanities, history, science and medicine."[38] At the age of 34, he became the head of the prestigious Institute for the History of Medicine in Leipzig.

Sigerist moved to Johns Hopkins University in 1932 to head up its medical history program. For a European immigrant to America,

Sigerist played an unusually important and visible role in health politics. He was able to do so because of his impeccable European qualifications and erudition, in part the result of his privileged background, as well as his considerable personal charisma and drive. The years Sigerist spent in the US were arguably the most productive of his life, although he wrote relatively little medical history during that time. He was evidently caught up in the reformist milieu of American medical liberalism and in some senses had the good fortune of being the right person in the right place at the right time. The range of his accomplishments over those fifteen years is astonishing. At Johns Hopkins University he reformed the American Association for the History of Medicine, and founded the still-important scholarly journal, the *Bulletin for the History of Medicine*. He was a gifted teacher and mentor, with a devoted following among a generation of young North American physicians and public health experts. Sigerist emboldened and gave voice to self-identified health radicals, including Mindel Cherniack Sheps and Cecil Sheps, who became part of a group whose members would privately refer to themselves as "careniks."[39] Many of them were Jewish. At a time when anti-Semitism was a reality in North American medicine, Sigerist's inclusion of Jews in his inner circle was notable.[40]

It was not his reputation as a medical historian that drew Douglas to Sigerist, however. In the last half of the 1930s, Sigerist was better known in political circles and to the broader public for his advocacy of "socialized medicine" in the US and his opposition to a private medical marketplace. It was this profile, and the response to *Socialized Medicine in the Soviet Union*, that landed Sigerist on the cover of *Time* magazine in 1939.

Not surprising for someone who advocated a strong state role in health care provision, Sigerist was an aficionado of rational health care planning and delivery. His book, *American Medicine*, written in the early 1930s before he arrived in the US, praised the country's scientific and technological dynamism, but criticized its "outdated, irrational, and disorganized" delivery. Sigerist taught health planning to his students at Johns Hopkins University, instructing them in his seminar, for example, to make detailed studies of health conditions and socio-economic and health data in each of the Maryland counties, and then to develop an ideal plan for a health system that would deliver health care to all the population. Students were to cost out the plan as well.[41]

Sigerist's high level of expertise in health planning, organization, delivery, and financing (essentially health policy) has been de-emphasized by historians. Yet he should be seen not only as an advocate of socialized medicine and a talented medical historian: Sigerist also taught himself the political economy of health care in both capitalist and communist societies. Like those of his cohort in the US such as Alan Gregg and I.S. Falk, who lobbied for a federal role in health care, and all of the younger physicians and health economists they trained, Sigerist became familiar with the woolly intricacies of health organization and planning. This passion for detailed policy debate would become one key attribute of the movement for socialized medicine.

For Sigerist, health care in a capitalist society would always be constituted by the "deficiencies of a compromise." He was very clear on the distinction between socialized medicine and state health insurance—a distinction that commentators have since effectively blurred. Even in countries like the UK and France, which had moved towards a larger state role in health provision, medical service was fragmented among "state medicine, insurance medicine, charity medicine and private medicine." Only in the Soviet Union, Sigerist argued, was there no fragmentation caused by the compromises of capitalist medicine; rather, the health system was "rational, logical, and clear."[42] Soviet medicine's key features were universally available free care, a focus on prevention, and centralized control and planning. That Sigerist chose to ignore, or was not aware of, the fragmentation and competing interests that plagued Soviet health care is perhaps not surprising. In his mind, the need for central planning and control was the lesson to be learned: "One need not be a military expert to know that unity of command is essential for the success of a campaign. And yet there is not one capitalist country that has achieved unity of direction in its health work."[43]

Sigerist's discussion of Soviet health care delivery begins with reference to the situation in the US, quoting the recommendations of the Committee on the Costs of Medical Care (1932) at length, especially its conclusion that medical care should be delivered by multidisciplinary teams of providers in group practices organized around a hospital. He then goes on to make a very interesting observation about the ubiquitous appeal of the health centre model of delivery:

> The Committee submitting the majority report recognized also that individual practice is bound to be inefficient in a highly specialized industrial society, and, in suggesting that medical service be given to the population through organized health centres, it recommended the very form of medical practice realized in the Soviet Union. I do not think that the American Committee was inspired by the Russian example. It came to its conclusion independently, after a long and painstaking investigation of conditions prevailing in America. The fact that many experts in capitalist America, as well as all experts in socialist Russia, recognized that medical service can be given most efficiently by groups organized in health centres is arresting evidence in support of the theory that group practice is the form of medical service best adapted to modern industrial society and to modern medical science.[44]

This is followed by a detailed discussion of Soviet health centres in urban areas, which especially impressed Sigerist, as they had Newsholme and Kingsbury.

Sigerist, like others, was fascinated by the Soviet Union because it was a valuable testing ground for the specific policies that would make up a socialist health care system: an actually existing socialism, not merely an ideal. It was the *only* state-run universal health care system in the world; as such, it was a unique health policy petri dish. *Socialized Medicine in the Soviet Union* is generously embellished with superlatives and jargon-laden slogans, much of which now sounds naïve and politically unsophisticated. For this, Sigerist was deservedly criticized. His book was neither an objective nor dispassionate assessment of the Soviet experiment. Sigerist himself, however, would not have claimed to be objective; his belief in the need for a socialized system was never hidden. And his book was far from superficial. It contains nearly four hundred pages of detailed explication of the functioning of Soviet health care: administrative and political structure; financing; medical education and research; delivery mechanisms; and health outcomes. This expert knowledge was to be put to use in the war against conservative forces in health care.

Sigerist's ideas about socialized medicine, and the knowledge of health services organization that he gained during two extended visits to the Soviet Union, eventually made their way directly to Saskatchewan. Additionally, the Soviet journeys of two prominent Canadian physicians, Frederick Banting and Norman Bethune, played their own role in promoting Soviet achievements in Canada. They were among those hundreds of physicians who made the journey to the Soviet Union in the summer of 1935 to attend the International Physiological Congress, the first such meeting to be held in the Soviet Union. At home, Banting and Bethune contributed to public and political debate about reforming the country's health care system and held up the Soviet Union as a model of what might be achieved by the state. Both men returned to Canada praising Soviet health care as superior to the state of health care provision in their own country. They spoke out in newspaper articles, in speeches to medical organizations, and to political groups such as the League for Social Reconstruction. Their contribution to the influence of Soviet ideas in Canadian health care activism was significant.

Like Sigerist, neither Banting nor Bethune was a confirmed radical before his engagement with the Soviet Union. They would seem to fit Sheila Fitzpatrick's description of those visitors who were experts in their fields, and who went to the Soviet Union to learn something about what was happening in their field of specialization, rather than out of an ideological commitment. As Fitzpatrick explains, "the Soviet Union was worth the trip in professional terms: it was not delusory to suppose that interesting things were going on, for example in the area of state organization of science, economic planning, experimental theatres and the mass dissemination of high culture."[45]

Yet, the lasting significance of their visit went beyond observation and curiosity. Like Sigerist, both men were deeply moved and excited by the possibilities Soviet medicine represented for the future. After their return to Canada, the men ultimately took very different political paths. Bethune's Soviet visit in particular led to lasting and dramatic political engagement: a commitment to communism; health activism in Montreal; journeying to Spain to serve the Spanish Republican Army; and, finally, his time in China serving as a surgeon with Mao's army resisting Japan, which led to his death from sepsis in November 1939. Banting's passion for radical medicine was shorter lived. At the outbreak of World War II, he worked with the Royal Canadian Air Force, investigating the physiological problems of flight. He died after an air crash in Newfoundland in 1941, where he was en route to England to test a new pilot suit for high-altitude flight. However divergent their lives, both men publicly emphasized the value of Soviet approaches to science and medicine, and raised the possibility that a state-led system of health care could do a better job of guaranteeing health than the current system of capitalistic medical care.

Norman Bethune's North American ancestors on the paternal side were fur traders, clergymen, doctors, and businessmen. His great-great-grandmother, Louisa McKenzie, was the daughter of a fur trader and a Woodland Cree woman. According to Bethune's biographers, Roderick and Sharon Stewart, his childhood hero was his surgeon grandfather, after whom he was named. Educated in Toronto and in the medical schools of London and Edinburgh, Norman's grandfather was for a time a very successful professor of surgery at Trinity College in Toronto, before his alcoholism lost him his position and his family. Norman's father, Malcolm Bethune, had a difficult early life after his mother left with four of the couple's five children and returned to her family home in Scotland. He married a religious woman, Elizabeth Ann Goodwin, whose family had also been devastated by alcohol addiction. Malcolm experienced Christian salvation and became a Presbyterian minister.

Malcolm Bethune's first congregation was on the edge of the Muskoka district of Ontario, in the small community of Gravenhurst. It was logging country; Gravenhurst had seventeen sawmills, which earned it the title "Sawdust City." Reverend Bethune was a fundamentalist, an evangelical, and a temperance advocate, as was his wife. Henry Norman was born to the couple on March 4, 1890, the middle child of three. He was "hyperactive, highly intelligent ... insatiably curious," and rebellious as he grew up; a competitive risk taker with strong personal convictions and opinions. Although Norman's relationship with his strict, overbearing, and perhaps emotionally unstable father was a difficult one, the Stewarts argue that Norman also learned a strong sense of justice from his Christian upbringing, suggesting that "the need to serve became as ingrained in his character as his rebelliousness."[46]

The family moved frequently from the time Norman was three years old, from congregation to congregation, many in small, remote resource communities. No engagement lasted long. His father's health was poor, and the family had little money. Norman left home immediately upon graduating high school and put himself through university. In 1907–1908, he worked in construction camps in the Algoma District, on lake boats on Lake Huron, and as a village schoolteacher. He saved enough to enter the University of Toronto in 1909, but he struggled in his courses. Rather than enter medical school, in 1911 he took a position at Frontier College, which sought to educate workers in remote work camps in Ontario. He became a "labourer-teacher" at a lumber camp on Lake Panache. In the evenings, after a day of punishing physical labour in the bush, Bethune "gave classes to his fellow workers in English, Canadian history and geography, arithmetic, letter writing and hygiene."[47] He worked there for the winter, and then began medical school in Toronto in fall 1912, where he worked in a restaurant to pay his expenses. His academic performance was mediocre, except for clinical surgery.

When war broke out in summer 1914, Bethune enlisted almost immediately and was assigned to the Second Field Ambulance of the Canadian Army Medical Corps. He saw action in one of the most brutal of battles on the Western Front, the Second Battle of Ypres in April 1915, when chlorine gas was used as a biological weapon by the German army for the first time. Bethune was a stretcher bearer, until he was injured by shrapnel in his leg. He was declared medically unfit for combat and sent home to resume medical studies in an expedited program designed to generate physicians for the armed forces. He was mobilized again towards the end of the war, this time into the Royal Navy, and faced the most serious medical crisis of his career when influenza broke out aboard his vessel, infecting 107 of the 207 crew members, including Bethune himself. He developed potentially deadly bronchial pneumonia, a common complication of the influenza virus, and spent three weeks desperately ill. Bethune was fortunate to have received good medical care, and survived where so many others did not. Bethune graduated with his medical degree in December 1916. He made an impression on his classmates as a "distinct individualist" and an "enigma."[48] One of these classmates at the University of Toronto was Frederick Banting, although the two men do not seem to have been friends.

After the war, Bethune remained in Britain for a time, working and enjoying life in a large metropolis. He met his Scottish wife, Frances Penney, whom he would marry and divorce twice. In 1922 he became a fellow of the Royal College of Surgeons of Edinburgh. There was little evidence of Bethune the radical during his time in London, when he cultivated expensive tastes in clothes, food, art, and company. Money became a major preoccupation. He returned to North America with his new wife and started to build a practice in Detroit, then a booming car manufacturing city. It was in Detroit that he contracted pulmonary tuberculosis. He spent about a year in the Trudeau Sanitorium in Saranac Lake, where he underwent artificial pneumothorax, which involved collapsing the diseased lung in order to allow it to heal by injecting air into the chest cavity. In Bethune's case, the results were dramatic, and he was able to leave the sanitorium. For some time, however, he needed pneumothorax "refills." He eventually performed these on himself.[49]

Scholars have speculated about how the disease affected Bethune's life. One of the first scholarly evaluations of Bethune, written by Gabriel Nadeau, was published in the *Bulletin of the History of Medicine* in October 1940, less than a year after Bethune's death in China in November 1939. Henry Sigerist was the journal's editor at the time. The piece described Bethune as "one of the most brilliant and versatile men of our generation," and explored the possible linkage between tuberculosis and Bethune's creative, restless, and impatient nature. Certainly, he had faced the possibility of death. Bethune himself said that his time at Saranac deepened his intellectual and spiritual life. Professionally, tuberculosis "made a thoracic surgeon of him," as he would learn the surgical technique that had saved his life.[50] He moved to Montreal to work under Edward Archibald at the Royal Victoria Hospital; Archibald had himself been a patient at Saranac. After three years at the Royal Victoria, as relations cooled between himself and Archibald, Bethune took an appointment as Chief Thoracic Surgeon at Hôpital du Sacré-Coeur de Montréal. In 1934, he was elected to the executive council of the American Association for Thoracic Surgery.

Bethune's biographers are careful to note that Bethune was a complex, difficult, and sometimes dysfunctional man and physician. Bethune's personal life was often dramatic and messy, with problems fueled by alcohol abuse. His two marriages and divorces to Frances were especially destructive to his stability and health. He could be callous and cruel to friends, lovers, and colleagues alike. He was mercurial and occasionally violent. Although he was ambitious and appreciated and desired a life with material comfort and cultural richness, he ridiculed bourgeois values and frequently the wealthy themselves. Works written about Bethune depict a man who was simultaneously charismatic and difficult to like. Professionally, despite his successes, there were questions about his judgment as a physician and surgeon. Some believed he took unnecessary risks; mortality rates among his patients were at times high, although he cared deeply for them. There is also evidence that his heavy drinking affected his performance. Ideas, however, flew off him like sparks. His most recent biography suggests Bethune may have suffered from bipolar disorder.[51]

Bethune had reached the heights of his profession as a surgeon. Health politics, however, were starting to interest him. Beginning during his time at Saranac, and intensifying by 1933, Bethune's attention turned to the social origins of tuberculosis. Roderick and Sharon Stewart argue that his time at Sacré-Coeur played a role in Bethune's growing belief in the social aspects of disease, especially the role of poverty, poor housing, and lack of access to medical care. From being a man with conservative political tendencies—at times anti-labour and opposed to socialism—Bethune's views evolved during his years treating working-class patients, and through his friendships in Montreal's artistic circles. Larry Hannant has argued

that the disease itself radicalized Bethune, and that "his dissatis-
faction with existing tuberculosis treatment began to stir in him
a new political conscience."[52] He sought a new audience beyond
fellow physicians, who Bethune tended to view as conformist and
disinterested in the "great problems of our age."[53] In 1933, he wrote
a short radio play, *The Patient's Dilemma*, which he submitted to
the Canadian Tuberculosis Association. He began to speak publicly
about the relationship between tuberculosis and social conditions,
particularly in the province of Quebec, where tuberculosis mortality
was twice as high as the national average. His prescription for change,
however, remained very much focused on medical screening and
treatment. Addressing income inequality itself was not Bethune's
focus at this stage.[54]

In early 1934 Bethune began attending meetings of the League
for Social Reconstruction (LSR). At an LSR meeting, he met
George Mooney, who ran the YMCA in Verdun. By the fall of 1934,
Bethune had offered to help provide free medical care at a clinic
he established and attended once a week. It was through Mooney
that Bethune became actively interested in the Soviet Union, when
Mooney invited him to attend a lecture by Maurice Hindus, an
American journalist who had recently visited the USSR. According
to the Stewarts, Bethune was deeply skeptical of Hindus's claims
that Soviet medicine was superior to North America's, and it was
out of curiosity to see for himself that he made the decision to attend
the 15th International Physiological Congress.

Little in-the-moment documentation exists of Bethune's trip to
the Soviet Union, apart from a few letters he wrote to Marion Scott,
the wife of Frank Scott, with whom he was in love; and speeches
he gave about his impressions. No diary has survived of his journey. Nevertheless, when Bethune returned to Canada, he began to
speak publicly about the politics of medicine. He was enthusiastic
about the Soviet Union. He was one of four Montreal physicians
who had attended the International Physiological Congress and were

invited to speak to the Montreal Medico-Chirurgical Society about their impressions of Soviet Russia. Bethune's speech, "Reflections on Return from 'Through the Looking Glass'" was printed in the Society's journal. In his speech, Bethune states that his purpose in visiting Russia was "primarily to look at the Russians, and secondarily, to see what they were doing about eradicating one of the most easily eradicable of all contagious diseases, namely, tuberculosis."

Bethune's short speech to this room full of physicians is fascinating. It is poetic and passionate, clever and nuanced. The speech is organized around Bethune's reading of Soviet communism through Lewis Carroll's *Alice in Wonderland*. While the world "through the looking glass" may seem wrong and everything appears upside down, it is a world of possibilities:

> That it's "Jam tomorrow and Jam yesterday but never Jam today," might be taken as the complaint of those workers who are impatient of what they may think is the slow progress of improvement in living conditions, and the White Queen's remembrance of things which happened the week after next, as an example of the unlimited optimism and the faith that the Russians have in their own future. And it would also be true of Russia today to use the White Queen's reply to the protest of Alice, who said: "Oh, I can't believe that"/ "Can't you?" said the Queen. "Try again; draw a long breath and shut your eyes."[55]

Alice finds that the fire in the fireplace is no illusion, but is real. "So I shall be as warm here as in the old room, warmer, in fact, because there will be no one here to scold me away from the fire." The Soviet health system, it seems, was the fire that warmed. Bethune said that witnessing the Soviet experience was as contradictory as a man observing a woman giving birth; she is beautiful but also pitiful; she is absurd but also magnificent and sublime. "Russia presents today the most exciting spectacle of the evolutionary, emergent and heroic spirit of man ... To deny this is to deny our faith in man..."[56]

Soon after his Soviet journey, Bethune joined the Communist Party of Canada, although he turned down the offer to become chairman of the Montreal branch of the Friends of the Soviet Union. Bethune wrote to Marion Scott that he wasn't sure why the organization wanted him as chairman, because "since my trip, my expressions have not been entirely complimentary in some quarters (depending of course on my audience!—enthusiastic to the reactionaries, minimizing to the radical.)" He expressed his mixed views to Marion:

> I explained my attitude frankly to Mr K—saying definitely that though in theory I am entirely in agreement with the ideology of this modern religion. Yet I was disturbed and rather deeply disturbed, in some of its aspects in practice. In short, that I did not believe that communism as practiced in Russia today was a suitable technic for the Anglo-Saxons (predominately Anglo-Saxon, at heart) of this country. Their attempt to discover some method of herd (?) living suitable for their new concepts of equality and justice is a machine age. But that basically—not immitatevily [sic], in detail, I was in deep sympathy with Russia. To my surprise he agreed with me.[57]

Bethune was convinced the Soviets had much to teach Canadians about health care, and he used the Soviet example as a launching pad for his reform agenda. In the fall of 1935, he delivered another speech to the Medico-Chirurgical Society, this time a harsh critique of health care in Canada, and against for-profit medicine. "Take Private Profit Out of Medicine" was delivered at a symposium on medical economics in April 1936, and was published in the *Canadian Doctor* in January 1937. Bethune argued that medicine is a capitalistic profession, "operating as a monopoly on a private profit basis." In "the people versus the doctors," the people were losing, and Canada, along with the rest of the capitalist world, suffered from "poverty of health in the midst of scientific abundance of knowledge of disease."

Adequate medical care for all is available, but only for those who can pay. "We are selling bread at the price of jewels," Bethune argued. He proceeded to give a class analysis of Canadian society, arguing not only that poverty caused ill health, but also that poverty was the cause of lack of access to medical care. Here, Bethune drew upon American documents that had shaped New Deal demands for universal health care, such as the report, *Committee on the Cost of Medical Care* (1932). The quality of Bethune's economic analysis of access to care indicates how engaged he was during this stage in his life with issues of public policy and the role of the state in health care.[58]

The economics of health care, he argued, put physicians in a difficult position. The high price of medical education mandated young physicians to make money, while the accumulation of scientific knowledge made individualistic practice impossible to do well. Bethune opposed fee-for-service (which he saw as morally problematic) and supported group practice as the only realistic way for physicians to provide good care to patients. Bethune, not unlike many health advocates in the North Atlantic world in this period, connected a radical economic critique (poverty causes ill health) with a specific critique of public policy and demands for a reformed health care structure (lack of efficient access to medical care causes ill health). He advocated changes to the way health care is organized; while also arguing, "the best form of providing health protection would be to change the economic system which produces ill-health." Bethune elaborated:

> The practice of each individual purchasing his own medical care does not work. It is unjust, inefficient, wasteful and completely out-moded. ... In our highly geared, modern industrial society there is no such thing as private health—all health is public. ... Socialized medicine and the abolition or restriction of private practice would appear to be the realistic solution of the problem.

Let us take the profit, the private economic profit, out of medicine, and purify our profession of rapacious individualism. ... Let
us re-define medical ethics—not as a code of professional eti-
quette between doctors, but as a code of fundamental morality
and justice between medicine and the people.[59]

Bethune's speech addresses the importance of multidisciplinary
health care and the need for co-operation between health professionals—a touchstone of many radical health agendas during this
era. "Medicine must be entirely reorganized and unified, welded into
a great army of doctors, dentists, nurses, technicians and social service workers, to make a collectivized attack on disease and utilizing
all the present scientific knowledge of its members to that end."[60]

Bethune had by this point gone past a call for reform. He was
careful to distinguish between his call for socialized medicine and
universal health care insurance schemes, which he characterized as
"bastard forms of Socialism produced by belated humanitarianism out
of necessity."[61] His definition of socialized medicine was as follows:

Socialized medicine means that health protection becomes public property, like the post office, the army, the navy, the judiciary
and the school; 2nd: supported by public funds; 3rd: with services available to all, not according to income but according to
need. Charity must be abolished and justice substituted. Charity
debases the donor and debauches the recipient; 4th: its workers to
be paid by the State, with assured salaries and pensions; 5th: with
democratic self-government by the Health workers themselves.[62]

Thus, socialized medicine was not only to be state funded, it was
also to be democratically controlled. These sorts of principles were
widely held by advocates of socialized medicine during the 1930s.
Democratic control, multidisciplinary practice, salaried remuneration, and the rejection of a private charity-based model of health care
and universal provision were often lynchpins in a prescription for

health care that advocated a deeper reform than government health insurance would imply.

Beyond giving speeches, Bethune wanted action. As he wrote to Marion Scott after his return from the Soviet Union: "I feel a tremendous impulse to do, to act. I hate to be thought one of the intelligentsia who talk and talk and talk and believe their words. You feel their hearts are cold and it's only an intellectual conundrum. A game."[63] Although Bethune's passion for action took him far beyond Canada's borders, his desire to *do* rather than just talk and write were common among the doctors, nurses, and public health practitioners who attempted to create socialized medicine. Whether as public advocates or state employees, they struggled to square their radical views about health with the realities of changing public policy and the way that health care and medicine were organized in their own time and place.

In the fall of 1935, Bethune brought together a multidisciplinary group of health practitioners, including "physicians, surgeons, dentists, nurses, social service workers and statisticians," which would eventually become the Montreal Group for the Security of the People's Health (MGSPH). An open letter to Montreal's political candidates in the 1936 Quebec provincial election stated the group's purpose was to study "the relationship of present day medicine to the people and to the state, in all the civilized countries of the world."[64] The group was small, never more than twenty people, and included Libbie Rutherford (later Park) and J. Wendell Macleod, who have written and published extensively about the experience and their views on Bethune.

Libbie Park was a nurse. She would go on to do a post-graduate degree in public health nursing at the University of Toronto and serve in Europe with the United Nations Relief and Rehabilitation Administration. In the postwar era, she became secretary to the Health Division Toronto Welfare Council and secretary of the Toronto Peace Council and the Canadian Congress of Women.[65] She was the co-author of two books: *Bethune: The Montreal Years* (with Wendell Macleod and Stanley Ryerson) and *The Anatomy of Big Business* (with Frank Park). She and Bethune met at the end of October 1935 when he spoke about his Soviet journey at a meeting organized by Friends of the Soviet Union at Strathcona Hall in Montreal. Park did not come from a political or labour background, but became involved on the left as a result of her work as a nurse during the 1930s:

> I began to do voluntary work in the out-patient department of the Montreal General Hospital and there we were constantly reminded of the depression by over-crowded clinics, over-worked doctors and nurses, helpless patients waiting, endlessly it seemed, for attention, and it was there that I became aware of what the depression could mean. ... I had begun going to left-wing lectures and meetings. I attended some LSR meetings ... some of the Peoples Forum meetings held in the Unitarian church on Sherbrooke Street.[66]

In her recollections, Park describes Bethune as a compelling speaker, but also notes that he was far from the only physician to be interested enough in the Soviet Union to visit. She cites comments by prominent physician and historian of military medicine, Andrew MacPhail, that the Soviet Union had "no poor, no rich, no unemployed, no Communists," to explain the context for Bethune's support for Soviet medicine. Bethune's speech that night drew attention to Soviet efforts in tuberculosis care and control.

She and Bethune became friends and fellow health advocates. Despite Bethune's reputation as a sexual libertine, Libbie Park did not view him as sexist towards women:

> I liked his attitude towards women. He had none of the stereotyped male attitudes, and did not speak of women in derogatory sense. A woman was a person, her mind not the mind of a "woman" but of a person. In argument he was never patronizing,

never appeared to make allowances; if he disagreed with a woman he would not spare her. He respected women.[67]

Park recalled works they both were reading that year: Anna Louise Strong's *I Changed Worlds*, Julius Hecker's *Moscow Dialogues*, Marx and Engels' *Communist Manifesto*, and other works by Frederick Engels. Their intellectual milieu, she notes, was "oriented towards New York. That was where the most stimulating writing, painting and acting was going on. We were watching Roosevelt and making comparisons with Mackenzie King and Bennett."[68]

Libbie Park recalled a project Bethune worked on with visual artist Fritz Brandtner after his Soviet visit, which she referred to as a "Model City for tuberculosis patients." Arriving at Bethune's Fort Street apartment one day, she discovered the two men working on a sketch of the Model City:

> It was a delicate drawing in pastel colours, done in great detail, of a centre for patients ready to leave hospital but who should not return to their homes, to the environment where they had contracted the disease, until they were in good enough health to resist re-infection themselves and not to infect others, and able to take part in normal activities. The centre included everything needed for full rehabilitation—clinics, living accommodation, recreating centres, parks, shops and workshop where the patient could learn a trade or craft, or practice his own.[69]

The design for the Bethune/Brandtner Model City seems not to have survived, but the plan sounds very similar to ideas for tuberculosis care in London, England drawn up by the Soviet émigré architect Berthold Lubetkin, who designed the one of the first state health centres in London, the modernist Finsbury Health Centre, completed in 1939 (see chapter 2).

According to Park, Bethune was frustrated to discover a lack of interest from his medical colleagues in his model. She herself saw the plan as "utopian and too elaborate for a time of unemployment."[70] Although Bethune seemed to reject this criticism, he perhaps took some of it on board, as he turned his attentions to formulating an "overall health scheme."[71] He continued to look for international expertise on the subject, writing to Dr. Isadore Falk, for example, a US bacteriologist, medical economist, and member of the Committee on the Costs of Medical Care who played a key role in formulating health policy during the Roosevelt administration. Bethune began collecting information on health systems in Europe, Britain, and the US and invited others to join him.[72]

Wendell MacLeod welcomed the opportunity to participate in the group, because he shared Bethune's frustration at the complacency of his fellow physicians in Montreal. Having spent time in St. Louis and at Washington State University, where debate about health care policy created "considerable ferment," MacLeod was happy to be back in the thick of it.[73] MacLeod, too, was involved in the LSR and was impressed by the study of low income and health being conducted by Leonard Marsh.[74] Marsh was the director of social research at McGill University. The project assessed the nutritional status of 25 families in Montreal who had been living at "a relief level of income" for five years. Using school health records, they analyzed the heights and weights of 1800 boys according to socio-economic level.[75]

An informal gathering at first, the MGSPH studied the health systems of other countries, each member doing research on specific countries and aspects of health delivery, in order to develop a health program for Canada. Bethune's tendency was to push for a socialized model, but this perspective was not universally shared by the group. According to Park:

> Perhaps the majority of our group would have supported socialized medicine in one form or another, but we were trying to work out a practical health and medical programme, one that could

be brought into being within the existing framework of society and by putting pressure on governments that certainly were not socialist.[76]

Writing some decades later, Park argued that what Bethune meant by socialized medicine in his speeches on the subject was not entirely clear. Did socialized medicine mean a medical system under socialism? Or was it a form of state medical care within a capitalist system? In 1936, the group released its first and only major public statement, which was circulated in various venues, including the *Canadian Medical Association Journal*, and as an open letter to all Montreal candidates in the Quebec election. The document offered both critique and solutions the group perceived as possible in the current context, within a broader argument that the state should accept responsibility for health as it did for education, policing, the military, and fire protection. The MGSPH took the view that the political economy of health care had created contradictory dynamics in health care delivery, which was characterized by a "poverty of purchasing power in the midst of plenty," and "uneven distribution of the products of scientific knowledge and research." The majority of the population could not afford medical care, and charity provision was inadequate to the task, with poor quality care, and an "appalling lack" of prevention and "hygienic measures." Doctors were squeezed between the demands of their profession and increasingly specialized medical knowledge, and the pressure to provide medical care for patients who could not afford to pay. This, the MGSPH argued, contributed to an "economic crisis of medicine" and "a lowering of altruistic principles and the high morale of the profession."[77]

Just prior to the election, the City of Montreal had created an Unemployment Medical Relief Commission; elements of the MGSPH program were written specifically in response to this initiative. The open letter urged the continuance of medical care for the city's unemployed, but also the establishment of a City Medical

Planning Board, which would employ physicians on a per-capita payment system (no fee-for-service), and provide dental treatment, home nursing, and hospital care for the unemployed. The group also recommended that the government mount four different experimental health programs in selected areas of the province, to be "used as controls to each other in a proper scientific manner." These were: municipal medicine; compulsory health insurance; voluntary hospitalization health insurance; and health care for the unemployed on a fee-for-service basis. Of these four suggestions, only municipal medicine and compulsory health insurance are outlined in any detail, municipal medicine being the most fully described. This is also the most radical of the four proposals for study, and the one most closely in line with the features of socialized medicine held in common by transatlantic advocates.

Briefly outlined, the municipal medical system was to be made up of health units, achieved through an expansion of existing provincial public health units, with a full-time multidisciplinary team of providers including physicians, dentists, nurses, and specialists (such as gynecologists and obstetricians). Each municipality would have a "small modern hospital" and the health unit would focus on disease control, prevention, and treatment for the entire population. All staff were to be paid salaries. The costs of the scheme would be raised through municipal taxes and provincial grants to municipalities.

The immediate political impact of the MGSPH's position paper was minimal. With the election of Maurice Duplessis, hopes for reform in Quebec dwindled. In fall 1936, Bethune left for Spain, and members of the MGSPH would go on to other projects. Wendell MacLeod, Kay Dickson, and Grant Lathe went to work with Dr. Grant Fleming, Director of the Department of Public Health and Preventive Medicine at McGill University, to gather data for Leonard Marsh's study, *Health and Unemployment*. By 1938, the Bethune group had dissolved.

Bethune returned to Canada from Spain in June 1937. He began a national fundraising tour with the Committee to Aid Spanish Democracy, making public appearances and speeches in support of Spanish anti-fascism, the mobile blood transfusion unit he had founded for the Republican side in the Spanish conflict, and refuges for Spanish children. Bethune drew large crowds—when his train arrived at Montreal's Windsor Station, 1000 people were waiting. When he spoke at the Mount Royal Arena the following night, the audience was 8000 people. Among former friends and colleagues, he was greeted home less enthusiastically. Many were alienated by his radicalism, and he had burned his bridges with most of the medical community in which he once had held a prominent role. Bethune, perhaps suffering from post-traumatic stress given the horrors he had witnessed in Spain, was physically frail and drinking heavily.[78]

A grueling speaking tour followed. He arrived in Winnipeg on July 19, 1937. According to Bethune's most recent biography:

> Despite the lateness of the hour—it was 1:30 AM—a band and a jubilant welcoming party of five hundred were waiting on the platform for the train. As the band struck up, Bethune was lifted into the air and carried, clenched fist held high, through the cheering crowd to a waiting taxi which took him to the Hotel Fort Garry. In the afternoon he spoke at the Ukrainian Labour Temple and in the evening in the Walker Theatre, where some of the audience had to be seated on the stage to accommodate the overflow crowd of two thousand.[79]

Bethune's speech in Winnipeg called for unity among progressives in Canada, and class unity between professionals—such as doctors like himself—and labourers. During his speaking tour, Bethune talked about socialized medicine:

> In my practice I hated the two, five and ten-dollar bills that came between me and my patients. Many other doctors feel

the same way. I believe that doctors should be civil servants and that treatment should be free to the public and paid for out of general taxation.[80]

A young Cecil Sheps, who had graduated from medical school a year before, heard Bethune speak in Winnipeg. According to his son, Sam, Cecil was moved by Bethune's speech, in which he pointed out "the callous indifference to human suffering in Spain and elsewhere by the medical and governmental institutions of the day."[81] Bethune's conception of what being a physician could mean had influence on this young doctor from a Jewish socialist background.

At the time of his visit to the Soviet Union, Banting was probably Canada's most famous medical scientist, having won (with John Macleod) the 1923 Nobel Prize in Physiology for the discovery of insulin treatment of diabetes, making them the first Canadian Nobel laureates. Adulation followed Banting the rest of his life. Michael Bliss described his biography of Banting as "a study in the problems of being a hero."[82] The early 1930s was a difficult period for Banting. By then over 40 years of age, he had not been able to replicate the medical research success of his earlier career. He published little, and instead oversaw the research of others in the Banting Institute at the University of Toronto. In 1934 he was knighted, but in Bliss's estimation he was depressed and wanted only privacy. Banting, a veteran of the First World War, was also concerned about future peace. He travelled extensively in Europe in 1933; by the time he returned, he was convinced there would be another war.

Michael Bliss's *Banting: A Biography* pays relatively little attention to Banting's political views, but it does portray him as a man with deep egalitarian tendencies, socially and in his laboratory. Despite his fame, he did not associate with Toronto's social elite and disliked ostentation, and possibly the rich themselves. Like Bethune, he had close relationships with visual artists who were on the political left—in his case, the painter A.Y. Jackson of the Group of Seven, with whom he had a long friendship. There is no evidence that Banting had direct involvement in electoral politics or activism, but he was not uncritical of his own society. Banting, like others of his time, was curious about the Soviet Union, and when the opportunity to attend the International Physiological Congress presented itself, he took it.

Writing just before the fall of Soviet communism, in the final years of the Cold War, Bliss is dismissive of Banting's admiration for the Soviet Union. But Banting's views on the USSR should be more fully contextualized. Banting equated the USSR with the new. Even before his arrival he described it as the "new land of great promise. I go to observe the progress of the greatest experiment of all time."[83] About a month later, Fred Banting wrote to A.Y. Jackson from the Soviet Union. His admiration for the country was apparently genuine:

> I have though[t] of you very often in various places on this trip, and often wished that you were here with the little box and the colours. I think you could do something with it but I could not. I have not even made pencil sketches.
>
> I am sure you would like the life of Russia. They are doing things. I have never had a more interesting and enjoyable trip in any country. On every side there is building of houses, roads, factories. University buildings, parks. Science and art have never so flourished since the days of the Medici (?) family in Italy.[84]

Banting extended his stay in the Soviet Union by a couple of months, and spent this time touring the Soviet Union—over 10,000 kilometres of travel, Banting estimated—during which time he became an avid supporter of Soviet medicine, and came to praise its commitment to science.

Banting kept a daily journal of his Soviet visit, which was later transcribed into 70 pages of typed record. It isn't clear whether he edited his journal after returning home to Canada, although the typed journal entries are remarkably coherent and written in elegantly crafted sentences, so it is likely that some revision was made to his initial in-the-moment thoughts. The journal begins on Saturday, June 22, 1935, as he boarded the USSR *Smolny*. Aboard the ship made note of his companions:

> The crowd aboard is varied. A professor of the University of Toronto, and his wife, two girls from Australia, sisters, one interested in music and art, the other in eugenics, socialism, primitive races, social science. These are all I have met. There are many Jews, some French, some Germans and some Russians. Jews predominate. Many English and many internationals. American twang is frequently heard. [85]

Banting was relieved that no one on board, except the professor from Toronto, knew who he was. He saw the journalist Alexandrine Gibb from the *Toronto Star* onboard but believed she didn't recognize him. On arrival in Leningrad, however, Banting was paired with Gibb by the Soviet tourist agency, Intourist. "That cursed paper is here to pest me even at this distance," Banting observed.[86] "She is a typical *Star* reporter," he complained.

While on board, Banting educated himself by reading an orthodox Soviet text on Marxist political economy by Lev Abramovich Leontiev, *Political Economy: A Beginner's Course*, which was first published in 1935. "The book is most readable and clever," Banting noted.[87] He claimed that he had often felt antipathy toward the Soviet Union—"fear of the place and fear of the Communist Movement," as he put it. Nonetheless, many of Banting's musings on the Soviet system were jarringly positive and unrealistically optimistic. In fact, he appears to have held rosy views about communism in the Soviet Union well before he arrived there—unless his journal has been entirely re-written from the perspective of afterthought. "In Russia man cannot exploit man, but a man can exploit the work of his own brain. The Russian system is built upon a plan, a theory, a philosophy ... Leaders in Russia do not command or dominate. They are chosen because of the brain, judgment and integrity," he wrote, while still on the Baltic Sea.[88] He praised Marx and Lenin as among the "greatest philosophers" and the "greatest minds."

Upon arrival, Banting's first priority was to attempt to meet Ivan Pavlov, Russia's great physiologist. Banting's diary entry for June 28th tells the story of how he secured his visit with Pavlov as a farcical exchange with evasive, somewhat dishonest, and inefficient Soviet officials. On the first day in Leningrad, Banting and several others negotiated through Intourist for an appointment with Kupavlov and Rosenthal of the Institute of Experimental Medicine. At first, the group's request was refused as Pavlov was elderly and allegedly in poor health; then, Banting alone was granted permission to visit Pavlov's laboratories, and perhaps see Pavlov. Banting was given a tour of the laboratories where experiments were performed on dogs, but then was told that Pavlov had been at his country home for a couple of weeks. After further delays, they were eventually driven to Pavlov's home, where they had a short visit.[89]

Banting's journal says relatively little about the structure of the Soviet health care system. In this sense his diaries have a very different perspective from published works on Soviet medicine by authors such as Sigerist and Newsholme. As he was toured around the country, he recorded impressions of all of the workplaces, schools, daycares, courts, and other places that he saw, as well as thoughts about the natural beauty of the countryside, art, and architecture. One topic on which he does write extensively in his journal is gender relations in the Soviet Union, for the most part expressing the view that Soviet women enjoyed greater gender equality, work and educational opportunities, and relative freedom from child-care responsibilities. He was also clearly impressed by the apparent availability of birth control and abortion. Birth control was available free of charge. In early July, his group visited an abortion clinic in

Moscow, a 180-bed facility that had performed nearly 14,000 abortions, according to Banting. He described the treatment women received there and the rules for abortion procurement. A woman seeking an abortion was required to bring certificates from her doctor, her workplace, and her "home"—presumably, her father, husband, or male partner. Abortion was not free, but rather charged on a sliding scale based on income. If the women had a chronic illness such as tuberculosis or diabetes, or was "poor," she was treated for free. According to Banting, only first-trimester abortions were allowed. Abortions were performed without anesthetic (a fact on which he made no comment), although women who were "neurotic" might be given morphine. "Russian women stand it well without anesthesia," he claimed. "Young, old, ugly, pretty, well made and otherwise, all were here."

Banting was also careful to disconnect birth control from eugenics. After describing the free availability of birth control, Banting noted that "sterilization is not compulsory for feeble minded but may be done on request or advice." He then goes on to describe pro-maternal policies, such as two months leave with pay before birth and two months after, along with pre-natal clinics, maternity care, and nurseries. He observes the freedom with which Soviets can co-habit and divorce. Banting accepted quite blindly the Soviet treatment of prostitutes and indeed argued, implausibly, that Soviet society had virtually eliminated prostitution: "the government has made wives, marriage and divorce so easy that each man lives with a woman and has no need of a prostitute." His party toured an "institution for the care of deposed prostitutes" in Moscow, which housed 350 women who worked for their room and board and the medical treatment they received.[90] It does not seem to occur to him that this "clinic" might have had a carceral function.

Banting's journal is more plausible on the subject of his own interactions with his Soviet guides. He constantly recorded biting commentary in his journal, and from the outset is highly frustrated by Soviet bureaucracy, and even more so by the purported Russian lax sense of time. He immediately resented Intourist and was annoyed by the high level of supervision and control over his visit. However, little of this critical commentary made it into his public statements on the Soviet Union after his visit ended. During August and September of 1935, Banting became a public spokesperson for Soviet medicine. This seems all the more surprising if we accept Bliss's claim that Banting loathed the press as a result of his experience with press attention to the discovery of insulin, the Nobel Prize, and media scrutiny of his marital breakdown.[91] An interview with Britain's *Sunday Mail* on September 1, 1935, as he was returning to Canada from the Soviet Union quoted Banting:

> Russia, declared Sir Frederick, is one of the leading countries in medicine. She has a State medical service, of course, and that commands the interest of every doctor. They are doing great things in the Soviet Union, not only in medicine, but in industry. It is definitely a country for the young, although there is great opportunity for everyone. … Please make care, he added, that I was allowed to go about just as I wished. There is, indeed, more freedom in Russia than anywhere else in the world—and I've been all over the world.[92]

He argued that the way in which health services were organized in the Soviet Union was rational and equitable:

> The worker comes first in the Soviet Union and every factory has its medical health unit, first aid stations for quick treatment in case of accident, hospitals for the care of the sick, and clinics where not only the worker may go free of charge, but also his or her dependents. Each factory has its group of consultants for special cases, eye, ear, nose and throat, tuberculosis, surgery, and all other cases where the attention of a specialist is necessary. They are attached directly to the factory staff.[93]

Given the accessibility of free medical treatment, Banting reasoned, illness was treated earlier and more effectively.

Apart from media interviews, Banting wrote his own article for *Canadian Business* magazine in February 1936, entitled "Science and the Soviet Union." The article summarized what Banting viewed as "stupendous" progress towards industrialization and modernization, with scientific and educational achievement at the centre of Soviet achievement. Marshaling impressive statistics, Banting argued that the Soviet Union had more than tripled its number of physicians, and 10,000 new physicians were being educated per year. These physicians were part of "almost universal hospitalization of all sick people."[94] But it was the Soviet embrace of science and its commitment to medical science and research that most impressed Banting: "The government of the Soviet Union gave 15,698,398 rubles in 1933, 31, 517,418 rubles in 1934 and 35,780,748 rubles in 1935 to the All-Union Institute of Experimental Medicine, for the purpose of Medical Research."[95]

Banting also lauded progress made in biology, mineralogy, physics, chemistry, and botany, and expressed his support for the way in which science was applied, and the work of scientists who, he noted:

devoted themselves assiduously to the problems of the state. Their scientific knowledge was applied to the development of electric power, mining, industry of all kinds, and particularly to agriculture. … Today scientific research and the application of science to industry is the most impressive activity in the Soviet Union. There is no country in the world that is progressing so rapidly in this regard.[96]

This notion of science serving the people was a potent one in the 1930s; it struck a chord with scientists like Banting, who found the possibility of social relevance and honour appealing.[97] This may be viewed as a form of idealism, but it also spoke to a commonly shared critique of what Bethune and others would come to call capitalistic medicine, and a desire to perform socially relevant and useful work.

It is true that Banting's understanding of the Soviet Union was limited, not least by the manipulations of Intourist and Soviet agencies who shepherded him and others through their Soviet visits. He also wanted to see the best and did not ask hard questions. The more difficult question to answer is: why? The image of Soviet health care and medical science presented to western political travellers was so appealing because it tapped into desires and aspirations held in common—desires for greater social equality, for health care provision, and for an opportunity to serve the people and demonstrate social commitment. These aspirations have been, for the most part, historically silenced .

The place occupied by Soviet health care in the transnational imaginary of socialized medicine is multifaceted. Some of those who viewed it as an exemplar had knowledge of the structure of the Soviet system as detailed as it was realistically possible for a foreigner to have—commentators like Arthur Newsholme, John Adams Kingsbury, or Henry Sigerist might fall into this category. Their publications on Soviet medicine were well known across the boundaries of nation states; Sigerist would play an especially important role in the history of Canadian medicare. Political travellers like Banting or Bethune were much less knowledgeable; nevertheless, their views became important in the context of late-1930s political debates in Canada.

Although not colleagues, comrades, or friends, Banting and Bethune shared certain commonalities: both were iconoclasts and loners of a certain type and occupied the unusual position of being both leaders of the medical research community, yet somehow outside the medical establishment. They were roughly the same age; they attended the same medical school; they had both experienced the Great War and the Great Depression; they both had a passion for visual art and were themselves amateur artists. Both were apparently appealing to women, both their marriages had failed. Neither man came from leftist political backgrounds, yet they both became interested in medical politics in the 1930s. Both should be considered "ideas" men (as Bliss refers to Banting); perhaps idealists, but perhaps such a term is too pejorative. While Banting was the more famous at the time, both men enjoyed a public platform from which to articulate their ideas about Soviet health care and the need for reform at home.

The Soviet experience was not merely reflected back, unmediated or undigested, by Soviet medical travellers like Banting and Bethune. It was translated into specific local contexts. Red medicine served two functions in the Canadian context. The first was to expose the deficiencies of Canadian health care policy and the conservatism of the Canadian medical profession. The Soviet Union, a society barely out of feudalism, could and did do better. It was a useful discursive tool. Second, aspects of the Soviet approach to health care were incorporated into already circulating radical visions for health organization and politics, and they were elevated into an ideal to which radical reformers could aspire. While there was no single definition of what constituted "socialized medicine," elements included full state provision (as opposed to a health insurance model), the idea of the polyclinic or health centre providing a variety of health services close to home, and the melding of public health and preventive care with curative medical carethe blurring of the care/cure boundary. While these ideas were not purely Soviet, Canadian health advocates saw the value in the Soviet model and said so publicly. Thus, Soviet-Canadian transnational dialogue belongs in the history of Canadian socialized medicine.

The role of Soviet medicine as inspiration came amidst a growing awareness during the 1930s of the failures of countries such as Canada, the US, and even Britain (which already had a combination of voluntary provision and state health insurance, however inadequate) to meet the health needs of their populations. When visitors such as Banting and Bethune came home to their native countries, they spoke enthusiastically about Soviet developments, and argued that the Soviet experiment could point the way for reform at home. In this sense, although Banting and Bethune and others like them did not go to the Soviet Union as communists, their journeys radicalized them. Their voices joined those of others who argued that a Soviet vision of socialized health care and prevention of disease highlighted both the failures of public policy in Canada and an actually existing alternative set of state policies from which to borrow and learn. Understood within this context, Canadian political travellers who journeyed to the Soviet Union to witness its health care system were participating in a political moment occurring all over the western world, far beyond Canada's national borders.

ENDNOTES

1   Sydney Webb and Beatrice Webb, *Soviet Communism: A New Civilization?* (New York: C. Scribner's sons, 1935).

2   I am indebted here to the work of Kirk Niergarth. See http://blogs.mtroyal. ca/kniergarth/canadianvisitorstoussr/ Accessed 15 June 2018.

3   Roland Fairburn McWilliams and Margaret McWilliams, *Russia in 1926* (London and Toronto: J.M. Dent, 1927).

4   Michael David-Fox, *Showcasing the Great Experiment: Cultural Diplomacy and Western Visitors to the Soviet Union, 1921-1941* (New York: Oxford, 2012), 1.

5   Paul Hollander, *Political Pilgrims: Travels of Western Intellectuals to the Soviet Union, China and Cuba, 1928-1978* (New York: Oxford University Press, 1981); Ludmila Stern, *Western Intellectuals and the Soviet Union, 1920-40: From Red Square to the Left Bank* (London: Routledge, 2007).

6   David-Fox, *Showcasing the Great Experiment*, 2.

7   Sheila Fitzpatrick and Carolyn Rasmussen, eds., *Political Tourists: Travellers From Australia to the Soviet Union in the 1920s-1940s* (Carlton, VIC: Melbourne University Publishing, 2008).

8   David-Fox, *Showcasing the Great Experiment*, 25, 3.

9   David-Fox, *Showcasing the Great Experiment*, 72.

10 Susan Gross Solomon, "Foreign Expertise on Russian Terrain: Max Kuczynski on the Kirghiz Steppe, 1923-24," in *Soviet Medicine: Culture, Practice, and Science*, ed. Frances L. Bernstein, Christopher Burton, and Dan Healey (DeKalb, Illinois: Northern Illinois University Press, 2010), 86 note #1.

11 Peter Kuznick, *Beyond the Laboratory: Scientists as Political Activists in 1930s America* (Chicago: University of Chicago Press, 1987).

12 Susan Gross Solomon, "The Expert and the State in Russian Public Health: Continuities and Changes Across the Revolutionary Divide," in *The History of Public Health and the Modern State*, ed. Dorothy Porter (Amsterdam: Rodopi, 1994), 184.

13 Michael Bliss, *Banting: A Biography* (Toronto: McClelland and Stewart, 1984).

14 Kuznick, *Beyond the Laboratory*, 145.

15 Tricia Starks, *The Body Soviet: Propaganda, Hygiene, and the Revolutionary State* (Madison, Wisconsin: University of Wisconsin Press, 2008), 3.

16 Sally Ewing, "The Science and Politics of Soviet Insurance Medicine," in *Health and Society in Revolutionary Russia*, ed. Susan Gross Solomon and John F. Hutchinson (Bloomington and Indianapolis: Indiana University Press, 1990), 69–73.

17 Solomon, "The Expert and the State in Russian Public Health," 201, 203.

18 Neil B. Weissman, "Origins of Soviet Health Administration: Narkomzdrav, 1918-1928," in *Health and Society in Revolutionary Russia*, ed. Susan Gross Solomon and John F. Hutchinson (Bloomington and Indianapolis: Indiana University Press, 1990), 97.

19 The goal of its "own medicine" is referred to by Weissman, 98. For Soviet medical education and research in social hygiene see Solomon, "The Expert and the State."

20 Weissman, "Origins of Soviet Health Administration," 98.

21 Ewing, "The Science and Politics of Soviet Insurance Medicine," 70.

22 Weissman, "Origins of Soviet Health Administration," 102.

23 Weissman, "Origins of Soviet Health Administration," 104–6.

24 Solomon, "The Expert and the State in Russian Public Health," 197, 196.

25 Quoted in Solomon, "The Expert and the State in Russian Public Health," 196.

26 Solomon, "The Expert and the State in Russian Public Health," 203.

27 Solomon, "The Expert and the State in Russian Public Health," 202.

28 Christopher Williams, "The Revolution from above in Soviet Medicine, Leningrad 1928-1932," *Journal of Urban History* 20, no. 4 (August 1994), 515–19.

29 Williams, "The Revolution from above in Soviet Medicine," 522–24.

30 Susan Gross Solomon, "Social Hygiene and Soviet Public Health, 1921-1930," in *Health and Society in Revolutionary Russia*, ed. Susan Gross Solomon and John F. Hutchinson (Bloomington and Indianapolis: Indiana University Press, 1990), 191.

31 Mark G. Field, *Soviet Socialized Medicine: An Introduction* (New York: The Free Press, 1967), viii.

32 Arthur Newsholme and John Adams Kingsbury, *Red Medicine: Socialized Health in Soviet Russia* (Garden City, New York: Doubleday, 1933).

33 John M. Eyler, *Sir Arthur Newsholme and State Medicine, 1885-1935* (Cambridge; New York: Cambridge University Press, 1997), 371.

34 Newsholme and Kingsbury, *Red Medicine*, 9–10.

35 Newsholme and Kingsbury, *Red Medicine*, 231.

36 Field, *Soviet Socialized Medicine*, x. "Sigerist's books ... were well-intentioned, sympathetic, but rather uncritical (if not somewhat ax-grinding and Pollyanic) views of Soviet medical organization and public health. These views were influenced, no doubt, by Sigerist's enthusiasm for the *principle* of socialized medicine which, as a historian of medicine, he felt was *the* medicine of the future, and by his politically naïve conceptions of Soviet society, even during the worst years of Stalin's totalitarianism and terror."

37 Eyler, *Sir Arthur Newsholme and State Medicine*, 372.

38 Elizabeth Fee and Edward T. Morman, "Doing History, Making
    Revolution: The Aspirations of Henry E. Sigerist and George Rosen,"
    in *Making Medical History: The Life and Times of Henry E. Sigerist*, ed.
    Elizabeth Fee and Theodore M. Brown (Baltimore and London: Johns
    Hopkins University Press, 1997), 277.

39 Donald L. Madison, "Remembering Cecil," in *Cecil G. Sheps Memorial
    Volume*, ed. Donald L. Madison (University of North Carolina at Chapel
    Hill: Cecil G. Sheps Center for Health Services Research, 2005), 11.

40 For anti-Semitism in the life of George Rosen, whom Sigerist mentored, see
    Fee and Morman, "Doing History, Making Revolution."

41 Elizabeth Fee, "The Pleasures and Perils of Prophetic Advocacy: Socialized
    Medicine and the Politics of American Medical Reform," in *Making
    Medical History: The Life and Times of Henry E. Sigerist*, ed. Elizabeth
    Fee and Theodore M. Brown (Baltimore and London: Johns Hopkins
    University Press, 1997), 201, 211.

42 Henry E. Sigerist, *Socialised Medicine in the Soviet Union* (London: Victor
    Gollancz, 1937), 83.

43 Sigerist, *Socialised Medicine in the Soviet Union*, 95.

44 Sigerist, *Socialised Medicine in the Soviet Union*, 289.

45 Fitzpatrick and Rasmussen, *Political Tourists*, 24.

46 Roderick Stewart and Sharon Stewart, *Phoenix: The Life of Norman
    Bethune* (Montreal and Kingston: McGill-Queen's University Press, 2011),
    7, 13.

47 Stewart and Stewart, *Phoenix*, 24.

48 Stewart and Stewart, *Phoenix*, 28.

49 Stewart and Stewart, *Phoenix*, 76.

50 Gabriel Nadeau, "A T.B.'s Progress, the Story of Norman Bethune,"
    Bulletin of the History of Medicine, 8 (1940): 1144–45.

51 Stewart and Stewart, *Phoenix*, 104, 95-96, 101-102.

52 Larry Hannant, *The Politics of Passion: Norman Bethune's Writing and Art*
    (Toronto: University of Toronto Press, 1998), 34.

53 Quote from Hannant, *The Politics of Passion*, p. 71.

54 Stewart and Stewart, *Phoenix*, 107.

55 Hannant, *The Politics of Passion*, 91.

56 Hannant, *The Politics of Passion*, 92.

57 Library and Archives Canada (hereafter LAC), R2437-0-2-E, Marion Scott
    fonds, Vol 14, File 20 Bethune, Letter to Marion Scott, October 8, 1935.

58 Hannant, *The Politics of Passion*, 97–99.

59 Hannant, *The Politics of Passion*, 100.

60 Hannant, *The Politics of Passion*, 101.

61 Hannant, *The Politics of Passion*, 102.

62 Hannant, *The Politics of Passion*, 102.

63 LAC, R2437-0-2-E, Marion Scott fonds, Vol 14, File 20, Bethune, Letter to Marion Scott, October 8, 1935.

64 Osler Library Archives (hereafter OLA), P156, Norman Bethune Collection, Box 372, Acc. No. 512, "An Open Letter to All Political Candidates Seeking Election in Montreal," August 1936.

65 Wendell MacLeod, Libbie Park, and Stanley B. Ryerson, *Bethune: The Montreal Years* (Toronto: James Lorimer & Company, 1978), 12.

66 MacLeod, Park, and Ryerson, *Bethune: The Montreal Years*, 76.

67 MacLeod, Park, and Ryerson, *Bethune: The Montreal Years*, 98–99.

68 MacLeod, Park, and Ryerson, *Bethune: The Montreal Years*, 97.

69 MacLeod, Park, and Ryerson, *Bethune: The Montreal Years*, 102.

70 MacLeod, Park, and Ryerson, *Bethune: The Montreal Years*, 102.

71 MacLeod, Park, and Ryerson, *Bethune: The Montreal Years*, 103.

72 LAC, MG30, Norman Bethune fonds, B55, File 1-6, "Various Commentaries on Health Insurance and Medical Economics."

73 MacLeod, Park, and Ryerson, 61.

74 MacLeod, Park, and Ryerson, 104.

75 MacLeod, Park, and Ryerson, 67.

76 MacLeod, Park, and Ryerson, 108.

77 OLA, P156, Norman Bethune Collection, Box 372, Acc. No. 512, "An Open Letter to All Political Candidates Seeking Election in Montreal," August 1936.

78 Stewart and Stewart, *Phoenix: The Life of Norman Bethune*, 215–16. The assessment that Bethune may have been suffering from post-traumatic stress is my own, not that of the Stewarts.

79 Stewart and Stewart, *Phoenix*, 220.

80 Stewart and Stewart, *Phoenix*, 226–27.

81 Donald L. Madison, ed., *Cecil G. Sheps Memorial Volume* (University of North Carolina at Chapel Hill: Cecil G. Sheps Center for Health Services Research, 2005), 71.

82 Bliss, *Banting: A Biography*, 10.

83 Thomas Fisher Rare Book Library (hereafter TFL), Frederick Banting Papers, MSS Coll 76, Box 30, File 7, Diary, June 22, 1935.

84 TFL, MSS Coll 76, Frederick Banting Papers, MSS Coll 76, Box 2, Letter to A.Y. Jackson, July 29, 1935.

85 TFL, MSS Coll 76, Frederick Banting Papers, Box 30, Diary, June 22, 1935.

86 TFL, MSS Coll 76, Frederick Banting Papers, Box 30, Diary, June 27, 1935

87 TFL, MSS Coll 76, Frederick Banting Papers, Box 30, Diary, June 23, 1935.

88 TFL, MSS Coll 76, Frederick Banting Papers, Box 30, Diary, June 25, 1935.

89 TFL, MSS Coll 76, Frederick Banting Papers, Box 30, Diary, June 28, 1935.

90 TFL, MSS Coll 76, Frederick Banting Papers, Box 30, Undated diary entry written either June 30 or July 1, 1935.

91 Michael Bliss argues that Banting's dislike of journalists was quickly entrenched. Bliss, *Banting: A Biography*, 110–11.

92 TFL, MSS Coll 76, Frederick Banting Papers, Box 48B, Scrapbook, "Russia for Youth: Famous Doctor's Views," *Sunday Mail*, Glasgow, Sept 1, 1935.

93 TFL, MSS Coll 76, Frederick Banting Papers, Box 48B, Scrapbook, "Science Replacing Quackery in Soviet," 95.

94 Sir Frederick Banting, "Science and the Soviet Union," *Canadian Business* (February 1936), 15.

95 Sir Frederick Banting, "Science and the Soviet Union," 15.

96 Sir Frederick Banting, "Science and the Soviet Union," 15.

97 See Kuznick, *Beyond the Laboratory*.

CHAPTER 2

A SMILE IN THE MACHINE

British Labour and London's Interwar Health Centre Movement

The "Social Insurance and Allied Services Report," more commonly known as the Beveridge Report, is often referred to as the keystone of the National Health Service (NHS). Historians of Canadian medicare consider it influential to the development of Canadian health care policy debates during and after World War II.[1] Yet Beveridge's report, released in November 1942, was just one, rather liberal, contribution to long-standing discussions about improvements to health care provision in the UK. Beveridge proposed essentially a contributory insurance model for social services, including health care. At the time, the health centre model remained at the centre of health-policy debates, where it had been for nearly twenty years. Just as in the US and the Soviet Union, health centres represented many of the aspirations and plans for the medical and political left.

In 1920, Lord Bernard Dawson, chair of the Lloyd George (Liberal) Government's Medical Consultative Council and author of the Dawson Report, proposed that health centres form the nucleus of primary care delivery in a state health system.[2] The Labour Party had advocated primary care delivery at health centres as early as 1919, when its Advisory Committee on Public Health issued a report endorsing them. The Labour Party's Public Health

Advisory Committee made two intersecting proposals for health reform in the early 1920s. The first was that health centres would form the "foundation" of a national health service, "dispensing free curative and preventive care from the grass-roots up." The committee also recommended, based on the input of physician Somerville Hastings, that in a socialized system of health care, physicians should be employed full time by the state and paid a salary. "With these proposals, Labour had, even in the 1920s, a radical alternative in health planning."[3]

As Virginia Berridge has pointed out, early support for the health centre model was "in part inspired by the revolutionary changes in health care in the Soviet Union ... after the October Revolution."[4] During the interwar years, awareness of Soviet medicine grew in Britain. The British edition of Henry Sigerist's *Socialized Medicine in the Soviet Union* (1937), which argued for health centres with a full range of coordinated preventive and primary services, had a significant impact in the UK. Fabian reformers Sidney and Beatrice Webb wrote the forward for the British edition.[5] Sigerist's book had been preceded by several years by Newsholme and Kingsbury's *Red Medicine* (briefly discussed in the previous chapter), which argued that "a marvelous reformed and extended medical service had been organized in Russia, the methods and procedures of which the rest of the world would do well to study."[6] Newsholme's biographer, John Eyler, reveals that by the end of the 1920s, Newsholme had developed a transnational understanding of health care systems by "systematically studying Continental and American medicine."[7] Newsholme was invited to the United States in early 1926, by the Milbank Memorial Fund, where he visited rural health demonstration projects in New York State funded by Milbank. Newsholme was asked by John Kingsbury to undertake a study of European health systems in order to help Milbank make the case in the US for fundamental health reform. Newsholme visited thirteen countries in Continental Europe in 1929 and 1930, out of which came the three-volume publication, *International Studies on the Relation Between the Private and Official Practice of Medicine* (1931), and then his influential book, *Medicine and the State* (1932). According to Eyler, Newsholme was not an uncritical observer, but nonetheless believed that Europe's experience had an important lesson for America. Newsholme argued that the need for state involvement in health was an inevitable outcome of the "advancement of civilization and the development of moral sensibility."[8] State health insurance was not a flawless model, however: Newsholme saw that insurance could generate waste and emphasize treatment over prevention. He also worried that insurance on its own would generate a "doctor-seeking habit."[9]

Newsholme's final collaboration with Milbank came through a 1932 invitation from John Kingsbury to journey to the Soviet Union. Newsholme was initially skeptical that anything could be learned from the Soviet experiment. But he did agree to go with Kingsbury, and the two of them spent four weeks in the Soviet Union in fall 1932, travelling over 9000 miles from Kazan to the Caucasus. Like other prominent visitors, the two were provided resources by the Soviet state, including a car, interpreters, and special visits to points of interest including Pavlov's lab, polyclinics in Leningrad and Gorky, sanatoriums in Yalta, and other health organizations. They were aware that they were being shown the best of Soviet health care, and that information from interpreters and interviews was partial and biased. Still, Eyler argues, Kingsbury and Newsholme "trusted their ability to sift the evidence they were shown and to arrive at a good understanding of the nation's health and health care provisions."[10]

Kingsbury and Newsholme did not have identical views on Soviet medicine; Eyler argues that Kingsbury was the more uncritical admirer of the two and pressured Newsholme to reduce his criticisms as they prepared their study for publication. He urged Newsholme to leave out his moral qualms about Soviet policies on divorce and abortion, for example. More so than his co-author, Kingsbury viewed

Red Medicine as essentially a political intervention in favour of social-ized medicine. His priority was to publish a book that was accessible and with broad public appeal in the US and Britain—hence the pro-vocative title and high-quality photographs illustrating the book. Kingsbury hired the documentary photographer Margaret Bourke-White, who was then the staff photographer at *Fortune* magazine. (She would later join *LIFE* and shoot their first cover in 1936.)[11] In 1930, she was the first western photographer to document the Soviet Five Year Plan. Bourke-White travelled to the Soviet Union (where she visited three times in the 1930s) with Kingsbury's list of sug-gestions and photographed rest homes, hospitals, the Tuberculosis Institute at Tiflis, and the Cardiac Sanatorium in Georgia, among other sites, which illustrate *Red Medicine*.

The book's preface begins, "When a Russian becomes ill the Government does something about it. ... Soviet Russia has decided that the health of the individual is the concern of society as a whole."[12] The comment reflects not just image manipulation by Soviet agencies (discussed in the previous chapter), but also the political perspec-tive of these authors. Descriptions of Soviet life, politics, industry, agriculture, marriage, divorce and family life, and abortion occupy nearly 200 of the book's 300 pages. Although intentionally written with few statistics to enhance its accessibility, the book takes the sociological approach popular at the time among advocates of social medicine in the West. The last third of the book outlines Soviet medical treatment, organized into a system of state-run dispensaries, polyclinics, and hospitals: "every doctor in Soviet Russia is a State official," Newsholme and Kingsbury explain. They praise the Soviet system for aiming to eliminate the isolation of the individual phys-ician in private practice and for "securing the complete unification of medical work." Soviet medicine emphasized the "collective and environmental treatment" of the patient, understanding their health in a broader context of work and community—what we would call today the social determinants of health.[13]

Dispensaries and polyclinics had similar structures and aims. Dispensaries were the smallest unit of medical service at the local level; the polyclinics tended to be larger, included a greater number of specialists, and often acted as training sites for nurses and physicians. Both served residents of a defined local area, providing preventive and curative medicine to everyone in the population; in most cases, care was free of charge, although according to Newsholme and Kingsbury some clinics did charge fees. *Red Medicine* described a large polyclinic known as the "ambulatorium" in Leningrad, which employed 128 doctors from all branches of medicine, where workers were treated for free either at their homes or after being transferred to a hospital or specialized institution such as a tuberculosis sanatorium. Some Soviet polyclinics, such as the one in Kharkov, were special-built facilities clearly designed to be showcases for Soviet medicine. Newsholme and Kingsbury were deeply impressed by the resources brought together at Kharkov:

> This particular polyclinic is situated in a workers' district and is intended primarily to give gratuitous medical aid in the factories of Kharkov.
>
> The polyclinic is a great multiform dispensary, serving some 40,000 workers and their families. It is controlled by the Department of Health of the Kharkov City Soviet and is supported out of insurance funds. The new building consists of four floors. ... The first floor comprises surgical urological, and orthopedic departments, a chemical and bacteriological laboratory, a dispensary for children under four years old, offices for the physicians, for inquiry, and for reception.
>
> The second floor has a therapeutic department and a special department for the treatment of workers in dangerous industries, a department for consultations on physical culture, a psycho-neurological dispensary, a dispensary for anti-narcotic treatment, a dispensary for prenatal and gynecological care and

for consultation on questions of sex and marriage, a department for electric and light-radiating treatments, and a hall for corrective gymnastics.

On the third floor is the ophthalmic department and the department for ear, nose, and throat disease, an inhalatorium, a sanitary consultation, a dental department, and a dispensary for young children.

There are in addition four old pavilions, a tuberculosis dispensary, a mild-food kitchen, a dietetic dining hall, a pharmacy, and diagnostic wards with ninety beds and physiotherapeutic wards with sixty beds.

The above enumeration gives an imperfect idea of the elaboration and completeness of the arrangements for every branch of medical or hygienic needs; nor does it express the completeness of the arrangements for co-operation between these various special departments for the benefit of patients.[14]

The Kharkov polyclinic was located near a tractor factory with 16,000 workers, which had its own on-site polyclinic and 400-bed hospital. Newsholme and Kingsbury were enthusiastic about this dazzling polyclinic as a model.

Red Medicine was not an entirely uncritical book and Newsholme was no starry-eyed Soviet acolyte. He tended to praise aspects of Soviet medicine that echoed his own call for reforms in British health. In his 1919 book, *Public Health and Insurance*, Newsholme emphasized the need to integrate preventive and curative medicine and the value of physician teamwork in a salaried health service. *Red Medicine* applauds the provision of free medical care in the Soviet Union, and the country's attempts to eliminate gaps and lack of coordination in health care provision. The book's conclusion argues that, in these ways, Soviet achievement outpaced health care in either Britain or the US.

Writing on the history of medicine in Britain, Dorothy Porter refers to an "international social medicine movement," which was at the same time an intellectual approach to health problems facing countries like the UK. Influenced by Soviet social hygiene, western social medicine sought to analyze health and illness in their social contexts, and to bring social science techniques to bear on finding solutions to the problem of health inequality:

> The interdisciplinary program between medicine and social sciences would provide medicine with the intellectual skills needed to analyze the social causes of health and illness in the same way as the alliance between medicine and the laboratory sciences had provided new insights into the chemical and physical bases of disease. But these developments took place within, and were inherently bound to, the international debate concerning the establishment of socialized medicine and the eradication of health inequalities.[15]

Proponents of social medicine in interwar and World War II Britain intended it to be more than a set of prescriptions. They sought to politicize medicine and to involve medical professionals in contemporary debates about social and medical reform and the role of the state. These debates intensified during the economic crisis of the 1930s and in wartime discussions about the need for a national health service and access to services without financial barriers.

Labour's program for health reform was enlivened by discourse on the medical left. Radical physicians who became active in the Labour Party argued in favour of a re-organized system of socialized medicine with health centres at its heart. The re-organization of health services was badly needed in Britain. Health spending and services grew significantly in the interwar years, but health care was poorly coordinated among a number of programs and services. Primary care was available to employed male members of the workforce via the National Health Insurance Act (1911), while the poor law dispensed hospital and long-term institutional care to the most impoverished. In 1929, the Local Government Act introduced greater support for municipal health services.[16] The national government funded maternal and child welfare clinics, and the counties allocated funds for tuberculosis care. Despite these overall improvements in health and health provision between 1900 and 1930, benefits were "inequitably distributed and linked with features such as social class background, gender, age and geographic area," Steven Cherry argues.[17] According to Charles Webster, "The services themselves, including hospitals, were frequently stigmatized for being unnecessarily bureaucratic and inhumane."[18]

The health centre model became a key element of the political left's response to these inequities. By the early 1930s health centres featured prominently in the health policy proposals of the Socialist Medical Association (SMA), the Medical Practitioners' Union, and the Labour Party at national and local levels.[19] The SMA was founded in 1930 and formally affiliated to the Labour Party the following year, but remained a distinct organization. Historian John Stewart has argued that the SMA had influence within Labour disproportionate to its size and played a key role in the creation of the National Health Service (NHS) after the war. Some of its influence was due to the commitment of the SMA's first president, Dr. Somerville Hastings, a man his fellow socialist physicians praised as having lived a "remarkable life" and as "quietly efficient, persevering, shrewd and kindly," "a shy man without personal ambition ... greatly revered by his colleagues in the Labour Party."[20] Hastings was also a highly accomplished physician. Trained at University College, London and Middlesex Hospital, Hastings became a Fellow of the Royal College of Surgeons in 1904 and served as the President of the Laryngology Section of the Royal Society of Medicine in the late 1920s. Hastings served in both world wars as part of the armed forces medical services. He retired from private practice in 1945.

Hastings was a central figure in a generation of politically active members of the medical left in Britain. According to Stewart, "Hastings saw himself as a Christian Socialist and was active ... in the Fabian Society and the Independent Labour Party" in the early twentieth century. He was elected Member of Parliament (MP) for Reading in 1924 and 1929–1931, and he was elected to London County Council (LCC) representing Mile End from 1932 to 1946, during which time he served as Chair of the LCC's Hospital and Medical Services Committee. From 1945 to 1959 he was the Labour MP for Barking. Like Arthur Newsholme, he had a transnational perspective on health care reform. Hastings participated in the founding meeting of the International Socialist Medical Association at Carlsbad in 1931. The same year, he visited the Soviet Union with his physician friend and Labour colleague, Bermondsey's MP Alfred Salter. The two men had much in common. Five years older than Hastings, Salter was born in 1873 in Greenwich. He took his medical training at Guy's Hospital, London, was awarded a scholarship in public health, and was appointed a bacteriologist at the Lister Institute of Preventive Medicine soon after completing his medical training. Like Hastings, whose father was a Reverend, Salter came from an intensely religious family, who became Plymouth Brethren. Salter's biographer, Fenner Brockway, says that Salter was speaking at street-corner Salvation Army meetings by the time he was 15. Salter was politicized during his time at Guy's, "overlooking the slums of Bermondsey," and went to work at a Methodist settlement house in the district. There he met Ada Brown, his future wife and future Mayor of the Borough of Bermondsey.

Hastings published his impressions of this visit as *Medicine in Soviet Russia*, and the influence of the Soviet health centre is clear in his reform program, *The People's Health*, published by the Labour Party in 1932. Hastings adopted from the Soviet model several principles for socialized medicine: the importance of multidisciplinary teamwork in health organization; the value of good record keeping; and the Soviet integration of preventive and curative medicine under one roof. Hastings also emphasized popular control over health services as fundamental in a democratic society.[21] According to John Stewart, the Soviet system inspired Hastings' vision for health: "a service where all functions revolved around one focal point, and where the anarchy, overlap and class discrimination of the existing British system was done away with."[22]

These were years of increasing optimism in England's medical left. Socialist reformers saw the chance to reform public health services at the municipal level as a result of the Local Government Act, which turned poor-law health services over to the county and county borough councils in England and Wales. The Act was important to the expansion of publicly funded hospital care in the interwar years.[23] Combined with other legislation such as the Maternity and Child Welfare Act (1918), the Public Health (Tuberculosis) Act (1921), and the Midwives Act (1936), the law also created an opportunity for progressive borough-level governments to develop integrated health programming for tuberculosis prevention and treatment, maternal and child welfare, school medical services, dentistry, school meals, sanitation, and infectious disease control that was based in principles of equity, and did not segregate care for paupers and non-paupers.[24] These programs were to form the basis for an incipient health centre movement, which was especially successful in London.[25]

Health centres were intended to coordinate local services, develop a broader range of health care than was normally available from the local borough (to include the treatment of common diseases like rheumatism, for example), and make care available in a single location. London's health centres demonstrate the innovation possible in public health and medical care provision at the municipal borough level by the late 1930s, even in absence of a national health service. In London, for example, expanded and improved state hospital services were key to Labour's platform in the 1934 London County Council (LCC) elections. Labour's health care commitments contributed to their virtual electoral sweep of the city. At the same time, Labour-dominated local borough councils within Red London began to reimagine primary and preventive health care in their districts. The London boroughs of Bermondsey (1935), Finsbury (1936), Southwark (1936), and Woolwich (1938) built landmark health centres in the years leading up to the outbreak of the World War II.[26]

Not all Labour boroughs in London constructed health centres during this period, but some Labour councils undertook ambitious programs for health reform. The 1930s saw few political successes for Labour at the national level, and this contributed to a greater focus on local government. Historians of Labour in the interwar years have argued that local party activists built political success by showing "the relevance of socialism to everyday life"[27] and its commitment to "offer alternatives to daily insecurities."[28] The interwar slogan of the Woolwich Labour Party, for example, was: "the Labour Party is not politics—it is life. Do you belong?"[29] According to John Stewart, in the mid- to late 1930s, Labour demonstrated a growing awareness of health care as an issue of significance to its electoral success.[30]

The majority of credit for this political focus on health care as relevant to the daily lives of working-class people must be given to the long-standing activism of Labour women. When elected to maternity and child welfare committees and public health committees, they played a key role in promoting local health initiatives. Labour women worked, where possible, with progressive medical officers of health to make medical care and auxiliary services available to borough mothers and children. As Pat Thane, Patricia Hollis, Pamela Graves, and others have argued, politically active women in Britain from the late nineteenth century on were more likely to give issues of social welfare prominence in their work than were men, including Labour Party men.[31] When and where local Labour councils worked to expand social provision, as Duncan Tanner has noted, "It was often prompted to consider such ideas by its own women's sections."[32]

By the First World War, women were being elected to the boards of poor-law guardians and rural and urban county and borough councils across the country, where they served on education, library, and relief committees. Although little electoral ground was gained for women nationally after the franchise was granted in 1918, locally it was another story, as hundreds of women successfully campaigned to join local councils, boards of guardians, and the magistrate's bench.[33] In 1934, there were 729 borough councilors elected in London; 150 of them were women—over 20 percent. Women were active on the maternity and child welfare committees (where they were sometimes in the majority) and public health committees of the London borough councils in which health centres emerged. These women politicians pushed local committees and councils to act within the full scope of permissive welfare legislation.

Labour women claimed a place at the political table based upon their specific knowledge of the health, educational, economic, and child welfare needs of working-class women. They argued forcefully that health issues were best represented by women of their own class.[34] This is not to say, however, that they did not push boundaries of class and gender in their local government capacities. As Pamela Graves has noted, there were meaningful differences in the approach of Labour women to health and welfare issues compared with that of their conservative male opponents. Pamela Graves's interview with Jessie Stephen, elected to the Bermondsey Board of Guardians in 1921, reveals that Ms. Stephen argued for the dignity and comfort of the poor who needed state support:

> One of her first acts was to get rid of the rituals of deference which obliged old people to stand up when a guardian entered the room. "Neither I nor my [Labour] colleagues, could stomach this kow-towing to elected representatives and it must cease." Finding the inmates eating on benches, she ordered proper chairs and tables and a greater variety of food.[35]

Jessie Stephen also opposed the stigmatization of poor mothers and children and argued against the segregation of unmarried mothers in poor law institutions. Stephen, like other Labour women in this period, argued that working-class and poor recipients of state programs were entitled to equal treatment, and quality services. These values found their way into Labour's program for health reform.

After growing electoral successes, Labour-led borough councils in London made access to health care a priority and began to enact a transformation of mainstream medicine. As we have seen, a number of London boroughs built landmark health centres in the years leading up to the outbreak of the Second World War, as did several suburban boroughs. Local councils in Camberwell (1938) and Kensington (1939) proposed centres whose construction was prevented by the outbreak of war. London's health centre movement sought to provide an integrated range of preventive public health and primary care, under popular control, centrally housed, and built to a high standard. Health centres reflected a new assertive and innovative approach to the health problems of the urban working class and poor.

The most publicly celebrated of the new borough health centres was Finsbury. The Finsbury Health Centre opened in 1936. In the late 1930s, Finsbury was known as one of the most politically radical boroughs in London. Described by some as The People's Republic of Finsbury, the borough erected a monument to Lenin in the 1940s. In the early 1930s the Finsbury Borough Council was less radical, but solidly Labour. In 1938 it elected as mayor Dr. Chuni Lal Katial, an Indian émigré. Katial and Councilor Harold Riley were the leading forces in the campaign to build the Finsbury Health Centre. Katial was both Mayor and Chair of the Public Health Committee and worked closely with the Soviet émigré architect, Berthold Lubetkin, to design their innovative new centre. Lubetkin was an outspoken leftist in addition to being a highly regarded

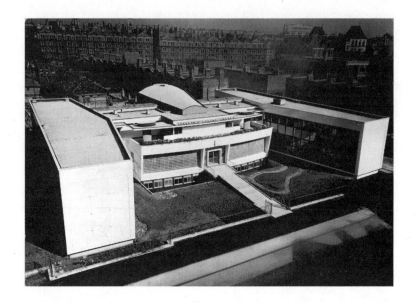

Finsbury Health Centre
COURTESY RIBA

architect. According to his biographer, John Allan, for Lubetkin "architecture was the ideological means to a social end," a "social weapon" in the struggle for mass emancipation.[36]

The Finsbury Health Centre, on Pine Street in Clerkenwell, still stands today. It is a Grade I listed heritage building, because of its architectural significance to British modernism. When it opened in 1936, visitors and clients approached the building between two "opening arms"[37] (the outer wings of the building) and entered into a large, formal lobby, painted in sky blue and Tuscan red, "furnished with glamorous custom-designed chairs and lamps," and further decorated by educative murals and a colorful map of the borough.[38] The lobby was bathed in the soft natural light filtered through the exterior walls of glass brick. Patients walked out of the slums of one of the poorest boroughs in London, and into a nurturing, warm space in a state-of-the-art modern building. It was the Finsbury Labour Party's landmark public building, which opened with great fanfare and political pride, a key plank in local Labour's program of social transformation and renewal.

The health centre built upon the existing backbone of borough health care, mainly in maternity and child welfare provision and tuberculosis prevention and care. Services for mothers and children in Finsbury were delivered at two borough maternity and child welfare centres that attended to the health needs of women, babies, and children to age 5. Lectures, clothing clubs, and sewing classes were organized at the centres. The borough did not run its own birth control clinic, but it did advertise the services of the Goswell Women's Welfare Centre, which provided birth control to Finsbury women. The borough employed seven health visitors, who made house calls to expectant mothers, infants up to a year old once a month, and older children less often. Programs included a dental clinic for mothers and their children, a special clinic for Italian immigrant families in the district, an artificial sunlight clinic, massage treatment for children, and free dinners for expectant and nursing mothers and toddlers up to age five. The borough provided milk either at cost or for free, and home visiting to expectant mothers. In conjunction with the LCC, arrangements had been made for children under age five suffering from ear diseases to be treated at a specialist clinic.

Women and their children could receive home nursing paid for by the borough, delivered by the nurses of the Metropolitan Nursing Association. Illnesses such as measles, whooping cough, diarrhea, pneumonia, and tuberculosis were treated. The nurses also treated maternity cases and apparently delivered babies. Finsbury instituted a midwifery scheme in 1930, directly employing municipal midwives. In 1932, some adjustments were made to this scheme, wherein the borough no longer directly employed its own midwives, but rather contracted with St. Bartholomew's Hospital, the City of London Maternity Hospital, and the Royal Northern Hospital, which would provide midwives and institutional care in more complicated cases. In 1936, with the passage of the Midwives Act, this program was taken over by the LCC. The 1937 annual report of the borough's health department indicated that almost all births in the district were either attended by public midwives or took place in hospital. Very few confinements were attended by private practitioners.[39] The borough also had a program of "home helps" for the ante-natal, confinement, and post-natal periods. Home helps were not nurses, but women hired to help in the running of the household as women dealt with pregnancy, birth, and recovery.

A health centre for Finsbury was first proposed in 1935 and received loan approval (after considerable negotiation) from the LCC in 1936.[40] Finsbury Health Centre cost £62,000 to build; £7,000 over budget. It housed a dental surgery clinic, a tuberculosis clinic, a solarium for light treatment, a bacteriological laboratory, and a reception house with "male and female wards, bathrooms and sanitary accommodation, and a communal kitchen, for cases of disinfestation and infectious disease." This facility was to house individuals and families while their homes were being disinfected. In the basement, accessed by an entrance separate from the rest of the clinic, were a disinfecting station, a cleansing station, and a mortuary. The mortuary was equipped with a waiting room and viewing chapel. The new health centre provided a wide array of services, including physiotherapy, massage, and electrical therapy. With the opening of the centre came new services provided by the borough, including a foot clinic and a clinic for women "subject to 'change of life' diseases" that also treated minor gynecological conditions.[41] On the second floor of the building were housed the offices of the public health department, and at the back of the building was a large lecture theatre that could hold 70 people, where the borough planned to host health lectures, films, and slide presentations to the public. There was also a roof terrace for the use of the staff.

Other boroughs such as Bermondsey built new health centres as part of a broader package of municipal reforms aimed at "safeguarding health."[42] Led by a Labour majority through the 1920s and 1930s, the borough developed a number of innovative local government initiatives while enjoying consistent grassroots support. Bermondsey Labour has been described as "a highly organized, active party, but supremely pragmatic in its politics."[43] Labour women in Bermondsey were especially well organized. Their political strength was, in part, the work of Ada Salter who had been organizing working class women there for decades.[44] Ada was married to Alfred Salter, a borough councilor, who was elected as Member of Parliament for Bermondsey West in 1922, its first Labour MP. Ada Salter, a Quaker and a socialist, was elected as a poor law Guardian in 1919, then to Bermondsey borough council in November 1922. Labour won the majority of seats in this election, and Ada Salter became mayor of Bermondsey, London's first woman mayor. By 1928, Bermondsey had the greatest number of women elected to office of any town or city in Britain.[45]

Despite the borough's deep poverty, the council undertook an extensive program of beautification. In the 1920s, the Beautification

Committee planted nearly six thousand trees, cared for by the council. As Mayor, Ada Salter hired a full-time gardener for the borough and launched the "Brighter Bermondsey Movement," which brought clubs, playgrounds, and music to the borough, performed by the borough choir, or the Bermondsey Municipal Orchestra.[46] She also spearheaded the replacement of over-crowded tenement housing in the borough, preferring the construction of small cottages with gardens. One such project, the Wilson Grove Estate, opened in 1928.[47]

Led by Ada's husband Alfred Salter (who retained his seat on Bermondsey Council even while an MP) the borough expanded services such as public baths, maternal and child health clinics, and tuberculosis care. A solarium opened in 1926, where cases of tuberculosis (especially non-pulmonary), rheumatism, rickets, skin diseases, and more general "debility" were treated in over 25,000 attendances per year. By the late 1930s, the borough also paid to have approximately 30 residents per year with intractable cases of tuberculosis sent to a sanatorium at Leysin, Switzerland.[48] The Bermondsey Public Health Centre, opened in November 1936, was the first of its kind in the country.[49]

The need for a health clinic (later referred to as a health centre) was first formally identified by the borough council as early as 1928. In November, it considered a report authored by D.M. Connan, the medical officer of health, which proposed that the borough construct a new facility "for the early diagnosis, supervision and treatment of acute rheumatism, arthritis and cancer." Connan made the argument that there was no adequate provision for dealing with these issues in the borough, where the health problems associated with unemployment, poverty, and poor housing were especially prevalent. The centre would also house a children's clinic for the diagnosis and treatment of sick children, in addition to tuberculosis and maternity and child welfare services already provided elsewhere by the borough. In Connan's view, it made economic sense to house a number of different clinics together in one building, centrally located.[50] The budget for the proposed centre was initially over £96,000.[51] Despite a public inquiry held by the Ministry of Health, and a lengthy debate with LCC officials lasting into 1931 over the expanded arrays of services at the proposed clinic, the plan failed to obtain loan support at this time from the LCC or the Ministry.[52]

The borough council continued to press the question, however, and in 1933 again approached the LCC, this time with plans for a more modest building, housing slightly more limited services, at a cost of £44,125. The required financial support came in 1934, after Labour gained control of the LCC. However, it was not clear sailing. Yet again, progress stalled, this time hinging upon the borough's intention to have an x-ray apparatus in the health centre's tuberculosis clinic. The county medical officer of health, Frederick Menzies, disapproved of the provision of x-ray services at the borough level. He and other county officials viewed this as an unnecessary duplication of expensive services already available elsewhere, either at public or voluntary hospitals.[53] The question was ultimately resolved in favour of the borough, but not before considerable rancour, and the intervention of Ada Salter, by then a member of the LCC.

The Bermondsey Public Health Centre was opened in November 1936. Unlike Finsbury, its more famous cousin, the Bermondsey Centre attracted little attention in architectural circles. The relatively functional building was designed by the council's architect, H. Tansley. Under the clinic's roof were consolidated a number of health programs already provided by the borough, and some new services. These included a foot clinic, a range of infant, maternal, and women's health clinics (including gynecological care), a tuberculosis diagnosis and treatment centre, an x-ray department, a laboratory, an "electro-medical" department providing light treatment, and a dental clinic.

The importance of Labour's willingness to push the boundaries of borough health programming is perhaps even more clearly suggested in the example of Southwark, where Labour had won the 1919 elections, lost in 1922, and did not regain power until 1934.[54] Under Municipal Reform Party control in the intervening years, there was little expansion in health services, and local people relied upon voluntary and poor-law agencies.[55] The borough was criticized by the health ministry for its lack of vigour in areas such as tuberculosis care and prevention.[56] After 1934, the Labour council worked to expand maternity and child health services, including maternity and home nursing programs and convalescent services. One of the first tasks Labour undertook after the 1934 election was the creation of the new standing Public Health and Sanitary Committee, which undertook a "complete investigation of the public health problems of the borough." This investigation found that the borough lacked the administrative and clinical capacity to fulfill the needs of a modern public health service and set off a process of expansion in health programming.[57]

In July 1936, the borough council laid the foundation stone for a new health centre in a public ceremony. A new building would result in better coordination and convenience, drawing together programs that had been housed in disparate and inadequate spaces. When the centre, which cost £50,000, opened in September 1937, *The Lancet* praised the borough council for having "wisely decided that the building shall have a pleasing appearance and by the brightness of its interior give a cheery welcome."[58] The building was attached to an existing municipal complex housing the town hall and the public library. It was an attractive modern building of red brick, three stories high and air conditioned. Statuary decorated the Walworth Road entrance, depicting "the functions of the new building with relation to family health—motherhood, various stages of childhood and the spirit of healing."[59] This statuary reveals the continuing centrality of maternal and child health to the vision and mandate of local borough councils, and the emphasis on women's reproductive health issues as a primary area of concern. The clinic gave a new home to the tuberculosis dispensary and the maternity and child welfare department. It housed new equipment, such as an x-ray department and laboratories, and boasted of the only illuminated colposcope in the country for its women's health clinic. Other services included a dental clinic, a solarium, and a health education department. The borough intended to extend its services to include clinics for menopause, breastfeeding, and rheumatism.

Bermondsey and Southwark aimed to house as many borough health services as possible in the new health centre building. The history of the Woolwich health centre, however, shows that even with the goal of a comprehensive centre in mind, some compromise and flexibility might prove to be necessary. Woolwich Borough Council was dominated by Labour in the post-World War I era. The party first came to power in November 1919, and with the exception of a hiatus from 1931 to 1934, Labour consistently held the majority of council members and significantly shaped the borough's social policy development. In January 1937, a special meeting of the Public Health and Housing Committee (which was made up of the same individuals as the Maternity and Child Welfare Committee) of the borough council, chaired by Mrs. E.L. Reeves, met to discuss the creation of a central health centre.[60] Built at a cost of £18,066, it was the least expensive of the four centres.[61] Like Bermondsey's, it was built by direct labour (that is, labour hired by the borough) under the direction of the borough's own architect and engineer.

In promoting its new centre, the borough emphasized it had been working to provide integrated services throughout the 1930s, first with Eltham Centre (1931), which provided school medical care and maternity and child welfare services, "the first municipal centre in London" to "make possible the coordinated care and treatment of children from birth until they left school."[62] The new Woolwich Central Health Centre went further in providing a broader range of services available in a single location. Opened in 1939, it housed maternity and child welfare services, health services for school-age children, an orthopedic clinic for children under the age of 5, a dental clinic, a massage clinic, and an electro-therapy clinic. Adult clinical treatment was available, such as sunlight treatment, a foot clinic, and rheumatism care. The borough took over children's orthopedic care and treatment of chronic rheumatism from the Woolwich Invalid Children's Aid Association and the British Red Cross Society, respectively. Under the recommendation of the Maternity and Child Welfare Committee, the decision was taken by council to include them in the new central site.[63]

The borough's health care programming was not all concentrated in the health centre, however. Tuberculosis care in the borough was not moved into the new health centre, as it had been in Bermondsey and Finsbury. Woolwich Borough Council operated main and branch tuberculosis dispensaries at separate locations. The main dispensary had been renovated and modernized as recently as 1934, and the borough provided a comprehensive service for tuberculosis sufferers still living in the community, including home visits by nurse specialists, outdoor shelters for home use, additional nourishment for the poor, home nursing care when needed, and free dental treatment. Thus, while providing a similar level of tuberculosis care as other boroughs, Woolwich compromised on the "all-in-one" model. The new building housed neither the public health department as a whole nor a department of health education. Nor did it have a theatre in which to show health education films. These were generally shown in the borough's museum or town hall, adjacent to the health centre. Thus, while Woolwich was committed to building an impressive public space with a full range of local health services, it also adopted a flexible and pragmatic approach to the new building, integrating it where appropriate with existing services and placing it in close proximity to other public spaces including the town hall and the public library, in a strategy similar to Southwark's.

Considering these boroughs together, a more detailed understanding of the health centre model emerges. At multiple levels, borough councils sought to push the boundaries: those between disciplines and skills, between prevention and cure, between disease and the environment. Taking this into consideration, we can read beyond the "efficiency" embodied by the all-in-one health centre to reveal the way in which the health centre represented a social and political analysis of health. If we can understand London's borough health centres as representative of a broader health centre movement, that movement was based upon certain central characteristics: a seamless integration of preventive and curative health services; care delivered by multidisciplinary teams; accessibility; health education; democratic and local governance; and a notion of health improvement as linked to broader social transformation and greater economic equality.

The health centres were generally part of a package of borough spending that included new or refurbished municipal facilities— the town hall, public baths, the public library, green space, and new housing. Bermondsey, for example, constructed "two marble-lined swimming pools, full communal laundering and washing facilities, with Russian, Turkish and Finnish Baths."[64] The borough council's building program was the largest undertaken by any municipal council in London, with 2700 new housing units created in this era. Bermondsey considered the "beautification" of the borough just as important to healthful living as the provision of medical services, creating a specific council committee to initiate the "greening" program.[65]

More and better housing provision was desperately needed in these inner-London boroughs in the 1930s. Bermondsey, Finsbury, and Southwark had among the most severe overcrowding problems in metropolitan London, despite the fact that they also experienced depopulation in this period.[66] Housing for working families and the poor was often dark, damp, poorly constructed, and infested with vermin. Many accommodations lacked amenities such as sanitation, electricity, and hot running water. Walls were crumbling, and roofs leaked.[67] On the day of the health centre's public opening Arthur

Gillian, chair of Southwark's public health committee, noted the connection between housing and health: "slums were being cleared, overcrowding was being overcome by new housing plans, and Southwark was now one of the healthiest boroughs of London."[68]

Finsbury Borough Council's relationship with Berthold Lubetkin and his firm, Tecton, had resulted in the "Finsbury Plan," a comprehensive program of social transformation, with generous social facilities, including the health centre, educational and recreation facilities, open and green spaces, and housing. The borough's plan highlighted a commitment to communal spaces and facilities, which would provide the necessities of life, in the broadest sense, for the people of the borough, while encouraging social interaction and pleasure.[69] Flats were to be surrounded by parks, public paths, and play areas for children. Neil Bullock has argued that the Finsbury Plan should be understood as a statement of class equality and entitlement: "even local authority tenants would be able to enjoy the kind of benefits and convenience that in the 1930s had been reserved for the affluent."[70]

Woolwich, although not classified as "severely overcrowded" by the Registrar-General's standard, undertook an extensive housing and slum clearance program in the interwar years, constructing over 2000 dwellings from 1929 to 1938.[71] It also invested in public utilities such as electricity, and sold appliances to residents of the borough at a reasonable cost. During the borough's health exhibition in 1934, visitors received a pamphlet extolling the health benefits of electric light and heat, now affordable for working-class residents: "in the all-electric home, dirt, dust and fumes do not exist, and furthermore, the ease with which household tasks are accomplished, gives more time for leisure and the enjoyment of the open air, so essential to good health."[72]

These boroughs had a common vision of communal life in which physical health interacted with social life in the broadest sense. Bermondsey and Woolwich also used their extensive housing and beautification programs as economic levers to provide well-paying, unionized jobs to the unemployed men of the boroughs. Thus, public spending in housing projects addressed several pressing social issues at once: unemployment, low wages, and housing availability and quality. Paying above-market wages was a politically controversial measure. The borough councils, however, viewed health as related to questions of social inequality and inadequate wages, even in as much as they acknowledged the impact of poor environmental conditions—dampness, overcrowding, inadequate fresh air and light—that characterized working-class life.

Particularly in Finsbury and Bermondsey's health centres, the housing of public health and disease prevention in the same space as curative medical and nursing services signaled the importance placed upon crossing the prevention–cure divide. Everything from sanitary inspection to tuberculosis care, midwifery services, treatment for rheumatism, or health propaganda was organized and delivered from the health centre. In Woolwich, integration was reflected somewhat differently. Preventive-health facilities were housed outside of the health centre proper, although in the vicinity. But the borough's committee structure reflected the intersection of prevention and cure. Woolwich's approach to democratic organization suggested an awareness of the importance of social conditions to health. The Public Health and Housing Committee was responsible for constructing the new health centre, and the members of this committee also constituted the Maternity and Child Welfare Committee, which oversaw services for women and children in the borough. This level of coordination and overlap between political decision makers in child welfare, housing, and health programming established clear lines of communication as the borough council moved forward on a holistic model.

Health centres housed a multidisciplinary team of staff, led by a medical officer of health. Woolwich Central Health Centre, for example, employed an array of health professionals and auxiliary staff, including five part-time medical officers, four assistant medical officers, six consultants (mostly for obstetrics cases), one anesthetist, six part-time vaccination officers, three part-time dental surgeons, one part-time public analyst, seventeen sanitary inspectors, twelve health visitors (nurses), three tuberculosis visitors (nurses), sixteen clerks, and one dispenser (for tuberculosis medications). This configuration of staffing was standard in the health centres discussed here. The majority of these staff members were on salary with the borough council—the exceptions were the six obstetrics consultants. Although the practice of putting doctors on salary was a controversial one within the medical community in this period as it would be in the future, the London health centres were apparently not, judging by the numerous physicians they employed, hampered by medical opposition to it. This may have been because in working-class districts of London during an economic depression, medical jobs providing a steady income were very attractive to local physicians. In many cases, medical officers who worked in maternity and child welfare were women, whose position within mainstream medicine was still marginal and subject to gender discrimination.

As Labour women had long argued, working-class women faced overwhelming difficulties in seeking out care for themselves and their children, including issues of transportation, child care, and the demands posed by domestic labour in poor housing conditions. Improved access, if it was to be meaningful, required a health system that was more responsive to the practical needs of working people, men, and women. Small details were seen to make a significant difference. For example, the maternity clinics in Bermondsey operated by appointment so that mothers could avoid long waits. Babysitting for a mother's other children was provided. There were evening clinics scheduled for borough residents. This was particularly important in order to attract to the clinic men and women who normally worked during the day. Bermondsey also stressed the privacy and confidentiality of its services to patients. The new tuberculosis clinic, for example, provided two "soundproof" consulting rooms.[73] At the gynecological clinic the council stressed, "it is hardly necessary to add that all consultations are private and confidential."[74]

Health centres promoted a move towards universally accessible health care, regardless of economic status. The goal was that anyone in the borough could receive treatment, not only the most destitute. The availability of general medical services for men (some of whom were covered by the National Insurance Act provisions), not just women in their reproductive years and children, was one of the distinguishing features of Bermondsey Health Centre, establishing its importance on the leading edge of British social welfare. Finsbury also intended to extend access to the health care centre's services to non-residents who worked in the borough.

The comfort and security of patients and families was also considered important in the planning of health centre buildings and services. This was most obvious in the case of Finsbury. The modernist design of the Finsbury Health Centre was considered a model of efficiency, but its interior design was not cold and clinical. Lubetkin believed that his building should be welcoming to all of its clientele. Patients entered the clinic through the warmly lit glass brick lobby, and visited a reception desk. There were comfortable chairs for people waiting for appointments. These small amenities were not the norm in other health care settings. As another example, patient mobility was taken into consideration. All medical clinics in the Finsbury Health Centre were located on the main floor. The building's entrance was approached via a ramp, not steps, making it easier for the disabled and the elderly, and for parents pushing strollers, to access the building. In 1946, the Islington Communist Party praised some of these elements of the Finsbury Health Centre. It contrasted Finsbury with the overcrowded outpatient clinic at Archway Hospital, where patients waited "hour after weary hour, sitting on the hard benches":

How different it could be! A Health Centre in the middle of green lawns and flower beds. Modern, well-ventilated buildings. We wait in a cheery waiting room, with a fire, and flowers on the table. A nursery to leave the youngsters in. A rest-room for us when we have seen the doctor.[75]

Thus, health centres carried a message about the dignity of the ordinary people living in these districts of London. Borough health centres sought to provide care that was comfortable, respectful, and close to home.

In order for this new model of health care to be a success, borough residents had to embrace it. All four boroughs had very active health education programs. Elizabeth Lebas has described Bermondsey's pioneering forays in the making of health films, street cinema, public lectures, and other forms of health propaganda as a "new representation of individual responsibility for the body and the socialised means of practically assuring it."[76] In her analysis, socialized health care in boroughs such as Bermondsey was didactic in nature, and health education was meant to change individual behavior, such as to improve personal hygiene. This perspective is true in part, but it was perhaps also the case that health propaganda served a more pragmatic purpose: to guarantee the success of the health centres, which had become central to local Labour's political platform. Promoting them was essential.

Between 1923 and 1948, Bermondsey's health department made approximately 30 films—written by its own staff and filmed in its own studio—and was the first borough in Britain to do so. Southwark imitated Bermondsey's health education program through the use of "propaganda by slogans on posters, illuminated signs on street lamps, traveling cinemas"[77] and brochures advertising the borough's health services. It created space in the health centre for a Health Educational Department, which offered public lectures illustrated with films and permanent public health exhibits, as did the Finsbury Health Centre. Finsbury Borough Council advertised its social program through the "Finsbury Film," made by the council in 1931 to provide "a record of the work which is being carried on in the Borough on behalf of the inhabitants, with special reference to the Health Department's activities."[78]

Health centres had a clear political meaning to London's Labour Party activists. They were seen as vehicles for promoting municipal socialism to the public. Southwark Borough Council argued that their proposed centre would bring about better administration and efficiency, but also that "valuable propaganda will be effected by the fact that in course of time the public will become accustomed to regarding the proposed Health Services Department as a place to which they may immediately resort for information, advice or other assistance in any matter appertaining to public health."[79] The other target audiences for borough communications were health professionals, policy makers, and politicians, who were to be convinced of the wisdom of socialized medicine through the health centres's successes. These boroughs courted and received media attention, and their health centre projects enjoyed a considerable level of support from both the mainstream press and medical professional journals, such as *The Lancet*.[80]

The element of local control was key to Labour's interwar health policy. According to Abigail Beach, the Labour party's policy on health centres "stressed the importance of community responsibility for the service, operating through democratically elected, politically responsive local authorities."[81] In London, where there were both borough councils and a metropolitan London County Council, it was *which* local authority that became a potential sticking point. As Labour borough councils sought to significantly expand the margins of locally provided health services, upper levels of government attempted to assert their own control. This was a particularly serious barrier to the health centre model prior to Labour's LCC victory in 1934, but even during a period of Labour dominance, tensions existed between the LCC and the boroughs. Perhaps not surprisingly, the two levels of Labour government (and the bureaucracies they oversaw) each sought to maximize their own sphere of influence over health.[82] Overall, however, Labour supported the health centre model of care, and the principle of local control, into the period during which the Labour Party formed the national government.

The development of health centres in these four London boroughs contributed to realizing the goals of socialized medicine. Perhaps more importantly, they provided concrete examples of how health services should be organized and delivered in a socialized system.[83] London's health centres provided party activists and groups such as the SMA with an actually existing model for health care delivery that reflected their key priorities. Ironically, however, the closer Britain came to the introduction of a national health service during the war years, the less clear it was that this socialized health centre model would thrive in a new system. A mention of health centres was *de rigeur* in a variety of health reform proposals from across the political spectrum in wartime Britain. A political struggle emerged over the key features of a health centre model. In the process the concept was contested and obscured, despite (or perhaps because of) the success of experiments like the London Labour health centres.

The challenge to a *socialized* health centre model was evident in the "Model Health Centre" proposed by the Interim Report of the Medical Planning Commission (MPC) (1942), a committee struck by the British Medical Association.[84] The Interim Report suggested that "health centres" had become all things to all people— ranging from their conception in the Dawson Report (1920), which had envisioned primary and secondary care centres where general practitioners and nursing services treated patients with specialists as consultants, along with ancillary services such as radiography and laboratory testing, through to privately owned group practices

located in a common physical space called a "health centre." The
MPC undertook to develop its own concept for a "model health
centre." Not surprisingly, their model health centre was in essence
a counter-proposal to the socialized health centre model, adopt-
ing palatable aspects while preserving medicine's authority and
independence. The MPC's proposal was in essence a physician
group-practice setting, with the health centre *building only* provided
by the state. Physicians would be contracted to assume responsibility
for services then provided by local authorities, including midwifery
programs, infant and child welfare, school health programs, and the
like. Health visitors, nurses, and midwives would "assist" physicians
in delivery of antenatal, post-natal, and infant and child health care.
The MPC rejected any role for the health centre in specialized areas
of medicine, including the treatment of tuberculosis, venereal disease, "mental deficiency," orthopedics, and child guidance. Under
such a model, London's health centres would be stripped of several
significant elements of their model of care.

In response to the MPC and the publication of the Beveridge
Report, Labour worked through its Public Health Advisory
Committee (PHAC) to fine-tune its position in this shifting
health-reform landscape. Members of the SMA, including David
Stark Murray and Somerville Hastings (who was named Chair),
formed a strong and influential contingent on the PHAC, generat-
ing research, memoranda, and public documents on postwar health
planning. Harold Laski, secretary of the Labour Party's Central
Committee on Reconstruction, suggested that the PHAC write
a pamphlet, which appeared in 1943 as *National Service for Health*,
authored by Murray. The pamphlet reviewed the failings of the
current health system and concluded that Britain needed a "state
medical service." The pamphlet promoted health centres, salaried
physicians, and the integration of prevention and cure. It suggested that private practice medicine, while not abolished, would
"wither away" under a socialized health system. The hospital system

(voluntary and public) and health centres would be integrated through regions, overseen by local authorities to assure democratic accountability. The system as a whole, however, would be overseen by the national Ministry of Health. A tension between centralization and local control ran throughout policy statements issued by both the PHAC and the SMA. The SMA's *A Socialised Health Service*, issued in early 1944, argued "administration should be a vital and living thing; ... all trace of bureaucracy, red-tape and lack of freedom should be rigidly excluded."[85]

As planning for a potential national health service proceeded through the final years of the war, debates about the health centre model remained key to events. A February 1943 government memorandum on a comprehensive medical service suggested that general practitioners should work in health centres and be paid by salary. In October's revised document, salaried payment had been replaced by a capitation model. Labour members of the wartime coalition cabinet expressed frustration that health centres were becoming more marginal to government discussions, increasingly referred to as "experimental." They feared that the desire to placate medical opposition was influencing government health planners and the new Minister of Health, Conservative Henry Willink.

The government prepared a White Paper on health services in January 1944. Labour MP Clement Attlee objected to the White Paper's proposal to allow private practice to continue among public practice physicians, while Ernest Bevin spoke out for health centres, the discussion of which had been muted. The issue of salaried payment continued to cause disagreement. According to Stephen Brooke, Labour's commitment to health centres did have an impact on the final version of the White Paper, which supported the establishment of a national health service. Doctors working in health centres should receive salaries, while those working outside health centres would be paid through capitation. Labour MPs had pressed the war government hard to secure changes to the White Paper consistent with party policy, but had also compromised on a completely socialized, salaried service. For Labour, the White Paper represented a starting point; this, too, was Hastings' view.[86]

While the SMA mobilized its membership and the public in support of a national health service, the British Medical Association's (BMA) opposition to the White Paper grew firmer and more hostile, especially towards the SMA physicians. Resistance to any national health service based upon health centres was articulated through a Cold War discourse of anti-communism and, according to Frank Honigsbaum, elements of anti-Semitism. By 1945, "health centres had come to mean not only salary and municipal control—even worse, they spelled socialism and communism." The right-wing physician group Medical Policy Association (MPA) drew connections between the financial struggles of indebted general practitioners, "international financial control by Jews," and the close ties between "high finance and socialism."[87] The BMA's views looked moderate by comparison to the MPA, but the BMA's determination to preserve private practice and avoid a fully socialized health care system did ultimately prevail, even after Labour won the 1945 general election.

The Labour Party, led by Prime Minister Clement Attlee, held power in Britain from 1945 until 1951, when the Conservatives were returned to government under Winston Churchill. The National Health Services (NHS) was Labour's most significant social reform.[88] Introduced by the Welsh former miner, Aneurin Bevan, Minister of Health, the NHS Act carried the ambitious promise of a socialized system, as well as the enormous burden of expectation that it could fix the problems with existing health services. In some ways, starting from scratch may have been easier. The NHS did achieve what Bevan wanted most: it provided a collective societal solution to health care, based on health care free to all at the point of access. Bevan made compromises on and departures from Labour Party health policy that would have long-lasting consequences, beginning with the abandonment of salaried physician payment, after what Brooke describes as "tortuous negotiations" with the BMA. The NHS made the decision to pay general practitioners by capitation, not salary, and to allow the continuance of private practice. This was an agonizing decision, but one that Bevan believed was necessary to gain physician support for the NHS. Labour's experience in New Zealand was a cautionary tale. There, the implementation of free health care for all through the 1938 Social Security Act had been stalled by physician opposition to universal state coverage. Bevan was more prepared to compromise on payment model, than he was on his commitment to universality and the establishment of a health service free at the point of access. Indeed, Bevan resigned from the Labour government in 1951, when it introduced user fees for dentures and eye glasses.

Bevan faced criticism for his policy of nationalizing all hospitals (public and voluntary) in Britain, which created a highly centralized hospital sector. The loss of local government control over health care services was opposed by groups such as the SMA, and some within the Labour Party. Indeed, Bevan's framework for the NHS faced opposition on all fronts, as Patricia Hollis (biographer of Bevan's wife, Jennie Lee) has noted—from the SMA, from some Cabinet colleagues, from the BMA, and from the Conservative Party. The SMA, which had become increasingly peripheral to Labour's health policy development during and after the 1945 general election, communicated its evaluation of the NHS legislation in a press release, in which it argued that Bevan had made too many concessions to vested interests. John Stewart's careful research on the SMA has demonstrated that some of its members remained bitter decades later about how the NHS was implemented: in 1972, David Stark Murray referred to private practice within the NHS as a "bribe" to placate the BMA. Others viewed matters with regret, as a lost opportunity. Such public opposition from the medical left was difficult for Bevan to take, and it must have led to strained relations between Bevan and the SMA's leaders. Bevan privately referred to the SMA as "pure but impotent."[89] Stewart argues, "on taking up his ministerial post Bevan did not feel obligated to take particular heed of the SMA." Even before Labour formed government, there is evidence of the SMA's declining influence over the party's health policy. Theirs was not the only, or perhaps even the most important, voice attempting to influence decision making. Stewart notes the differences of opinion on matters such as local control between the SMA, the Trades Union Congress, and the Fabian Society as possibly indicative of a growing sense that the SMA's policy positions were insufficiently pragmatic.[90]

The NHS, which provided universal, free coverage at the point of access funded out of general revenues (rather than as a form of health insurance) was a radical program. But it was not the Labour program for socialized medicine that had been developed before the party took power. Tensions over the future of a health centre model persisted throughout Labour's term in government. It should be remembered that a number of elements of the health centre model, in addition to salaried payment, faced resistance from the BMA and its allies: the aim to create multidisciplinary teams and break down professional barriers; a delivery framework that would integrate preventive and primary care; and the principle of local democratic control. On the latter point, the NHS was criticized by the left for its apparent reversal of Labour's earlier commitment to local authority control and its overall centralization. As Martin Powell observes, "the desire to democratize the NHS has been a persistent theme of the left ever since."[91]

In the first few years after the passage of the NHS Act, primary care based in health centres still seemed a live option. The London County Council (LCC), for example, proposed building a network of health centres under the auspices of Section 21 of the NHS Act.[92] In its 1948 development plan, the LCC announced:

> It is the Council's intention that ultimately a comprehensive
> health centre (or a group of centres providing the same compre-
> hensive services) shall be provided for each health service area
> having a population of approximately 20,000, so sited that no
> residents will have to travel more than about a mile from their
> homes to the centre ... it is estimated that the county of London
> will be divided into 162 health service areas each of which will
> require a comprehensive health centre.

Each centre would provide services very similar in range to the pioneering borough council health centres: "general medical and dental
services, maternity and child welfare clinics, health education,
pharmaceutical services ... and office accommodation for the midwifery, health visiting, home nursing and other .... services."[93] The
LCC maintained the long-term desirability of such a plan, despite
a Health Ministry circular of March 1948 stating that no general
program for health centres could be undertaken until resources
improved. However, the LCC's ambitious plans for 162 London
health centres were never realized; nationally, few health centres
were ever constructed. Their place in 1940s health planning became
largely invisible to history.

Bevan appeared to have moved away from health centres even
in principle, but the evidence does not entirely suggest that he had
abandoned the concept. The Labour Government faced competing
demands and limited resources. By 1947, Britain was in an economic
crisis, which necessitated a re-assessment of spending priorities and
cuts to proposed spending. At the same time, Bevan suggested that
building health centres was less of a priority than addressing the
housing crisis: "the quicker we can provide enough decent houses
the less we shall need health centres," he argued in 1946.[94] A 1948
circular did promise consideration by the Ministry for health centre schemes with strong levels of local support. Michael Ryan has
noted that a subsequent letter attempted to soften the blow further

by encouraging local authorities with urgent need for health centres to inform the Ministry, while any new housing projects were to include in their plans space for future health centres. Bevan's Central Health Services Council, established in late 1948, created a Health Centre Committee that reported to Council in December 1950. This report recommended a limited health centre program be started immediately, with longer term needs to be assessed. The government planned to consult both local authorities and the BMA as a process to move forward. However, in 1951, Labour lost a snap general election. The Conservatives, reflecting the wishes of the BMA, supported private group practice over the health centre model. Whatever its commitment to health centres, Labour could do little when out of government.

The ideas and experiences that shaped the health politics of British Labour in the 1930s and during World War II were echoed in the health politics of Saskatchewan. Networks of knowledge and experience promoting the health centre model criss-crossed the Atlantic. Saskatchewan's history will also highlight, as does Britain's, how local people took ideas with international currency and applied them to their own situations and their own realms of possibility. Nonetheless, the health centre model was at the heart of debate on the left in both countries during this period. Potentially adaptable to local circumstances, the health centre model represented the transformative goals of an international movement for socialized health care.

ENDNOTES

1   Heather MacDougall, "Into Thin Air: Making National Health Policy, 1939-1945," in *Making Medicare: New Perspectives on the History of Medicare in Canada*, ed. Gregory P. Marchildon (Toronto: University of Toronto Press, 2012), 56–58.

2   Frank Honigsbaum, *The Division in British Medicine: A History of the Separation of General Practice From Hospital Care, 1911-1968* (London: Kogan Page, 1979), 64–68; Abigail Beach, "Potential for Participation: Health Centres and the Idea of Citizenship 1920-1940," in *Regenerating England: Science, Medicine and Culture in Interwar Britain*, ed. C. Lawrence and A.K. Mayer (Amsterdam: Rodopi, 2000), 208; Virginia Berridge, "Health and Medicine," in *The Cambridge Social History of Britain, 1750-1950*, ed. F.M. L. Thompson (Cambridge, UK: Cambridge University Press, 1990), 227. The Dawson Report recommended essentially a version of group practice by general practitioners, and was non-committal on the issue of local governance. It lacked some of the elements of the health centre model discussed in this study.

3   John Stewart, "Socialist Proposals for Health Reform in Inter-War Britain: The Case of Somerville Hastings," *Medical History* 39, 3 (1995): 348; Stephen Brooke, *Labour's War: The Labour Party During the Second World War* (Oxford: Clarendon, 1992), 134–35.

4   Virginia Berridge, "Polyclinics: Haven't We Been There Before?," *British Medical Journal* 336 (2008): 1161.

5   Peter Kuznick, *Beyond the Laboratory: Scientists as Political Activists in 1930s America* (Chicago: University of Chicago Press, 1987), 146–49.

6   Arthur Newsholme and John Adams Kingsbury, *Red Medicine: Socialized Health in Soviet Russia* (Garden City, New York: Doubleday, 1933), Introduction.

7   John M. Eyler, *Sir Arthur Newsholme and State Medicine, 1885-1935* (Cambridge; New York: Cambridge University Press, 1997), 358.

8   Eyler, *Sir Arthur Newsholme*, 362.

9   Newsholme quoted in Eyler, *Sir Arthur Newsholme*, 362.

10   Eyler, *Sir Arthur Newsholme*, 366.

11   Eyler, *Sir Arthur Newsholme*, 366.

12   Newsholme and Kingsbury, *Red Medicine*, vii.

13   Newsholme and Kingsbury, *Red Medicine*, 230–31.

14   Newsholme and Kingsbury, *Red Medicine*, 238–39.

15   Dorothy Porter, *Health Citizenship: Essays in Social Medicine and Biomedical Politics* (Berkeley: University of California Medical Humanities Press, 2011), 158.

16   An earlier version of this research on London health centres was published as Esyllt Jones, "Nothing Too Good for the People: Local Labour and London's Interwar Health Centre Movement," *Social History of Medicine* 25, 1 (2011): 84-102.

17   Steven Cherry, "Medicine and Public Health, 1900-1939," in *A Companion to Early Twentieth-Century Britain*, ed. C. Wrigley (Oxford: Blackwell Publishing, 2003), 405.

18   Charles Webster, *The Health Services Since the War*, Vol. 1 (London: Her Majesty's Stationery Office, 1988), 8–9.

19   Abigail Beach, "Potential for Participation: Health Centres and the Idea of Citizenship 1920-1940," in *Regenerating England: Science, Medicine and Culture in Interwar Britain*, ed. C. Lawrence and A.K. Mayer (Amsterdam: Rodopi, 2000).

20   Charles Brook quoted in Stewart, "Socialist Proposals for Health Reform in Inter-War Britain," 339.

21   Stewart, "Socialist Proposals for Health Reform in Inter-War Britain," 340.

22   Stewart, "Socialist Proposals for Health Reform in Inter-War Britain," 353.

23   For the London County Council's (LCC) efforts to improve access to hospital care see John Stewart, "'The Finest Hospital Service in the World?': Contemporary Perceptions of the London County Council's Hospital Provision, 1929-39," *Urban History* 32 (2005): 327–44; Alysa Levene, Martin Powell, and John Stewart, "Patterns of Municipal Health Expenditure in Interwar England and Wales," *Bulletin of the History of Medicine* 78 (2004): 635–39.

24   Berridge, "Health and Medicine," 228; Alysa Levene, Martin Powell, and John Stewart, "The Development of Municipal General Hospitals in English County Boroughs in the 1930s," *Medical History* 50 (2006): 3–4.

25   The history of health centres in England and Wales remains under researched. In future, any narrative that emphasizes central London as I have here may prove to be inaccurate.

26   LCC local approval was also sought for health centres in Camberwell (also a Labour borough) and Kensington. See London Metropolitan Archives (hereafter LMA) LCC/MIN/2376, Hospital Management Sub-Committee Papers, Dec 1, 1938; LCC/MIN/2215, Minutes of the Hospitals and Medical Services Committee, November 10, 1938.

27   Duncan Tanner, "The Politics of the Labour Movement, 1900-1939," in *A Companion to Early Twentieth-Century Britain*, ed. C. Wrigley (Oxford: Blackwell Publishing, 2003), 47.

28   Dan Weinbren, "Sociable Capital: London's Labour Parties, 1918-45," in *Labour's Grass Roots: Essays on the Activities of Local Labour Parties and Members, 1918-45*, ed. Matthew Worley (Aldershot: Ashgate, 2005), 195.

29 Weinbren, "Sociable Capital," 194.

30 John Stewart, "'For a Healthy London': The Socialist Medical Association and the London County Council in the 1930s," *Medical History* 42 (1997): 417–36.

31 Pat Thane, "Visions of Gender in the Making of the British Welfare State: The Case of Women in the British Labour Party and Social Policy," in *Maternity and Gender Policies: Women and the Rise of the European Welfare States 1880s-1950s*, ed. Gisela Bock and Thane (London: Routledge, 1991), 93–118; Pat Thane, "Women in the British Labour Party and the Construction of State Welfare, 1906-1939," in *Mothers of a New World: Maternalist Politics and the Origins of Welfare States*, ed. Seth Koven and Sonya Michel (London: Routledge, 1993), 343–77; Patricia Hollis, *Ladies Elect: Women in English Local Government 1865-1914* (Oxford: Clarendon, 1987); Pamela Graves, *Labour Women: Women in British Working-Class Politics 1918-1939* (Cambridge: Cambridge University Press, 1994).

32 Tanner, "The Politics of the Labour Movement," 46.

33 Graves, *Labour Women*, 154.

34 Graves, *Labour Women*, 170.

35 Graves, *Labour Women*, 171.

36 John Allan, *Berthold Lubetkin, Architecture and the Tradition of Progress* (London: RIBA Publications, 1992), 129, 133.

37 Jonathan Glancey, "A Vision Still Worth Fighting For," *The Independent*, March 29, 1995, 25.

38 Glancey, "A Vision Still Worth Fighting For," 25.

39 Islington Local History Centre (hereafter ILHC) Metropolitan Borough of Finsbury, Annual Report of the Public Health of Finsbury for the Year 1937.

40 ILHC, Metropolitan Borough of Finsbury, Annual Report of the Public Health of Finsbury for the Year 1935, 26-34; LMA, LCC/PH/PHS/4/17 London County Council Public Health Department Records, Tuberculosis, Finsbury Chest Clinic.

41 ILHC, Finsbury Health Centre Files, Pamphlet, "Opening of the Finsbury Health Centre."

42 Southwark Local History Library (hereafter SLHL) PC 613, "How Bermondsey Safeguards Health," *Municipal Journal*, September 27, 1935, 1721.

43 Sue Goss, *Local Labour and Local Government* (Edinburgh: Edinburgh University Press, 1988), 20. See also Fenner Brockway, *Bermondsey Story: The Life of Alfred Salter* (London: Independent Labour Publications, 1995).

44 Graham Taylor, *Ada Salter: Pioneer of Ethical Socialism* (London: Lawrence and Wishart, 2016), 184.

45 Taylor, *Ada Salter*, 185.

46 Taylor, *Ada Salter*, 191-92.

47 Taylor, *Ada Salter*, 201.

48 SLHL, Borough of Bermondsey, Report on the Sanitary Condition of the Borough of Bermondsey, 1928, 1936.

49 SLHL, Metropolitan Borough of Bermondsey, "Souvenir of the Opening of the Public Health Centre," November 7, 1936.

50 SLHL, Borough of Bermondsey, Public Health Committee Minutes, November 27, 1928, "Special Report by the Medical Officer of Health on the Provision of Facilities in Bermondsey for the early Diagnosis, Supervision and Treatment of Acute Rheumatism, Arthritis and Cancer."

51 LMA, LCC/PH/PHS/4/11, London County Council, Public Health Department Records, Tuberculosis, Bermondsey New Dispensary, 1929-1936, Letter from Borough of Bermondsey to Clerk of LCC, January 22, 1930.

52 "Bermondsey Council Fights the L.C.C. for Clinic Loan," *Southwark Recorder*, November 8, 1929, np. See also the correspondence in LMA, LCC/PH/PHS/4/11 between the borough, the LCC, and the Medical Officer of Health.

53 LMA, LCC/PH/PHS/4/11, London County Council, Public Health Department Records, Tuberculosis, Bermondsey New Dispensary, Memo From Dr. Hewat to Dr. Brander [St. Olave's], September 27, 1933.

54 Goss, *Local Labour and Local Government*, 18–19.

55 Goss, *Local Labour and Local Government*, 29.

56 SLHL, Metropolitan Borough of Southwark Council Minutes, "Report of the Special Committee re Health Services," June 27, 1934, 286–289.

57 SLHL, File 614.03, Metropolitan Borough of Southwark, "The Ceremony of Laying the Foundation Stone of the New Public Health Services Department," July 11, 1936. See also Borough of Southwark Council Minutes for 1935, which reveal the Committee's efforts to expand health provision.

58 "A Health Centre for Southwark," *The Lancet*, October 2, 1937, 826.

59 SLHL, File 614.03, Metropolitan Borough of Southwark, "Opening of the New Health Services Department, Official Programme," September 25, 1937.

60 Greenwich Heritage Centre (hereby GHC), Metropolitan Borough of Woolwich, Minutes of Proceedings, January 27, 1937.

61 GHC, Metropolitan Borough of Woolwich, "Opening of Central Health Centre," January 14, 1939.

62 GHC, Metropolitan Borough of Woolwich, "Opening of Central Health Centre," January 14, 1939.

63 GHC, Metropolitan Borough of Woolwich, Minutes of Proceedings, September 28, 1938, "Report of Maternity and Child Welfare Committee, September 7, 1938."

64 Elizabeth Lebas, "The Making of a Socialist Arcadia: Arboriculture and Horticulture in the London Borough of Bermondsey after the Great War," *Garden History* 27 (1999): 220.

65 Lebas, "The Making of a Socialist Arcadia," 221.

66 Ken Young and Patricia Garside, *Metropolitan London: Politics and Urban Change 1837-1981* (New York: Holmes and Meier Publishers, 1982), 192. The authors note: "The Registrar-General's 1931 standard defined overcrowded boroughs as those that exceeded the County of London average percentage of households living at more than two persons per room. Children were not counted."

67 Graham Towers, *Shelter Is Not Enough: Transforming Multi-Storey Housing* (Bristol: The Policy Press, 2000), 22.

68 "Health Services in Southwark," *The Times*, September 27, 1937, 17.

69 P. Coe and M. Reading, *Lubetkin and Tecton: Architecture and Social Commitment* (Bristol: Arts Council of Great Britain, 1981), 173.

70 Neil Bullock, "Fragments of a Post-War Utopia: Housing in Finsbury, 1945-51," *Urban Studies* 26 (1989): 47.

71 Young and Garside, *Metropolitan London*, 192; Weinbren, "Sociable Capital," 203.

72 GHC, W614, Pamphlet, "Woolwich Health Exhibition," 1934, 35.

73 SLHL, Metropolitan Borough of Bermondsey, *Souvenir of the Opening of the Public Health Centre*, November 7, 1936, p. 10.

74 *Bermondsey Labour Magazine*, November 1936, p. 4.

75 ILHC, L3L3.153, Islington Communist Party, "Wipe Out Ill-Health in Islington," n.d. (1946?)

76 Elizabeth Lebas, "'When Every Street Became a Cinema': The Film Work of Bermondsey Borough Council's Public Health Department, 1923-1953," *History Workshop Journal* 39, 1 (1995): 43.

77 SLHL, Southwark Council Minutes, February 27, 1935, Report of the Public Health and Sanitary Committee.

78 ILHC, Annual Report on the Public Health of Finsbury for the Year 1934-35, 92.

79 SLHL, Southwark Council Minutes, March 27, 1935, Report (No. 2) of the Public Health and Sanitary Committee.

80 See for example "Finsbury's New Health Centre Opened," *Islington Gazette*, October 23, 1938; "A Health Centre for Southwark," *The Lancet*, October 2, 1937.

81 Beach, "Potential for Participation," 210.

82 Young and Garside, *Metropolitan London*, 192. In regard to housing, they refer to Labour in Woolwich as "fiercely independent comrades," who desired to maintain their distance and autonomy from central London government, let alone the national Ministry of Health, regardless of whether these bodies went Labour.

83 Martin Powell, "Socialism and the British National Health Service," *Health Care Analysis* 5, 3 (1997): 190. Powell argues that the definition of the health centre was "unclear" in this period.

84 "Medical Planning Commission: Draft Interim Report," *British Medical Journal* 1, 4250 (June 20, 1942): 743–53.

85 John Stewart, *The Battle for Health: A Political History of the Socialist Medical Association, 1930-51* (Aldershot: Ashgate, 1999), 156.

86 Brooke, *Labour's War: The Labour Party During the Second World War*, 203–8; Stewart, *The Battle for Health*, 159.

87 Frank Honigsbaum, *Health, Happiness, and Security: The Creation of the National Health Service* (London and New York: Routledge, 1989), 274, 279.

88 Brooke, *Labour's War*, 337.

89 Stewart, *The Battle for Health*, 180.

90 Stewart, *The Battle for* Health, 173.

91 Powell, "Socialism and the British National Health Service," 191.

92 LMA, LCC/MIN/6575, Minutes of the Health Committee, May 4, 1948.

93 LMA, LCC/MIN/6575, Minutes of the Health Committee, May 11, 1948.

94 Quoted in Michael Ryan, "Health Centre Policy in England and Wales," *The British Journal of Sociology* 19, 1 (1968): 35.

CHAPTER 3

SASKATCHEWAN 1944

Building a Model

The movement for health equity extended well beyond the metropoles of Europe and North America. In Saskatchewan, a dynamic campaign for socialized medicine culminated in the 1944 Health Services Survey Commission Report (known as the Sigerist Report), which was commissioned by Premier Douglas immediately after the CCF's election victory. For almost a decade prior to the Sigerist Commission, however, health politics in the province had been shaped by the transnational perspective and effective grassroots activism of the State Hospital and Medical League (hereafter the League), which was founded in April 1936. Its first president was Charles Lionel Dent, a businessman from Prince Albert; its vice president was Frank Eliason, an activist in the Saskatchewan Grain Growers Association, the Saskatchewan Federation of Agriculture, and the United Farmers of Canada. At the August 1936 Prince Albert fair, the League operated a first-aid booth, where it sold memberships for 25 cents; clubs and municipalities could affiliate for $5.00. According to a history of the League written by Mrs. C. Serjeant, an active member:

> The object of the League was to promote in every way possible the socialization of the medical structure of the Province—to gather, tabulate, and compile information derived from worldwide sources; and to assist the government bodies of the Province in every constitutional way possible to promote this objective.[1]

At its inaugural convention, Charles Dent positioned the League as a forum for laypeople to influence political debate about health care through "much study and attention," and by promoting the goal of socialized medicine, which the League usually referred to as "state medicine." Over the next several years, the League's presence in Saskatchewan would grow. By the early 1940s the League had impressive broad-based support in the province not only from its several thousand individual members, but also from organizations including the Saskatchewan Wheat Pool, the Saskatchewan Federation of Labour, the Saskatchewan Teachers' Federation, homemakers' clubs, fraternal societies, co-operative groups, 120 rural municipalities, six cities, 24 towns, and 56 villages—and the provincial CCF, which at the party level embraced the League's program. The Saskatchewan Wheat Pool included League pamphlets in their mailings and its staff showed the League's film in rural communities.[2] This level of support allowed the League to engage in a very active public relations campaign to promote socialized health care, publishing numerous newsletters, pamphlets, and booklets, many of them written by its volunteer publicist, E.R. Powell, a Saskatchewan homesteader and an employee of the Wheat Pool.

Although political historians have recognized the importance of the League in building public support for socialized medicine, the organization's policy proposals have seldom received a close reading, despite the League's active research and publication program. The League's health care agenda was influenced by the confluence of local and transnational currents. In several regards, its definition of "socialized medicine" conformed to the transnational health centre model of care and drew inspiration from outside of Saskatchewan's borders. It also made important innovations to that model through its attempts to solve local problems in a mostly rural, sparsely populated province.

Promoting lay expertise and participation in policy development was consistently a part of League strategy throughout the 1930s and 1940s. The League asserted a claim on expert knowledge about health policy on behalf of laypeople. Its commitment to statistics, policy research, and tracing transnational developments in health were all designed not only to influence health politics in favour of socialized medicine, but also to make the point that laypeople were qualified to play a role in health care governance. Non-elite lay governance was frequently a key to the transnational health centre model. Thus, one of the first projects undertaken by the League, in 1936, was an ambitious survey of the health and medical needs of the province's residents. With the support of the Saskatchewan Wheat Pool, the survey was sent to every rural household. "The survey asked respondents to disclose their illnesses over the last five years, their durations, the various costs paid to doctors, nurses and hospitals, the number of medical visits and hospital stays, as well as the costs of these services and the amount of outstanding debt accrued."[3] Data from the survey was deployed in many of the League's publications over the next several years.

The League's commitment to lay input and governance was designed to counter the perceived disproportionate influence and power of organized medicine over decision making. For example, the League submitted a petition to the federal government in response to the Heagerty Committee's draft health legislation, arguing that the medical profession had undue influence over policy development, and calling for public input and consultation. Nevertheless, the League had a number of physicians in its leadership, including Dr. F.N. Morrie of Regina and Dr. W.H. Setka of Prince Albert, and it included other health care workers such as Joseph Thain, a former Welsh miner who was active in the Saskatoon City Hospital Employees' Union and was Vice President of the League's Saskatoon branch in the 1940s. Thain's recollections of the League emphasized both the transnational origins of his activism and the lessons of working-class health politics learned in coal-mining communities in his native Wales:

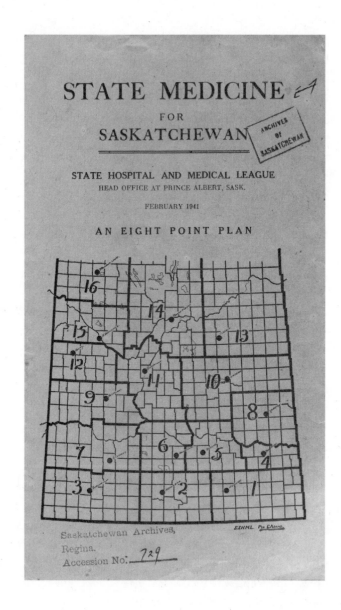

State Hospital and Medical League, *The Medical Quest* (1944)

SASKATCHEWAN ARCHIVES BOARD, R690.1.

Where I had come from the miners had already revolted and set up … what was known as the Tredegar Workmen's Medical Aid Society, paid for through contributions of their own and later by the Coal Company, that soon owned its own hospitals and paid its own doctors on a salary basis … the governing board *were all miners*, and their wives.[4]

Thain emigrated to Canada in 1928, but kept in close communication with his "fellow workers in Wales." When the League was formed, Thain claimed to have gathered information on British health care from Aneurin Bevan (future British Minister of Health), also a former Tredegar miner.

The League's first comprehensive statement in health policy, "State Medicine for Saskatchewan: An Eight-Point Plan," was published as a twelve-page pamphlet in February 1941.[5] This plan had been debated and passed at the League's October 1940 convention. The governance structure proposed by the League would have decidedly limited the influence of organized medicine over health planning and administration. The League promoted a ten-person provincial Board of Control, established by legislation, but separate and distinct in its operations from the provincial government. Four members of the Board would be chosen by municipal associations, two by the provincial government, and the remaining four board positions would represent physicians, nurses, and dentists. It is unclear from the document how representatives would be chosen; at times it refers to a process of appointment, at other times reference is made to election. Members of the Board were to serve three-year terms and could be paid no more than $7000 per year. This provincial Board of Control was meant to direct the health scheme through district boards of control, which presumably were to have a similar appointment structure.

The document proposed the creation of sixteen health districts and suggested geographic boundaries for them. The proposed health districts did not reach the northern end of the province, with boundaries ending at 55 degrees latitude. The League proposed that northernmost health districts were to "extend their services into the north" for the time being, until the "northland" became "sufficiently populated" to warrant the formation of new health districts. The League's publications, generated without Indigenous input and shaped by a colonialist mentality, viewed the north more or less as empty space, except where there were white settlers. They did not make any reference to Indigenous health, despite the fact that it lagged far behind that of the non-Indigenous community. The League's plan was therefore based not in complete health equity or universal access, but rather framed access to health care rights as accruing to non-Indigenous residents of Saskatchewan through their status as "citizens and ratepayers."[6] As non-citizens under Canadian law in this period, status Indians were seen as outside of the remit of socialized health care, at least in the League's published statements on the matter. Non-status peoples and the Métis were simply absent from the League's perspective. This was both a missed opportunity to formulate a health politics based on racial equality and a failure to join forces with Indigenous activists who were already struggling to improve health access.

As Maureen Lux has argued in *Separate Beds*, treaty Indians in Saskatchewan were active health advocates for their peoples, extending back to the treaty negotiation period. Treaty Six was the only one of the western Canadian numbered treaties (negotiated after Confederation to pave the way for white settlement) that made formal written reference to the "medicine chest"—a principle of government obligation to provide medicine that has become the heart of contemporary Indigenous claims to equal health benefits. Treaty Six, negotiated in 1876, covered Cree communities across the central and northern plains in Alberta and Saskatchewan. As was frequently the case with treaty rights, the federal government abrogated the obligations of the medicine chest and had to be challenged in court by

Treaty Six peoples. In 1935, George Dreaver, Chief of the Mistawasis Band, sued the federal government "to recover band funds that were spent on, among other things, drugs and medical supplies."[7] Between the signing of Treaty Six in 1876 and 1919, the federal Department of Indian Affairs had provided medicine and supplies to Mistawasis, but after 1919 had charged these costs to the band. The Justice in this case found for Dreaver and ordered the Department to reimburse the band $4500. Despite this victory, Lux argues, Indigenous peoples were expected to pay for medical care, as a signal of their successful assimilation into civilized society. As I discuss further in chapter 6, the lack of access to health care remained at the core of Indigenous activism in Saskatchewan, a key precursor to indigenous political resurgence during the 1960s. The League, however, remained distant from the cause of Indigenous health equity.

The League's plan proposed health services based on a "clinic" system at the local level, smaller hospitals in each district as needed, and district capital hospitals identified where more specialized medical services, including surgery and obstetrics, would be available. At the top tier of the district system were three larger clinics to be established at Regina, Saskatoon, and Prince Albert. According to the League, the plan should ensure an average of one doctor for every 1500 people, one dentist for every 2000 people, one nurse for every 500 people, and one hospital bed for every 300 people. The League identified a significant shortage of all health personnel in Saskatchewan, including physicians, but particularly nurses and dentists. A key factor in physician care in the province was doctors' urban concentration: over 60 percent of physicians practiced in cities or towns, while 75 percent of the province's population was rural. The League wished to see a re-distribution of medical resources so rural clinics could be served, and a two-tiered system of salaried payment for physicians—a $2000 annual salary for junior doctors, increasing annually by $500 until the regular physician salary of $4000 was reached. Specialists would be paid a maximum salary of

$6000 per year. The League's staffing model was multidisciplinary to
an extent, including doctors, nurses, dentists and, in larger centres,
pharmacists. A system of clinics and district hospitals in a rural and
sparsely concentrated population couldn't necessarily offer a bou-
tique of social workers, dieticians, child welfare nurses, and physical
therapists, but there is little evidence in the eight-point plan that professional hierarchies and the power imbalance between physicians
and nurses, for example, was being challenged. Doctors remained
very much in charge in this vision of care provision. There was no
suggestion that utilizing nurses to a greater extent could alleviate
the shortage of physicians outside of the north.

It was the League's position that all health care workers whose
services would be covered by the health plan, including dentists,
should receive salaried payment. The question of payment mechanism became a political flashpoint in the debate about socialized
medicine in Saskatchewan, as it had in Britain. This controversy over
physician salary has been written about extensively by historians of
medicare in Canada and is commonly assumed to have been the most
critical plank in the socialized medicine platform, the thing that
set socialized medicine apart from liberal insurance models, which
left fee-for-service intact. While accurate to a point, the emphasis
on salaried payment as point of cleavage fails to give full account
of other ways in which socialized care confronted both elite medical power and the primacy of the health care market. There is no
question, however, that from the 1940s on, salaried payment was to
become the flashpoint in medical opposition to socialized care, and
a fundamental rhetorical and political battleground, overdetermin-
ing debate and, from a historical perspective, glossing over a range of
ideas about payment that existed on the left and among physicians
themselves. C.L. Dent, the League's first president, advocated a balance between the rights and dignity of ordinary citizens, and the
"respect and trust" that should be afforded the medical profession.
For example, socialization for Dent did not mean the eradication

of physician private practice, which he argued would be "against the principles of British liberty." While sympathetic to the needs of physicians and nurses, who should be protected from financial insecurity, in a socialized system "the citizens must feel free to accept these services as citizens not as supplicants."[8]

The League placed considerable emphasis on prevention, referring to it as the keystone of its eight-point plan. This meant a focus on not only public health programming, such as vaccination, but also attention to the broader social and economic factors that influenced health—poor housing, working, and living conditions. The League echoed the housing reform agenda articulated by public health officials who since the early twentieth century had argued that overcrowding, lack of ventilation and light, and poor sanitary conditions would result in higher morbidity and mortality, as well as high rates of infectious diseases such as tuberculosis, measles, whooping cough, and diphtheria. Also, like reformers before them, the League explicitly associated overcrowded housing with "an increased incidence of delinquency."[9] The League's other main point of emphasis for prevention was industrial hygiene, by which it meant cleaner and safer working conditions, prevention of workplace accidents, and the elimination of conditions leading to the spread of communicable diseases. The League saw industrial hygiene as "a common ground of understanding between capital and labour," because the case could be made for its economic importance.[10]

This was a fairly conservative preventative agenda, lacking in controversy and consistent with the advocacy of mainstream public health experts such as the Canadian Public Health Association. Notably, the League said little about income inequality or poverty, except to argue that the poor should be provided with "better and more balanced foods" and carefully monitored by public health officials, especially school-aged children. There was no argument made that poverty generated ill health, or that the redistribution of wealth would lead to improved health outcomes. The eight-point plan did

not explain pragmatically how prevention and treatment were to
be integrated into the district health system. In this regard, the
integration of prevention and cure that characterized the health
centre model framework elsewhere was seemingly absent. Neither
did the League emphasize the self-care model of the London
Labour health centres, for example. Ironically, the prevention
section of the document is almost devoid of any sort of political
statement at all.

Yet, on other issues, the League's positions were prescient and
radical. It proclaimed that all private drug stores in the province
should be brought "partially" under the control of the state, and that
they be subject to price schedules and minimum stock requirements.
The League also advocated the creation of state-run drug dispensaries in each hospital, with a special schedule of prices "based on
service, rather than profit."[11] These dispensaries would be supplied
with pharmaceutical drugs by a government-owned wholesaler. This
was a step beyond the insuring of prescription drugs. It was a form
of quasi-public ownership and regulation of the retail side of the
pharmaceutical industry that would have alarmed drug retailers, and
pharmaceutical manufacturers as well, who would be selling drugs
not just to the local rural drugstore, but also the government itself—
hardly a free-market scenario.

The League calculated that its proposals would cost $8 mil-
lion annually and advocated the introduction of a simple 2 percent
"consumer tax," to be combined with a small portion of general government revenues to fund its plan. Municipalities would continue
to pay for the health costs of "indigent cases." The League argued
against a land tax as inequitable and made it clear that that any tax
ear-marked to fund the plan could not be voluntary, but must be
mandatory with no exceptions for individuals, groups, or compan-
ies. There would be no opt-out. Financial accountability for the plan
would be exercised through the provincial and district boards of control, which would be audited regularly by government. All hospitals

in the province would be leased or purchased by the provincial Board. "All hospitals and equipment in Saskatchewan shall be the property of the people of Saskatchewan," the League proclaimed, although it was quick to qualify this statement by saying that no one would be forced to sell their hospital to the state.[12]

A liberal discourse of rights and citizenship, including, at times, the individual rights of physicians, lay alongside prescriptions for total socialization of health. The pertinence of rights discourse is revealed even in the title of the League's 1943 booklet, *A Petition of Rights and a Bill of Health*, authored by E.R. Powell—a much more elegantly written document than the eight-point plan, and in some ways a more coherent one. And yet, the League did not see a contradiction between health "rights" and a fully socialized health system, advocating "state control" over health care provision and disease prevention. *Bill of Health* stated three central principles:

> First: ALL services must be provided including preventive and curative medicine and all other health services for ALL people regardless of the ability to pay. ...
>
> Second: The business administration of any health scheme to be successful must not be dominated by the medical profession. ...
>
> Third: (quoting the Canadian Federation of Agriculture) ... every opportunity should be given ... for the preservation and enlargement of ... providing services locally. Maximum efficiency and practicability should be sought, through local democratic participation of the people served.[13]

With tongue in cheek, *Bill of Health* stated confidently that the newly appointed federal Heagerty Committee would surely emphasize the inadequacy of contributory insurance in the countries whose health systems it examined: "Undoubtedly the experiences of New Zealand and Russia, where the most satisfactory results have been obtained, will received due consideration." It continued:

In Russia especially it should be noted that no half way measures have been applied. Contributory health insurance schemes
are out. The service is for all. They have struck at the root,
PREVENTION. Such minor considerations as "fee for service
or salaried doctors," "choice of doctor," "regimentation," "personal
or impersonal treatment" have not stopped the onward march
of progress.[14]

In 1944, the League issued its longest publication, Powell's 97-page
booklet, *The Medical Quest*. The most interesting aspect of this
booklet is its explicit transnational ambit. Chapters are devoted
to the Kaiser Hospitals in the United States, New Zealand and
Australia, and the USSR, in addition to analyses of health policy in
Saskatchewan and Canada. The chapter, "Socialized Medicine in
Russia," makes familiar arguments about the superiority of Soviet
medicine. Powell applauds its attention to prevention through health
programs such as sanitation, industrial hygiene, and labour protection, as well as through widespread social and economic change.
Relying mostly on Soviet government information, Powell accepts
uncritically the Soviet claim to have eliminated unemployment,
poverty, slums, and "the exploitation of man by man" (echoing ver-
batim the words of Frederick Banting).[15]

Health care in the Soviet Union was a source of inspiration for
the League in the first instance because health care in the Soviet
Union was free and universal and provided by the state:

The constitution of the USSR guarantees the working people of
the USSR the right to free medical services, security in old age,
maintenance in the event of loss of working capacity or illness, and
the right to state protection of the interests of mother and child.

All medical services—from the first aid to the most intricate
surgical operation—is rendered free of charge to the working
people of the Soviet Union.[16]

Viewing the Soviet Union in a positive light even as late as the mid-1940s was in keeping with the League's foundational premise that health equality could only come through a socialized system, planned and administered by the state. As the embodiment of what commentators referred to as the only fully socialized health system in the world, its supporters in the capitalist world tended to render it as nearly flawless. Even those more skeptical observers (like Arthur Newsholme) seldom focused on any specific problems with the operation of the health system in the Soviet Union, and instead chose to criticize the country's lack of civil or religious freedoms. Specific criticisms of Soviet health care would, in any case, have been very difficult without direct access to information not filtered through Soviet information agencies. The League's position on Soviet health and the tone of its commentary, then, were similar to those made by advocates of socialized medicine in Britain or the United States. It was neither more nor less laudatory or naïve on Soviet medicine than anything written by Henry Sigerist, Fred Banting, or Britain's Socialist Medical Association.

Like other supporters of Soviet achievements in health, the League stressed the country's commitment to scientific research, medical education, and efforts to make up-to-date knowledge and technologies accessible to general practice physicians and their patients. *The Medical Quest*, echoing other commentators, was impressed by how Soviet health care was organized. The Soviet provision of health care close to the workplace, in clinics Powell referred to as "health stations," helped create healthy working conditions, prevent industrial accidents, and provide medical treatment and referrals to specialist care or "health resorts, rest homes, and sanatoriums." Those needing specialist care would be sent to the district polyclinic. The polyclinic brought together large groups of general practice physicians, specialists, and ancillary services such as physiotherapy and laboratories. Powell explained the district organization of the polyclinic system, whereby each "therapeutist" at a polyclinic served a specific population in the surrounding district:

> [The physician] receives the people living in the zone assigned him in the polyclinic and visits them at home. But this family physician is in an incomparably better position than the former private practitioner of Tsarist Russia. He has all the latest achievements of medical science at his disposal … He can send his patient to any specialist in the polyclinic or call out a specialist to the home of the patient for consultation purposes; he can send the patient for a course of physiotherapeutic treatment and he can avail himself of the services of a well-trained staff of medical workers.[17]

The Soviets had also, in the League's estimation, vastly improved access to medical care in rural areas. In Tsarist Russia, "witch doctors and ignorant village midwives held full sway," Powell noted in *The Medical Quest*. This comment reveals the League's negative view of traditional healing and the role of female healers such as midwives, and its rather unquestioning embrace of mainstream allopathic care—what it would call scientific medicine. The League argued that the increased number of physicians and hospital beds in rural areas was impressive, but so too was the district system in the Soviet Union, which had established medical "centres" in rural areas, which might have hospital beds, clinics, first-aid stations, obstetrical departments, collective farm maternity homes, child and maternity welfare centres, nurseries, or departments for the treatment and prevention of tuberculosis, venereal disease, and malaria.[18] The central towns of rural districts would house larger hospitals and polyclinics. Soviet health policy attempted to draw physicians to rural areas by paying them higher salaries and offering them "material advantages," as well as re-training opportunities every three years, during which physicians would receive their full pay and an extra allowance.[19]

Directing the provision of medical care toward rural areas was made possible by the fact that all health care staff in the Soviet Union were employed directly by the state—something the League saw as deeply beneficial for both patients and doctors. *The Medical Quest* attempted to outline the benefits of this system for physicians, which included: ongoing training opportunities and access to the latest scientific research and advancements in medicine; the esteem and respect of the Soviet people; free tuition at Soviet medical schools; and the opportunity to work in an expanding and interconnected health care system, planned by the state. The lack of "co-operation" in medicine was a common complaint among advocates of a health centre model. Group practice, the League argued, was a step in the right direction. Individual practice constituted a "failure to co-operatively apply our medical science," which resulted in wasted resources and the duplication of investment in medical technologies, the cost of which was passed down to patients. "Why does not public opinion force into co-operative use and by specialists, if you please, ALL, not part here and there, but ALL the discoveries of medical science in strategically located centres?"[20]

Despite its rhetorical assertion in *Bill of Health* that issues such as physician payment or patient choice were minor ones, the League forcefully addressed these objections in its publications. Powell criticized the Canadian Medical Association's claim in its Report on Economics (1934) that patients freely chose when a physician's services were required, and that fees were arranged "on a personal basis" between the doctor and patient. The latter point, Powell noted, "seems farfetched," and the League questioned whether the sick individual should be forced to make a choice about whether or not to seek out (and pay for) medical attention. And, Powell argued, "the choice of a physician means little to nothing to our rural population where, in most districts, there is only one doctor."[21] At the same time, according to the League's calculations, 35 percent of Saskatchewan's doctors were already being paid a salary as municipal physicians at tuberculosis sanitaria and mental institutions. Fee-for-service

payment, Powell argued in *Bill of Health*, discouraged preventive medicine. Prevention was, as stated earlier, a key note in the
League's plan.

Bill of Health, unlike the earlier eight-point plan, did not outline
precisely how to finance socialized care, except to advocate funding through some form of taxation. The League's Supplementary
Brief to the Select Committee on Social Security in March 1943
argued for a manufacturing and processing tax, in part to spread the
potential burden placed on individuals through sales or consumers'
tax, or the agricultural sector through taxes on production. Specific
financing mechanisms, Powell argued, would need to be negotiated
with both municipal and federal levels of government. The League
attempted to explain why the success of contributory health insurance was impossible without state involvement and financial support:
neither private health insurance nor co-operative insurance schemes
could guarantee resources towards preventive care if they needed to
be actuarially sound. In addition, contributory insurance schemes
had two inherent problems, according to Powell. First, in order to
succeed, plans must include both those well-off enough to pay premiums and those who are currently healthy, not only those who are
likely to need services. This posed a challenge, as the healthy had
little incentive to purchase health insurance. Second, for the poor,
contributory insurance meant either inability to pay premiums (so
no coverage) or "neglect of dues and lapsed policies," leading to significant barriers to access. Thus, Powell argued, the state was in a
"unique strategic position in the matter of health services," able to
solve the inherent dilemmas of an insurance model efficiently, by
financing health care through general taxation.[22]

In *The Medical Quest*, Powell made a further critique of government health insurance as a failed model. His main example was the
British National Insurance Bill (1911), which, by tying health coverage to employment, had left the majority without access to care; in
1930, only 38 percent of the British population was insured. Powell

noted that "such half-way measurers are only temporary and must only be a stage leading to complete socialized medicine."[23] Australia's contributory method was criticized on similar grounds. *The Medical Quest* was more enthusiastic about New Zealand's health care policy, which was viewed by the League as taking steps towards full socialization of health care.

New Zealand's social security legislation was frequently referenced by western health reformers, from William Beveridge to the International Labour Organization (ILO) and the Heagerty Committee Report (1943) on federal health insurance.[24] As Bryder and Stewart have recently argued, New Zealand Labour's social policy, beginning with its 1938 Social Security Act, shaped British Labour's health politics and was closely monitored by the Socialist Medical Association (SMA). SMA physician David Stuart Murray, in his 1942 book *Health for All*, "argued that only two countries— New Zealand and the Soviet Union—had attempted to organize their medical services 'on a nation-wide basis.'"[25] This critique was consistent with the League's perspective, revealing how transnational networks in health politics circulated in multiple directions. Health activists in Saskatchewan, like their counterparts elsewhere, understood New Zealand to be a working example of what an elected democratic socialist government could achieve in health care, one that was superior to British policy at the time.

There was a straightforward reason for the League's enthusiasm for New Zealand's health program: it was not an insurance model. After the passage of New Zealand's Social Security Act in 1938, health coverage was added incrementally in 1940 and 1941, including "free general medical services," and hospital and pharmaceutical coverage. New Zealand Labour's health platform beginning in the mid-1930s stated that "services were to be universally available, resting on proof of citizenship, rather than proof of contribution."[26] Health care was financed through a combination of compulsory registration fees and general taxation, and free at the point of access.

However, the New Zealand case was not a clear victory for socialized medicine. According to the League, New Zealand's Labour government had failed to secure co-operation from the medical profession for an annual capitation fee in a panel system. "This proposal met with such strong opposition from the medical profession that the government switched to the consultation fee [fee-for-service] method."[27] Furthermore, Bryder and Stewart point out that the New Zealand Medical Association was opposed to universality and argued that government health programs should have an income limit for eligibility.[28] The Labour government's ongoing difficulties in bringing physicians on side significantly delayed the introduction of medical care coverage, and ultimately ended in concessions with which Labour's constituency was not happy. For this reason, Britain's Aneurin Bevan considered New Zealand's experience a cautionary tale about the need for relatively quick resolution of differences with the medical profession, even if doing so meant making painful compromises.[29]

All of the League's transnational explorations served to highlight the formidable challenges to socialized medicine put forward by organized medicine, from Auckland to London to Washington. Indeed, even private health insurance initiatives struggled to bring medicine's professional organizations on side. The Medical Quest included a discussion of two US private health insurance plans: Blue Cross hospitalization insurance, which operated on a not-for-profit basis and distributed the financial burden for hospitalization among subscribers; and Kaiser Permanente hospital and medical care, which at the peak of World War II provided health care for a quarter of a million workers and their families through prepaid group medical practice plans.

In the context of (failed) legislative efforts by the US Democrats to introduce a national health insurance plan, industrialist Henry Kaiser became "an instant expert on the nation's health because of the high visibility of his shipyard health plan."[30] Kaiser had made a fortune from New Deal contracts to build dams such as the Hoover and Grand Coulee, and owned Pacific coast shipyards and a steel plant that produced almost a third of the country's World War II cargo ships. Kaiser established the corporation's first medical program in 1938, contracting with Dr. Sidney Garfield to provide workers' compensation-related health care to about 5000 workers on the Grand Coulee Dam project. Garfield went further and created a pre-payment plan for the workers and their families, covering all non-work-related medical needs for about 50 cents per week. In 1941, this grew into the huge and ambitious shipyard medical programs for which Kaiser, and the Permanente foundations he and Garfield created, would become famous. In 1942, trustees of the Kaiser plan created a three-pronged set of health care institutions with financial assets accumulated during this period of expansion: the non-profit Permanente Foundation in northern California; Northern Permanente in Vancouver, Washington; and Kaiser Fontana Hospital Association.[31] Powell visited Northern Permanente on behalf of the League, and consulted with medical superintendent Dr. J.W. Neighbor and Superintendent Mr. F.A. Stewart to gather information for *The Medical Quest*. The Vancouver, Washington Northern Permanente Foundation Hospital, built during the war, had 330 beds and 30 doctors' offices—facilities built with $800,000 from the Foundation and $220,000 from the Federal Works Administration. Kaiser provided primary health care at his shipyards, organized along what Powell called the "clinic plan," built on teams of general practitioners, specialists, nurses, and technicians. Doctors worked on salary, earning between $4000 and $14,000 per year. It is easy to see why Powell was so impressed both by the project's ambitious scale and its delivery model. At the end of the war, when the shipyards' workforce had dwindled to fewer than 20,000, the Kaiser Foundation executive opened the Permanente Health Plan to the general public. Kaiser Permanente eventually grew into the largest Health Maintenance Organization (HMO) in the

United States, but in the 1930s and 1940s it gained the support of workers and unions as a "free enterprise alternative to national insurance and socialized medicine perpetually rejected by the nation's policymakers ... a prototype for health care reform within the limits of US politics and liberal economics, a masterpiece of ideological ambiguity and political consensus."[32]

The Kaiser program was also watched by health advocates because of Kaiser's very public battle against the American Medical Association (AMA) and its affiliated local medical societies. Organized medicine attempted to block physicians from participating in Kaiser's group practice pre-payment plans, which were alternately criticized as corporate or socialistic. State medical associations had considerable influence over the allocation of wartime medical human resources, which they exercised through their role on procurement and assignment committees. The California committee frequently threatened Kaiser physicians with armed-service mobilization. Political debate over the role of the AMA and local medical societies in managing wartime health manpower also led to a confrontation between Dr. Morris Fishbein, editor of the *Journal of the American Medical Association* (JAMA) and Garfield, largely over the issue of health care provision for workers' families, which Garfield, Kaiser Chief of Surgery Dr. Cecil Cutting, and others pointed out was completely inadequate.

Kaiser's historian Rickey Hendricks has argued that Kaiser's group practice physicians, led by Garfield, developed a collective identity and a distinctive medical-practice culture that reflected the geographic, economic, and social context of the Pacific west coast, including an assertive union movement based in the resource and waterfront industries.[33] The sheer size and resources of the Kaiser Permanente system during the war were also able to shield Garfield and his group practice colleagues, who shared with the broader medical left a commitment to prevention and a holistic approach to the health of the working-class patients they cared for. The liberal physicians who worked in the Kaiser system saw group practice as a positive model and apparently did not mourn the loss of fee-for-service payment.

This possibility of physician support for a group payment model providing care to working families was an important bulwark against the persistent opposition of the profession's public voices. For groups like the League, Kaiser's health program demonstrated that it was possible to bring physicians around to a different way of organizing health care. It was proof that not all physicians automatically shared the official views of their professional association about payment methods. The League found private insurance case studies useful for one additional reason: it allowed them to put forward a legitimate cost estimate for socialized health care in Saskatchewan. In *The Medical Quest*, the League pro-rated the costs of both the Kaiser and Blue Cross plans to generate per-capita estimates. A Blue Cross hospitalization plan would cost the province approximately $5 million per year; the "all-inclusive" primary and hospital care provided by Kaiser to its workers and their families would cost $11 million.

The organizing and propaganda work of the League certainly shaped health politics in Saskatchewan in the lead-up to the 1944 election. The organization had a very broad reach and had been a persistent voice in favour of socialized medicine and a modified health centre model for nearly a decade. Its influence upon the CCF's electoral platforms, however, is not entirely straightforward. Gordon Lawson's careful analysis of the CCF's position on physician remuneration, for example, indicates that the party did not publicly commit to salaried physician payment before it came to power in 1944, when it captured 47 of the 52 seats in the provincial legislature. An empowered CCF ambitiously promised to transform government:

> The people in the province have left no doubt in anyone's mind
> that they are ready for a new kind of government—and a new

kind of government is undoubtedly what they are going to get. It is going to be the first real "people's government" in the history of Canada.[34]

The "people's government" may have been more political rhetoric than concrete plan at the outset. Health care provision was the most important plank in the CCF's social services framework. According to the CCF's 1944 election platform, "Program for Saskatchewan," a CCF government would introduce "socialized health services ... with special emphasis on preventive medicine, so that everybody in the province will receive adequate medical, surgical, dental, nursing and hospital care without charge."[35] Access to health care, free at the point of delivery, was the main point of emphasis. The pamphlet, "Let There Be No Blackout of Health," highlighted free access and little else, apart from the pressing need that Saskatchewan residents had for affordable and better-quality care. Existing services were "belated and tainted with the stigma of charity," while both illness and its treatment were financially catastrophic for many. The CCF claimed that 90 percent of Saskatchewan residents "cannot pay for adequate medical services and so are forced either to do without them or depend on charity for them."[36] Election campaign literature stated boldly: "the CCF will provide every resident of Saskatchewan with all necessary medical and hospital care, regardless of his or her ability to pay." Public statements were ambiguous about how exactly this goal would be accomplished. There was no discussion in election literature of a funding mechanism or the introduction of government health insurance, how the system would be structured and governed, or how physicians would be paid—only the promise of consultation and co-operation with health professionals. The party would consult "specialists in public health administration," including the League as the main grassroots advocacy group in the province. On the other hand, the CCF attempted to assuage critics who argued that health decisions would be made for political reasons in a socialized system by committing to a "non-partisan, non-political administration."[37]

After forming government, the CCF had to transform the broad statements made on health during the election campaign into policy. On July 20, Premier Douglas cabled Henry Sigerist requesting him to lead a survey of provincial health services (the Health Services Survey Commission, hereafter referred to as the Sigerist Commission) and recommend a framework for the development of health services. Sigerist accepted almost immediately. Douglas also recruited Winnipeg physician and CCF school trustee and activist Mindel Cherniack Sheps to be secretary of the Commission; she and Sigerist played pivotal roles. Another member included Dr. J. Lloyd Brown, a Regina physician. Brown was born in Moosomin, Saskatchewan, graduated from McGill Medical School in 1928, and did two years of post-graduate work in pediatrics at the Montreal General Hospital and the Children's Hospital of Philadelphia. He returned to Saskatchewan to practice as a pediatrician in 1930. In 1940, he became President of the Regina and District Medical Society. Brown played a key role in the creation of Medical Services Incorporated, a private health insurer, serving as its president for four years. He was also Vice Chairman of the Health Insurance Study Committee of the College of Physicians and Surgeons. Another Sigerist Commission member, C.C. Gibson, was a hospital administrator and Superintendent of the Regina General Hospital. Gibson was a member of the American College of Hospital Administrators, and a past president of the Saskatchewan Hospital Association. He had served as Chairman of the Canadian Hospital Council's Provincial Survey Committee, part of the 1943 National Health Survey.[38] The two final Sigerist Commission members were Ann Heffel, a public health nurse, and J.L. Connell, a dentist.

The Sigerist Commission had a complex task, given the strength of local health care advocacy for socialized medicine and brewing medical opposition to the same. Although crucial to Douglas's

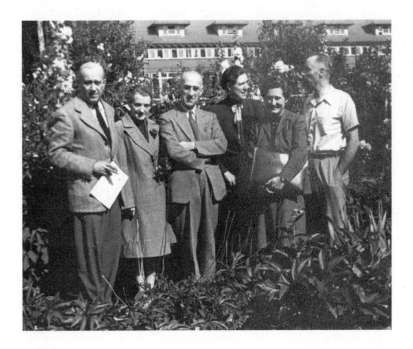

Henry Sigerist (far left), Mindel Cherniack Sheps (second from the right) and other members of the Saskatchewan Health Services Survey Commission, Prince Albert Tuberculosis Sanitorium, September 1944

IMAGE COURTESY OF THE ALAN MASON CHESNEY MEDICAL ARCHIVES OF THE JOHNS HOPKINS MEDICAL INSTITUTIONS health reform strategy, in the end the Sigerist Report said little that was entirely new. Many of its recommendations had been articulated for years by the League and others on the medical left. On July 13, 1944 Dr. Hugh McLean gave a speech to the CCF Convention that summarized the province's history of health services to date and suggested future directions for the newly elected government. The speech anticipated the key recommendations of the Sigerist Report. McLean had been a member of the CCF since the mid-1930s, radicalized by the events of the Regina Riot and the On to Ottawa Trek. According to medical historians Jacalyn Duffin and Lesley Falk, McLean was Douglas's main health policy advisor before 1944, and Douglas had asked McLean to lead his commission. However, McLean himself understood that he lacked the gravitas and public profile. Having run unsuccessfully for the CCF twice in Regina, he was known as a failed politician. He was also not a young man and had persistent health problems. Douglas's choice of Sigerist, and Sigerist's eagerness to participate in shaping events in the province, was a stroke of public relations genius. It ensured that the eyes of the world—at least the North American media—would be focused on events in the province. Sigerist played a pivotal role, as Duffin and Falk have noted, as distinguished outsider and catalyst.[39]

Duffin and Falk suggest that Sigerist's appointment brought political detachment to the Commission. This is open to question. Sigerist was an outsider with the credibility and clout of a Johns Hopkins University academic, but he was far from politically neutral; he was an outspoken public advocate of socialized medicine and a supporter of Soviet health care. He lobbied publicly for the passage of the Wagner-Murray-Dingell Bill, proposing a national system of health insurance, introduced in the US Congress in 1943. By the mid-1940s, in the context of postwar anti-communism, he was under investigation by the FBI as a potential fellow traveller and was eventually denied eligibility for government service in the US, after which he returned to Switzerland.[40] There was little question where Sigerist stood politically on the role of the state in health care provision.

Sigerist had visited Canada a few times during the early 1940s. Queen's University gave him an honorary doctorate in 1941, and the Canadian Association of Medical Students and Interns (CAMSI) played a role in bringing him to Toronto for a conference in November 1943. Its members "were interested in his work on Soviet medicine."[41] Sigerist's visit also drew the interest of the Canadian-Soviet Friendship Society and the Canadian Aid to Russia Fund, as well as the Health League of Canada.[42] Not surprisingly, those paying attention included the RCMP. Gordon Bates, Director the Health League, planned to bring Sigerist to Canada for a lecture series in February 1944. Sigerist was in high demand, traveling to Toronto, Ottawa, and Montreal. He spoke to the media in both French and English. He was a hit. The CCF began pursuing Sigerist one month after this tour. A CCF MP from Saskatchewan, A.M. (Sandy) Nicholson, had heard Sigerist speak during his second visit, and introduced Sigerist to fellow CCFers during his February 1944 tour. He suggested a country-wide tour for the party. Events overtook the federal CCF, however, when Douglas won the election in June 1944 with an overwhelming mandate. Instead of a CCF speaking tour, Sigerist went to Saskatchewan to head up the Health Services Survey Commission.

When Sigerist arrived in Regina in early September 1944, the Commission began a demanding agenda, hearing 88 briefs from members of the public in nine communities in nineteen days, completing public hearings on September 27.[43] After the Commission's whirlwind tour was done, Sigerist wrote his concise ten-page report quickly, submitting it to Douglas, who was both Premier and Minister of Public Health, for publication on October 4, 1944. The briefs to the Sigerist Commission came from a wide array of individuals and groups including: professional organizations (such as the College of Physicians and Surgeons and the Saskatchewan

Registered Nurses' Association) and hospital boards; the League; agricultural, labour, and women's groups; voluntary health plans and benefit societies; and over 20 municipalities.[44] These submissions have never received serious attention from historians of medicare, although they do give voice to the aspirations of ordinary people who had become advocates for socialized medicine. Several of these submissions are quoted at length in the following discussion.

The League's brief, submitted by W. Setka, began by explaining that the League had "predominantly a lay membership, a membership of thinking people," who discussed plans for future medical care in the belief that "the knowledge of medical science and its practical application must be made available to all, regardless of the individual's ability to pay."[45] Most of the arguments made by the League would have been familiar to anyone who had read their publications, including their detailed financial calculations on the amount of money spent annually on health care by governments in Saskatchewan, and the estimated per-capita cost of full health care provision. The League reiterated its position that socialized medicine would cost about $8 million per year, half of which was already being spent in various programs. The new CCF government, it argued, needed to raise $3.5–$4 million through some form of taxation. At the same time, "the ever-present worry and burden of large personal, Hospital, Medical and pharmaceutical bills would be abolished."[46]

The second part of the League's brief focused on organization and reiterated a number of key principles: lay governance and participation; more socially equitable access to medical education and the creation of a new medical school with "emphasis throughout the course to be placed on Socialized Medicine, in order to properly prepare the student for the Medicine of the future"; physicians to be paid a salary and provided with a public pension; a move toward publicly owned hospitals; drug coverage and government-run pharmaceutical medicine dispensaries; and a regional "clinic system" of treatment and prevention. The brief also proposed a system of mobile clinics for rural areas with sparse population:

> The mobile clinic will drive from one village to another on a regular route at regular intervals, carrying a physician, dentist, nurse and sanitary inspector giving medical, dental and nursing service, testing water supplies, inspecting living accommodations, giving prenatal instructions, nutritional instructions and ophthalmic services. When serious illness is encountered, the message is sent to the nearest regional clinic and the ambulance sent out. If private industry can send a cream truck out daily to collect cream, surely state enterprise can arrange for a mobile clinic to call and care for the health of the citizens.[47]

The League concluded by saying that its members, "men and women who look upon State Medicine seriously, as a religion and an ideal born of necessity," sought equal access for all to the benefits of science and modern medicine.[48]

Briefs to the Sigerist Commission were often detailed; like the League, authors frequently utilized the discourse of research, expertise, and knowledge to claim legitimacy to speak on complex matters of health policy, administration, and financing. Those from the rural municipalities (RMs), for example, drew upon several years' experience with municipal health care schemes and an awareness of their strengths and limitations. Several medical benefit associations (some of which referred to themselves as "medical co-ops") presented briefs, based on a different set of experiences than those of municipal medicine; however, both had well-developed financial and actuarial awareness about the costs of health care delivery and the impact of delivery models upon costs. Both groups, alongside professional associations and physician-generated private health insurance plans, had their own stake in the existing state of affairs. Some, however, were evidently more eager to see government expand its role in health care than others. The discussion here will focus for the most part on those groups that were generally supportive of socialized health care and attempt to tease out how they saw health care being financed and delivered under a new regime.

The RM of Pittville, in Hazlet, presented one of the most comprehensive rural briefs. Written by W.J. Burak, it included a summary of the RM's existing municipal scheme and a summary of the drawbacks of the plan, including insufficient preventive care, a shortage of specialists, and tensions around physician care (for example, concerns that unnecessary procedures were performed, or that patients too often sought out expensive specialist care—both of which were resolvable issues, according to Burak). The RM allowed private practice in addition to salaried work for the municipality. In his advice to the Commission, Burak cautioned that lack of physician co-operation could sink any proposed plan, again drawing on transnational knowledge:

> The failure of the Medical Profession to co-operate was mainly responsible for the defeat of British Columbia Health Insurance Act, for the defeat of National Health and Pension Insurance Act of Australia, for the shelving of Social Security Act of New Zealand, and for the defeat of the original health plan in France. Chile's Health Scheme has been inaugurated and has succeeded mainly because it received the co-operation of the Medical Profession.[49]

Burak's assumption seems to have been that medical co-operation could be secured with good planning; it is also apparent that his main focus was not physician remuneration, but the organization, financing, and feasibility of a provincial scheme. Having said that, for government health services, salaried remuneration was to be preferred. Burak suggested a system of major, minor, and travelling clinics, organized in a district system, with clinic doctors "paid a salary."

Briefs from labour could be more anti-physician in tone. "Fee for service is direct incentive for medical abuse," according to the

Saskatoon Trades and Labor Council. The Canadian National Railway Employees' Medical Aid Society was explicit about its negative experiences with physicians: "in numerous cases [they] are lax to co-operate, apparently taking the stand that our Society is endeavoring to chisel or doubt their diagnosis ... with further co-operation from the Medical Profession as a whole the affairs of the Society could be handled more satisfactory." The group also argued that physicians over-charged for medical and surgical care. The Society had praise for the College of Physicians and Surgeons, with which it had respectful dealings, but not for its individual members.[50]

Burak's brief emphasized the fact that the rural municipal system was largely organized and administered by laypeople, and that in a provincial scheme, laypeople should be considered for positions as directors of health districts. The importance of lay participation in administration and governance was similarly emphasized by the RM of Connaught, which argued that laypeople would pay for the plan and therefore should have a role in administering it.[51] A brief from the Regina Trades and Labour Council stated that "proper government control" was sufficient, leaving the details of governance and administration up to the CCF. W.H. Ansell of the Canadian Brotherhood of Railway Employees and other Transport Workers in Regina, on the other hand, specified what public administration of health care should look like:

> The actual administration of health insurance and public health services will mainly be in the hands of a Provincial Health Insurance Commission. The Chairman need not necessarily be a doctor, but, extreme care must be taken to insure against the possibility of the Commission being heavily weighted by those providing the services ... the economic and general aspects of administration are very definitely not matters on which the professions and other suppliers of services should have the deciding voice. The people who foot the bill should have control in the

administration. It is the Commission which will make the financial arrangements with the professions and the hospitals; if the Commission is to be predominantly professions, the process will be much too reminiscent of "Collective Bargaining" between an employer and a company union—the same people sitting on both sides of the table.[52]

The Saskatoon City Hospital Employees Federated Union further argued that workers should be considered for governance roles:

> There are groups such as orderlies, ward helpers, kitchen help, storekeepers, porters, dishwashers, office staffs, telephone operators and several others, who if given efficient instruction and supervision, can assist in the building of an efficient health plan. We also ask representation of labor of their own choosing on all Boards and Commissions.[53]

The brief presented by the Saskatchewan Federation of Agriculture, which represented producers' and consumers' co-operatives and the United Farmers Saskatchewan Branch, stated that a key principal of "state medicine" was "that laymen be in the majority on administrative health services boards."[54] Both the Saskatchewan Federation of Agriculture and the United Farmers of Canada (Saskatchewan Section) also endorsed the League program, as did the labour organizations presenting to the Commission. The League proposed a Board of Control appointed "on the basis of democratic representation of the various groups concerned with the giving and receiving of the services of the plan. Finance, labour, industry, agriculture, medical, dental and nursing professions should all be represented." Broad representation was intended to stifle potential criticism of government interference in health care, "and satisfy those who object to working under State control."[55] As the League was aware, their position on the role of the Board of Control ran counter to the views of organized medicine:

The doctors of this province at their annual convention felt that
the chairman of the Board of Control should be a medical man,
approved by the College of Physicians and Surgeons. The League
says that the Board shall select from among themselves a chairman and secretary. Labour says the medical profession must not
have too much power vested in its hands. So, being a democratic
group in a democracy, we of the League shall stick to our guns
and say "let them appoint a chairman from among themselves."[56]

This suggestion, however moderate, might well have been anath-
ema to the Regina Local Council of Women (LCW), who believed
the chairman of a provincial health commission—which would be
separate from any government department—should be a "qualified
medical practitioner who has been in active practice not less than 10
years." The professions and women "other than professional" might
also be represented, with "major groups of persons served," which
was not an endorsement of lay governance.[57]

International references were frequent in the briefs, revealing
the extent to which Saskatchewan residents had familiarized themselves with health policy and movements elsewhere. Again, advocacy
for socialized medicine was explicitly situated within a broader
rubric of the transnational. For example, the Saskatoon Trades and
Labour Council referred to positive developments in New Zealand,
Australia, and Russia. The Regina Trades and Labour Council,
represented by P.W. Haffner, proposed "evenly distributed health
centres" staffed by salaried doctors, similar to recent proposals
for Australia, and referenced the British Beveridge Commission
in support of "taking the medical benefits completely away from
the sickness insurance."[58] The brief presented by the League, which
was supported by several other organizations, began with specific
reference to "facts, figures and ideas gleaned through eight years
of research on the part of our organization. Information has been
obtained from all available sources, not only in this province, but

from various countries throughout the world."[59] Burak recommended that the province send members of an advisory committee to Russia, "to study the administrative and professional aspects of the scheme there. ... Russia is the only country where all services were made available to all people for a long time already, so much valuable information from the practical operation of the scheme may be obtained."[60]

Support for a district system of health centres, or clinics as they were sometimes termed, was widespread in the briefs, including from groups that may not have agreed with labour or the League on questions of governance or physician remuneration. However, what a health centre might look like was not always consistent. For some, it was essentially a physical space, either a stand-alone clinic or adjoined to a hospital, where support such as diagnostics, specialist care, or nursing was provided for general practice. For others, the health centre was more than a way of spatially ordering health care: it was a politics and a philosophy of health, meant to provide preventive and curative services delivered by multidisciplinary teams of providers, including not just nurses, but also midwives, social workers, dentists, pharmacists, and public health experts, all of whom would be salaried.

For example, the labour movement advocated full universal coverage for medical and hospital services, but also "complete preventive service," and "full and complete diagnostic and curative treatment, including dental care, chiropractic treatment and optometry" in a network of health centres. The need for multidisciplinary provision—not only physician services—was taken further by others, including the Provincial Council of Women (PCW) and the Saskatchewan Homemakers' Clubs, who advocated for a more central role for nursing and the importance of prevention and health education.

The submission from the PCW was developed by its Public Health Committee, and focused on the "Rural Health Problem":

Our study and interest has been directed along the lines of rural needs. ... First of all, realizing that most urban centres have much more adequate health facilities than many rural area [sic], we would emphasize that in any undertakings along this line, priority be given to the establishment of services in areas now unserved.[61]

The PCW's main stated points of reference were the Heagerty Committee Report, (which included detailed descriptions of health systems in several countries), the federal health insurance proposal, and municipal health plans in Saskatchewan. But one of the group's main conclusions was that health needs could best be met in rural areas with decent transportation infrastructure through the establishment of health centres located 40 to 50 miles apart, so that "no resident should be more than 25 to 30 miles from a centre." Health centres would be "strategically located" in "public health administrative areas," a variation on the League's proposed health regions. In parts of the province where transportation was poor, "emergency outposts" might be necessary, or specialized transportation be provided. The PCW was opposed to rural people having to travel long distances to receive care, but it also criticized the idea of travelling clinics as a method of serving rural people, which they characterized as "spasmodic" and "limited." Instead:

We would much rather see health services radiating from a well-staffed, centrally located hospital building, which could be a boon socially and economically, as well as physically, in a small town of from four to seven hundred population. The capacity could be 35 to 40 beds, and a dispensary, X-ray department and laboratory should be housed in the same building. A small attached wing could provide examination and consultation rooms for use of practitioners, as well as dental offices, which would benefit by proximity to operating room and hospital staff, for anaesthetic work.[62]

Although the PCW used "hospital" and "health centre" inter-changeably, which is somewhat confusing, their brief discussed to a greater extent than did many others a multidisciplinary team-based approach to rural health provision. In essence, the PCW suggested a central role for female providers such as nurses, social workers, and nutritionists. Their ideal staff complement had similarities to that of the London health centres, discussed in chapter 2. The PCW recommended that regional health centres/hospitals be staffed by a matron and nurses, a laboratory technician, an x-ray technician, a dentist, and a pharmacist. Their brief went further in suggesting that regional centres also employ a dietician, a public health nurse, a qualified welfare worker, and at least one or two members in an auxiliary home-nursing service. With such a well-staffed team, the PCW argued, fewer doctors would be required in rural areas. The PCW articulated an active role for nursing and social work in a rural health centre scheme, "advising and leading the people, always taking a full share in preventive work, immunization, and super-vision of home conditions of the pre-school and school child." The PCW also envisioned a form of home care, in which the "home-nurs-ing-housekeeper" could prevent the need for institutional care by supporting the aged and those with chronic conditions in their own homes.[63]

Like the PCW, the Saskatchewan Homemakers' Clubs expressed concern to the Sigerist Commission about the dispropor-tionate number of physicians practicing in urban areas. Under "most urgent present needs," their submission identified as a first prior-ity "more equitable distribution of doctors and nurses in relation to the population" and recommended that the government restrict the number of general practitioners in urban centres "on a popula-tion basis." They were supportive, however, of providing long-term inducements to health providers in rural areas, including a guaran-teed salary, comfortable housing and office space, and opportunities for post-graduate study.[64]

The Homemakers' Clubs made proposals similar to those made by the PCW for a multidisciplinary model with expansive duties for nurses and other female-led occupations. The group suggested that, in the short term, small health centres immediately be established by municipalities pooling resources, staffed by a doctor and a nurse, and also offering services such as housing home care, or what was referred to as a "nursing housekeeper service," which would "help in convalescent homes or who would be able to go into homes of convalescent or permanently ailing persons to give simple nursing care and to manage home duties."[65] Over the longer term, the province should be separated into divisions with health units staffed by a "medical health officer, public health nurse, nutritionist, sanitary inspector as well as general practitioner." These providers were key to enhancing prevention of illness and would administer enhanced services such as school lunch and physical fitness programs. Unlike the PCW, the Homemakers' Clubs were not opposed to the use of travelling clinics where necessary.

Neither of these women's organizations entered into direct discussion about physician remuneration. The PCW's brief did suggest a form of group practice in health centres, stating that doctors "could work together and also differentiate their work to some extent, one doing much of the surgery, one preventative medicine, and one internal work and obstetrics." Health centres should employ both experienced physicians and newer graduates who "might be required by their government to serve in specified places for a given time, in part payment for government assistance toward the cost of training."[66] A group-practice setting could, in the PCW's view, make rural practice more attractive to physicians by sharing the burden of on-call care, holiday coverage, and further training opportunities. A health centre model could also help equalize the distribution of physicians between urban and rural areas of the province.

The Homemakers' Clubs did not take a stand on how health services should be financed and did not specifically support a free-at-the-point-of-access service financed through taxation. Their submission avoided any discussion of health insurance per se. This may have been because the membership could not arrive at a shared position. The PCW, by contrast, advocated compulsory contributory health insurance covering all residents, but not a "free" health service financed through taxation. "Some opinions support the non-contributory basis," they argued, "but we contend that not only is self-respect a consideration here, but were residents who pay no taxes excused from paying the basic contribution, grave injustice would result."[67]

The melding of preventive and curative care and the importance of altering social conditions themselves in the pursuit of a healthier population were principal elements of socialized medicine emerging from many briefs to the Sigerist Commission. Organized labour stressed the material conditions that affected the health of working-class families, and the need to raise wages and incomes. The Canadian Brotherhood of Railway Employees and Other Transport Workers's brief quoted extensively from "National Service for Health," a pamphlet produced by the British Labour Party:

> If through a sound social and economic policy we can master poverty, we shall thereby do much to eliminate ill health; for poverty is one of the greatest single causes of ill health. If we secure for all, good conditions of work, with full employment and ample opportunity for leisure and exercise; if the citizen can obtain well built houses, with sanitation, water, clean and plentiful milk and other nourishing food, clean air, as much sunlight and possible, and freedom from injurious noises, then the health of the nation will benefit far more from these things than from much doctoring.[68]

Thus, the union argued, "the best of health services can produce their full effects only if they can operate in a healthy society." The Regina Trades and Labour Council brief, presented by P.W. Haffner, argued that the persistence of unsafe work and low wages made investments in health care stop-gap measures at best:

> it does not seem practical that when a worker becomes ill through conditions which exist at his place of employment or as a result of low wages and consequent lack of proper diet, that a medical health service should take that employee in, patch him, and send him back to the same conditions that originally made him sick. It would seem much like patching a leaky boat with an application of soft soap, knowing that the boat would soon need repairs again.[69]

Similarly, the Regina Labour Council of the Canadian Congress of Labour put the case that the Sigerist Commission should be addressing the broader context that caused disease:

> The underlying cause of unhealthy people is generally the way in which they are required to live. If the Canadian Nation is only going to supply a sub-standard living to a large section of the population, all the health services in the world will not result in a healthy nation. This Health Services Commission must of necessity deal, to some extent at least, with the economic conditions in the Province, with housing, food, clothing, etc. The raising of the living standard of the masses of the population will make immeasurable contributions to their healthy condition, which in itself is good and sufficient reason for advocating it. But, since the creation of a high standard of living will assist in maintaining a high level of production and consequently a high level of employment, it becomes not only the special interest of the labour and farm movements, but a national aim, a national objective which all Canadians will strive to achieve. Would therefore suggest that this Commission recommend, as a practical measure, that price floors under primary farm produce and minimum wages be set at a high level, which will guarantee a

living standard commensurate with our abilities to produce and one conducive to a healthy nation.[70]

The brief from the Melfort and District Mutual Benefit Association argued that medical education needed to convey greater awareness of these realities to young physicians:

> Greater emphasis must be placed upon the broad social and economic aspects of medicine: not only in the pre-med school, but throughout the whole school term. All student doctors should receive a general course in the social problems of the health of the people. Public health services, mechanics of public health administration as it exists should be compulsory. Contraversial [sic] social problems of health, health administration, group practice, clinical practice, research, all should be included. ... Dr. Sigerist, we believe that you will agree with us when we say that medical sociology should be compulsory.[71]

Rural presenters argued that health could not be improved without investment in basic infrastructure, particularly roads, and a lessening of isolation. For example, the Village of Lucky Lake explained to the Commissioners:

> This Village is situated on a branch of Canadian National Railways and is about 120 miles distance from the city of Saskatoon which lies to the North East and the city of Moose Jaw to the South East. We have no graveled highway within 30 miles of the town, no bus service and only a bi-weekly train service. The nearest other large point would be the town of Rosetown where there is a fairly good hospital, but roads to this point in the winter months are impassable. This Village is a center of a large district which has no Medical services other than those available at Lucky Lake and the only drug store for a radius of many miles is situated here. We have a small hospital

which was intended to accommodate seven beds, but has been made to accommodate ten at times.[72]

A letter to the Commission was received from Mrs. L.B. Anderson, Saskatoon, writing on behalf of the people of Shell Lake, located 70 miles west of Prince Albert:

> This spot in Saskatchewan is without a doctor, nurse, hospital, nursing home or druggist, and no conveyance of any kind except what the people beg off somebody who has a car. Three times in one day this need was great and refused to the last minute. Yes we have four large merchants with good cars and all refused assistance in time of need. Our nearest hospital is 70 miles and the pay of such comes from all our taxes and farms. ... The nearest nurse, doctor, and nursing home, also druggist is 35 miles. Roads are not passable in winter and a train three times a week. Bus in summer if no rain. No doubt you will find in your survey of Saskatchewan many such places but nearly all places at least have one car that can be called upon and used. But we have none, all we do have is our undertaker Mr. W.H. Wagner has a truck (small) that he has a glass top for to use as a hearse but he cannot go except the limit of 35 miles. He can go for a dead body but cannot take a live one 70 miles to the hospital. ... We as the people of Shell Lake do not ask for a doctor, nurse, hospital as it is well known there is a war on but we do ask for an ambulance (year round) so that we folks can know our loved ones can at least reach help and medical care.[73]

A brief from the Tisdale Board of Trade similarly emphasized the relationship between accessibility and the lack of adequate infrastructure, both physical and human: "It takes but little imagination to visualize the anxiety of the people, the difficulty of travel, the problem facing [the] doctors." The region's inhabitants experienced "poor, very poor accessibility" to health care, with 153 hospital beds and ten doctors serving 41,000 people.[74] The Saskatchewan Federation of Agriculture also made preventive recommendations to the Sigerist Commission, including the testing of drinking water and a supply of pure water where necessary (perhaps in response to the poor quality of well water in many cases), as well as testing of the healthfulness of the soil.

Several presenters pointed out in particular the lack of adequate prevention and health education under municipal medical plans. The Saskatchewan Federation of Agriculture observed that, although some municipal schemes might have childhood immunization programs in place, rural municipalities could not afford to provide school medical examinations and tests. The lack of prevention was acknowledged in Burak's municipal brief—there was no plan for ensuring immunizations—and was to be remedied through communicable disease prevention services. Neither was medical care insurance the answer on its own, according to the Federation, since it did not provide preventive medical care for the general public; again, Burak echoed this point, referring to the need for adult physical exams as a preventive health measure. The Canadian Brotherhood of Railway Employees and other Transport Workers argued that school medical services should be organized and delivered through health centres, along with child welfare services.

Prevention was especially emphasized by women's organizations; however, there were multiple understandings of what prevention entailed. In keeping with middle-class views on the average working-class (or rural) women's need for professional guidance, the LCW argued that leadership in prevention would be taken up by the public health nurse and child welfare worker, "advising and leading the people, always taking a full share in preventive work, immunization, and supervision of home conditions of the pre-school and school child. This home visiting service by nurse and social worker should be of inestimable value."[75] The brief presented by the president of the Saskatchewan Homemakers' Clubs similarly stressed the need for prevention and health education, and for more public health nurses. Supervision and expert professional guidance, however, was not the focus. Rather, the Homemakers' Clubs advocated for the availability of immunization to all children on a voluntary basis for diseases such as diphtheria, smallpox, scarlet fever, and whooping cough. While acknowledging that some members of the Homemakers' Clubs believed childhood vaccinations should be compulsory, the president argued that the "conscientious scruples of some persons in our population have to be considered."[76] The Homemakers' Clubs called for school lunch programs (urban and rural) and physical fitness. While these services were to be staffed by qualified personnel such as nutritionists, the emphasis was upon provision, not upon professional supervision. This represents a classic class-bound debate in the history of maternal and child health—while middle-class reformers emphasized the inadequacy of parental knowledge and the need for professional guidance, poor and working-class people focused on the need for meaningful supports and actual care provision, while maintaining parental authority.

Overall, briefs to the Sigerist Commission suggest a broad and very well-informed base of support for greater government action on the people's unmet health needs, but they also suggest that lay voices in Saskatchewan had an appetite for significant reforms. The level of knowledge evident in presentations from farmers, teachers, labour, women's groups, and municipal leaders was truly impressive. Many briefs emphasized the social causes of ill health and the need for a comprehensive approach that included prevention and public health. Saskatchewan residents made detailed recommendations on questions such as financing and organization and a number of briefs proposed a health centre model of care delivery, with which they seemed quite familiar. Certainly not all of the briefs discussed here, which shared a high level of commitment to immediate government action, agreed on all fronts. The League and labour proposed a fully socialized system, while others such as the PCW was happier with a contributory insurance model. The Sigerist Commission navigated these articulate calls for action in its final report, which was released in October 1944.

The Sigerist Report emphasized first and foremost the need to work towards greater health equity by providing "complete medical services to all the people of the Province, irrespective of their economic status, and irrespective of whether they live in town or country."[77] In the Report's analysis, inequality was both an economic and a spatial problem, which warranted special attention being given to reforming rural health delivery. The Sigerist Report recommended the creation of rural health districts as administrative units for both preventative and curative health services. These districts would be built upon rural health units, housed in rural health centres. They would be staffed by one or more physicians and a registered nurse and would have space for minor surgeries, a delivery room, and eight to ten beds. The municipal doctor would also act as a local health officer, handling immunizations, school medical services, and other public health measures in co-operation with district health centres. Sigerist encouraged the co-operation in establishing rural health centres of more than one municipality, to combat the strain on resources faced by municipal medical schemes.

Rural municipalities in Saskatchewan had been supporting physician services since the early 20th century. Beginning in 1916, rural municipalities were allowed by law to supplement physician incomes; by 1919, physicians could be hired on salaries up to $5000 per year. In 1935, legislation was introduced permitting municipalities to charge residents an assessment of up to $2 per head to finance physician services. By 1941, municipalities were allowed to pay physicians on a fee-for-service basis for the municipal work they performed. Often cited as a pre-cursor to medicare, the municipal doctor plans are seen by historians as a success story. The growth of rural municipal medical coverage attracted the attention of the US

Committee on the Costs of Medical Care (CCMC, discussed further in chapter 5). C. Rufus Rorem wrote a report on Saskatchewan municipal medicine for the influential committee. By the 1940s, there were over 100 municipal doctor plans in the province, serving about 210,000 people, one-quarter of the population.[78]

While laudatory of municipal doctors—"the backbone of all medical services"—the Sigerist Report expressed concern that municipal medicine was uneven, doctors were overworked and underpaid, and, in some cases, lacked proper infrastructure supports and expertise. To an extent, the establishment of health districts and rural health centres was meant to create a framework within which greater co-operation and coordination of rural resources could be achieved. The Sigerist Report did not suggest full provincial control over health services, but rather financial subsidies where needed through grants, and the creation of minimum standards of health care service.

The "seat" of each health district was to be the district health centre headed by a medical officer of health, who would administer public health services, but also "supervise and co-ordinate all medical services and all activities that tend to promote the people's health."[79] The district health centre was to be staffed in a multidisciplinary fashion, with sanitary officers, public health nurses, dentists, and specialists as needed. It would have its own laboratory and perhaps handle pathology. The Report suggested that the district health centre could be located on the premises of the major hospital of the district—alternatively, district hospitals themselves might serve as the health centre in towns where they are located. District hospitals were to provide medical treatment that could not be provided in rural health centres—major surgery and specialist treatment. Base hospitals in Saskatoon and Regina would provide the most complex and specialized care.

The model proposed by the Sigerist Report attempted to break down the boundaries between public health and medicine by having public health nurses and sanitation officers working with the regional medical officers of health, who would be located at district health centres. Sigerist attempted to be diplomatic about the state of public health programs in the province, but he saw the need for greater expertise in public health work, much of which was performed by general practitioners in rural areas. The Report argued that there was a "crying [public] demand for health education" across the province. Sigerist recommended involving schools in health education for children, and "civic organizations such as the Homemakers' clubs and the voluntary health organizations," which "must be mobilized permanently."[80]

Sigerist believed that urban health care was "less difficult and less urgent" than the situation in rural Saskatchewan, but there too he saw a lack of uniformity and uneven access to care.[81] Existing medical services plans and benefit associations, while beneficial to their members, reached only some and their benefits were not comprehensive. "The major problem is to bring complete medical services to all inhabitants of the cities, at a price they can afford," the Report observed. Sigerist's recommendation for immediate action on urban health was to gradually expand public health benefits to include maternity care and hospitalization through a system of compulsory health insurance. In the longer term, "final steps may have to wait until the Province can count on subsidies from the Dominion."[82]

The Sigerist Report did not discuss financing options to any significant extent, perhaps because how to pay for socialized care was not explicitly identified in the Commission's mandate. Sigerist's main preoccupation was how to plan and organize a system of socialized medicine: how to ensure that it was properly staffed and that it emphasized prevention; and how to ensure that it dealt with certain pressing disease issues, including tuberculosis, cancer care, mental health, venereal disease, and dental health. The Report was also focused on immediate action; it acknowledged that a full system of

socialized health care might have to wait until the federal government was prepared to contribute—something many observers hoped
would be imminent.

Elements of the Sigerist Report supported claims to democratic
lay governance raised by so many of those who presented briefs to
the Commission. The Report urged "the active participation of the
population" through the establishment of a health services commission associated with each rural health unit, consisting of "the
technical personnel, the teachers, and representatives of the rural
municipalities, towns and villages involved."[83] Representatives from
local health services commissions would constitute the district
health services commission, chaired by the district health officer.
Local and district health commissions would hold regular meetings
and conventions to discuss the health problems of their areas. The
Report did not make suggestions as to how the commission members would be chosen.

While Sigerist did not suggest abolishing private practice, his
Report clearly saw private practice as the undesirable outcome of the
inadequate incomes paid to municipal doctors and argued instead for
salaried remuneration—the future trend in health care. Municipal
doctors, he argued, "engage in private practice to make a decent living."[84] Sigerist recommended that the province set a minimum salary
for municipal doctors and future salaried physicians, which would
increase with years of service, annual vacations with pay, leaves of
absence for further training every few years, and a superannuation
fund. Health centres were to be publicly financed, with no overhead
cost to the physician, so that salary was net income.

The CCF came to office enjoying considerable public support for
its mandate to provide socialized health services. Numerous
briefs to the Sigerist Commission articulated a shared understanding
of the parameters of socialized medicine. The Sigerist Commission
Report was both a blueprint for the future and a reflection of a

shared politics of health. Influences upon it were myriad, inter-sectional, and multilocational. Sigerist's own support for socialized medicine and the Soviet model were evident, but so too was the influence of local health advocates active in the CCF and on the broader left, whose awareness of the international context placed their views in close proximity with those of Sigerist himself.

This vision for socialized medicine was not fully representa-tive or inclusive. The Sigerist Report's statements on health care in Saskatchewan's north and on "Indians" reflect a racialized and col-onialist view of Indigenous peoples. In this regard, little separated the Commission's views from those of physicians and public health experts who were not on the political left or supportive of a social-ized system. Echoing the League, Sigerist argued that the north was "sparsely populated" and that little could be done to provide better services there. Sigerist went further than the League's publi-cations, however, in pronouncing Indigenous peoples as a threat to the health of whites:

> The Indians, about 13,700 scattered throughout the Province, constitute a reservoir of disease. In 1941, close to ½ of all deaths of Indians, 174 out of 408, were due to infectious and para-sitic diseases. The tuberculosis death rate of Indians was 592 per 100,000 population, compared with 21 among the white population, in 1943. Ill health of the Indians is a menace to the health of the white population since the two races mix freely. The Indians would, in all probability, receive more medical attention if they could be included into the provincial system of rural health services. An agreement might be reached with the Dominion Government, under which the Province would assume responsibility for the health services of the Indians, and would be compensated for it by the Dominion Government. A similar agreement has already been made in the field of tuber-culosis control.[85]

On questions of race and disability, Sigerist cannot be applauded. The Sigerist Report recommended the institutionalization of "mental defectives" in a special "colony" with minimum capacity of 1500. Into the post-Nazi period, Sigerist remained a supporter of sterilization of the mentally "defective." The Sigerist Report argued:

> sterilization of mental defectives should be given careful consideration ... One should not be deterred by the fact that Nazi Germany has practiced sterilization in a brutal and wholesale manner, but should study the results obtained ... where sterilization has been practice humanely and cautiously with good results.[86]

He did not specify whether sterilization should be voluntary and require patient consent.

The Sigerist Commission ultimately had limited impact upon the development of health care during the first two Douglas administrations (1944–1952). The health centre model, at the heart of prescriptions for socialized medicine, was lost during the later 1940s and early 1950s. The purpose of this chapter, however, has been to establish its importance within a guiding set of shared principles and goals for a cohort of health advocates, including Sigerist himself, "outsiders" such as Mindel and Cecil Sheps, as well as local activists including the League and the Homemakers' Clubs. The health services model the Sigerist Commission advocated was a mix of the international and the local—an amalgam of existing public health services in Saskatchewan, such as municipal doctors and tuberculosis care, and a broader transformative framework for re-organization and growth. It attempted to work with the Saskatchewan context, while guiding the province towards a fully socialized system, the basic tenets of which were agreed upon.

The defining features of socialized health care were not unidimensional: socialized health care was not only salaried personnel; it was not only public state financing; it was not the absence of

contributory insurance in all instances. It was a model with iden-
tifiable moving parts, with a potential for adaptability to local
conditions, but nonetheless a coherent world view. That world-
view was distinct from health care insurance or medicare as we now
understand it: socialized or state medicine was more than health
insurance mandated by the state.

ENDNOTES

1   Saskatchewan Archives Board (hereafter SAB), R690.1, State Hospital and Medical League, File 7, "Summary of the History of the State Hospital and Medical League," by Mrs. C. Serjeant.

2   SAB, R690.1, State Hospital and Medical League, File 7, "Summary of the History of the State Hospital and Medical League," by Mrs. C. Serjeant.

3   Aaron William Goss, "Care regardless of the Ability to Pay : A Reconnaissance of Saskatchewan's State Hospital and Medical League," MA Thesis (University of Manitoba, 2013), 47.

4   SAB, R690.1, State Hospital and Medical League, File 8, "My Memories of the State Hospital and Medical League," by Joseph A. Thain."

5   SAB, R690.1, State Hospital and Medical League, File 18, "State Medicine for Saskatchewan."

6   SAB, R690.1, State Hospital and Medical League, File 18, "State Medicine for Saskatchewan," 3.

7   Maureen K. Lux, *Separate Beds: A History of Indian Hospitals in Canada, 1920s-1980s* (Toronto: University of Toronto Press, 2016), 163.

8   SAB, R690.1, State Hospital and Medical League, File 4.

9   SAB, R690.1, State Hospital and Medical League, File 18, "State Medicine for Saskatchewan," 9.

10 SAB, R690.1, State Hospital and Medical League, File 18, "State Medicine for Saskatchewan," 9.

11 SAB, , R690.1, State Hospital and Medical LeagueFile 18, "State Medicine for Saskatchewan," 10.

12 SAB, R690.1, State Hospital and Medical League, File 18, "State Medicine for Saskatchewan," 11-12.

13 SAB, R690.1, State Hospital and Medical League, File 9, "A Petition of Rights and a Bill of Health," 4-5.

14 SAB, R690.1, State Hospital and Medical League, File 9, "A Petition of Rights and a Bill of Health," 6.

15 SAB, R690.1, State Hospital and Medical League, File 10, "The Medical Quest," 33.

16 SAB, R690.1, State Hospital and Medical League, File 10, "The Medical Quest," 34-35.

17 SAB, R690.1, State Hospital and Medical League, File 10, "The Medical Quest," 39.

18 SAB, R690.1State Hospital and Medical League, , File 10, "The Medical Quest," 41.

19 SAB, R690.1, State Hospital and Medical League, File 10, "The Medical Quest," 42.

20 SAB, R690.1, State Hospital and Medical League, File 10, "The Medical Quest," 92.

21 SAB, R690.1, State Hospital and Medical League, File 9, "A Petition of Rights and a Bill of Health," 8.

22 SAB, R690.1, State Hospital and Medical League, File 9, "A Petition of Rights and a Bill of Health," 10.

23 SAB, R690.1, State Hospital and Medical League, File 10, "The Medical Quest," 19.

24 J.J. Heagerty, Chair, "Report of the Advisory Committee on Health Insurance," House of Commons, March 1943, 125-127.

25 Linda Bryder and John Stewart, "'Some Abstract Socialistic Ideal or Principle': British Reactions to New Zealand's 1938 Social Security Act," *Britain and the World* 8, 1 (March, 2015): 66.

26 Bryder and Stewart, "'Some Abstract Socialist Ideal or Principle,'" 57.

27 SAB, R690.1, State Hospital and Medical League, File 10, "The Medical Quest," 29.

28 Bryder and Stewart, "'Some Abstract Socialistic Ideal or Principle,'" 59.

29 Bryder and Stewart, "'Some Abstract Socialistic Ideal or Principle,'" 74.

30 Rickey Hendricks, *A Model for National Health Care: The History of Kaiser Permanente*, Health and Medicine in American Society (Piscatawney, NJ: Rutgers University Press, 1994), 7.

31 Rickey L. Hendricks, "Liberal Default, Labor Support, and Conservative Neutrality: The Kaiser Permanente Medical Care Program After World War II," *Journal of Policy History* 1, 2 (1989): 158.

32 Hendricks, *A Model for National Health Care*, 2.

33 *Hendricks, A Model for National Health Care*, 3.

34 Quoted in A.W. Johnson, *Dream No Little Dreams: A Biography of the Douglas Government of Saskatchewan, 1944-1961* (Toronto: University of Toronto Press, 2004), 3.

35 University of Saskatchewan Archives Special Collections (hereafter USASC), Sophia Dixon Fonds 224, "CCF Program for Saskatchewan," 1944.

36 USASC, Pamphlet/VF: JL197 .C75C7 #1.16. http://greatwar.usask.ca/islandora/object/usaskarchives%3A38718#page/2/mode/1up Accessed December 18, 2017.

37 USASC, Sophia Dixon Fonds 224, "CCF Program for Saskatchewan," 1944, 7-8.

38 SAB, R-251, Health Services Survey Commission, Box 1, File 12.

39 Jacalyn Duffin and Lesley Falk, "Sigerist in Saskatchewan: The Quest for Balance in Social and Technical Medicine," *Bulletin of the History of Medicine* 70, 4 (1996): 660. See also J.M. Duffin, "The Guru and the Godfather: Henry Sigerist, Hugh MacLean, and the Politics of Health Care Reform in 1940s Canada," *Canadian Bulletin of Medical History* 9 (1992): 191–218.

40 Elizabeth Fee, "The Pleasures and Perils of Prophetic Advocacy: Socialized Medicine and the Politics of American Medical Reform," in Elizabeth Fee

and Theodore M. Brown, eds., *Making Medical History: The Life and Times of Henry E. Sigerist* (Baltimore and London: The Johns Hopkins University Press, 1997), 216.

41 Duffin and Falk, "Sigerist in Saskatchewan," 663.

42 Duffin and Falk, "Sigerist in Saskatchewan," 664-665.

43 SAB, "A Checklist of the Records of the Saskatchewan Health Services Survey Commission (Sigerist Commission), 1944."

44 SAB, "A Checklist of the Records of the Saskatchewan Health Services Survey Commission (Sigerist Commission), 1944."

45 SAB, R-251, Health Services Survey Commission, Box 1, File 8, "Brief Presented at Saskatoon to Doctor Sigerist and the Personnel of the Health Survey Commission from the State Health and Medical League of the Province of Saskatchewan," 1.

46 SAB, R-251, Health Services Survey Commission, Box 1, File 8, "Brief Presented at Saskatoon to Doctor Sigerist and the Personnel of the Health Survey Commission from the State Health and Medical League of the Province of Saskatchewan," 5.

47 SAB, R-251, Health Services Survey Commission, Box 1, File 8, "Brief Presented at Saskatoon to Doctor Sigerist and the Personnel of the Health Survey Commission from the State Health and Medical League of the Province of Saskatchewan," 10.

48 SAB, R-251, Health Services Survey Commission, Box 1, File 8, "Brief Presented at Saskatoon to Doctor Sigerist and the Personnel of the Health Survey Commission from the State Health and Medical League of the Province of Saskatchewan," 14.

49 SAB, R-251, Health Services Survey Commission, Box 1, File 2, "A Brief Presented to the Health Services Survey Committee at its hearing in Regina, Sask, September 26, 1944 by W.J. Burak, Secretary-Treasurer, RM of Pittville, Hazlet, Sask," 6.

50 SAB, R-251, Health Services Survey Commission, Box 1, File 8, "Brief Submitted to Saskatchewan Provincial Health Survey Commission by the Canadian National Railway Employees' Medical Aid Society," 5.

51 SAB, R-251, Health Services Survey Commission, Box 1, File 2, "Memo for File re: Brief from RM of Connaught No. 457."

52 SAB, R-251, Health Services Survey Commission, Box 1, File 5, "Brief Submitted by Local Unions of the Canadian Brotherhood of Railway Employees and Other Transport Workers, Regina."

53 SAB, R-251, Health Services Survey Commission, Box 1, File 5, "Saskatoon City Hospital Employees Federated Union, Brief to be presented to Health Services Commission."

54 SAB, R-251, Health Services Survey Commission, Box 1, File 6, "Brief Submitted by the Saskatchewan Federation of Agriculture."

55 SAB, R-251, Health Services Survey Commission, Box 1, File 8, "Brief
    Presented at Saskatoon to Doctor Sigerist and the Personnel of the Health
    Survey Commission from the State Health and Medical League of the
    Province of Saskatchewan," 7.

56 SAB, R-251, Health Services Survey Commission, Box 1, File 8, "Brief
    Presented at Saskatoon to Doctor Sigerist and the Personnel of the Health
    Survey Commission from the State Health and Medical League of the
    Province of Saskatchewan," 7.

57 SAB, R-251, Health Services Survey Commission, Box 1, File 7,
    "Submission Presented to the Health Services Survey Commission on
    Behalf of the Provincial Council of Women," 3.

58 SAB, R-251, Health Services Survey Commission, Box 1, File 5, "Mr. A.
    Lovell, Saskatoon Trades and Labor Council;" "P.W. Haffner, Regina
    Trades and Labour Council," 2, 1.

59 SAB, R-251, Health Services Survey Commission, Box 1, File 8, "Brief
    Presented at Saskatoon to Doctor Sigerist and the Personnel of the Health
    Survey Commission from the State Health and Medical League of the
    Province of Saskatchewan," 1.

60 SAB, R-251, Health Services Survey Commission, Box 1, File 2, "A Brief
    Presented to the Health Services Survey Committee at its hearing in
    Regina, Sask, September 26, 1944 by W.J. Burak, Secretary-Treasurer, RM
    of Pittville, Hazlet, Sask," 8.

61 SAB, R-251, Health Services Survey Commission, Box 1, File 7,
    "Submission Presented to the Health Services Survey Commission on
    Behalf of the Provincial Council of Women," 1.

62 SAB, R-251, Health Services Survey Commission, Box 1, File 7,
    "Submission Presented to the Health Services Survey Commission on
    Behalf of the Provincial Council of Women," 1.

63 SAB, R-251, Health Services Survey Commission, Box 1, File 7,
    "Submission Presented to the Health Services Survey Commission on
    Behalf of the Provincial Council of Women," 2.

64 SAB, R-251, Health Services Survey Commission, Box 1, File 7, "Outline of
    Brief to be Presented to Health Services Survey Commission by Mrs. Eric
    Given, Provincial Presidents Saskatchewan Homemakers' Clubs," 1.

65 SAB, R-251, Health Services Survey Commission, Box 1, File 7, Outline of
    Brief to be Presented to Health Services Survey Commission by Mrs. Eric
    Given, Provincial Presidents Saskatchewan Homemakers' Clubs," 1.

66 SAB, R-251, Health Services Survey Commission, Box 1, File 7,
    "Submission Presented to the Health Services Survey Commission on
    Behalf of the Provincial Council of Women," 2.

67 SAB, R-251, Health Services Survey Commission, Box 1, File 7, "Submission Presented to the Health Services Survey Commission on Behalf of the Provincial Council of Women," 3.

68 SAB, R-251, Health Services Survey Commission, Box 1, File 5, "Local Unions of the Canadian Brotherhood of Railway Employees and other Transport Workers, Submitted by W.H. Ansell."

69 SAB, R-251, Health Services Survey Commission, Box 1, File 5, "P.W. Haffner, Regina Trades and Labour Council," 3.

70 SAB, R-251, Health Services Survey Commission, Box 1, File 5, "J.M. Toothill on behalf of the Regina Labour Council of the Canadian Congress of Labour," 3.

71 SAB, R-251, Health Services Survey Commission, Box 1, File 4, "Melfort and District Mutual Medical Benefit Association Ltd.," 10.

72 SAB, R-251, Health Services Survey Commission, Box 1, File 2, "Brief From the Village of Lucky Lake."

73 SAB, R-251, Health Services Survey Commission, Box 1, File 2, "Letter to Commission from Mrs. L.B. Anderson, Saskatoon, on behalf of people of Shell Lake."

74 SAB, R-251, Health Services Survey Commission, Box 1, File 2, "Brief Tisdale Board of Trade."

75 SAB, R-251, Health Services Survey Commission, Box 1, File 7, "Submission Presented to the Health Services Survey Commission on Behalf of the Provincial Council of Women," 2.

76 SAB, R-251, Health Services Survey Commission, Box 1, File 7, Outline of Brief to be Presented to Health Services Survey Commission by Mrs. Eric Given, Provincial Presidents Saskatchewan Homemakers' Clubs," 2.

77 Henry E. Sigerist, "Saskatchewan Health Services Survey Commission: Report of the Commissioner" (Regina: King's Printer, 1944), 4.

78 C. Stuart Houston, 36 Steps on the Road to Medicare: How Saskatchewan Led the Way (Montreal and Kingston: McGill-Queen's University Press, 2013) chapter 3, http://web.a.ebscohost. com.uml.idm.oclc.org/ehost/ebookviewer/ebook/bmxlYmt-fXzU5NTA5MF9fQU41?sid=8feb0b38-b418-4bf1-90ee-320f3c8498ec@ sdc-v-sessmgr05&vid=0&format=EK&lpid=ncx-11&rid=0.

79 Sigerist, "Saskatchewan Health Services Survey Commission," 4.

80 Sigerist, "Saskatchewan Health Services Survey Commission," 9.

81 Sigerist, "Saskatchewan Health Services Survey Commission," 6.

82 Sigerist, "Saskatchewan Health Services Survey Commission," 6, 4.

83 Sigerist, "Saskatchewan Health Services Survey Commission," 6.

84 Sigerist, "Saskatchewan Health Services Survey Commission," 5.

85 Sigerist, "Saskatchewan Health Services Survey Commission," 9.

86 Sigerist, "Saskatchewan Health Services Survey Commission," 7.

CHAPTER 4

DREAM OF A NEW WAY OF LIFE

Mindel Cherniack Sheps and Early Health Reforms in Saskatchewan

U pon the conclusion of the Sigerist Commission's work, Henry Sigerist returned to Baltimore. In early October 1944, Mindel Cherniack Sheps took up the task of implementing the recommendations of the Sigerist Commission. An influential woman in a male-dominated government and party, as assistant to the Minister (Premier Douglas) Mindel's role in driving the CCF's health policy has received very little recognition or analysis. Together with economist Thomas H. McLeod, Mindel provided the dynamism needed to push initial policy development through an inexperienced cabinet and a patronage-ridden civil service. She was the main drafter of the CCF's first health legislation, the Health Services Act (1944), which provided comprehensive health care for pensioners and widows, and created the Saskatchewan Health Services Planning Commission (HSPC)—the province's main health planning body. Mindel served as Secretary to the HSPC; at the end of the war, her husband Dr. Cecil Sheps became its first Acting Chair. The work of the HSPC was critical: it was meant to implement the regionalized health centre framework recommended in the Sigerist Commission Report and determine how to organize and finance district services.

Mindel's career as senior health advisor to Tommy Douglas was short-lived—less than two years. By the summer of 1946, she and Cecil had left Regina for New Haven, Connecticut, where Cecil earned a graduate degree in public health at Yale University as a Rockefeller fellow. The couple had expected to return to Saskatchewan, but their positions were not renewed by the Douglas government. At the time, their friends argued that the Sheps were "sacrificed" for the sake of peace with the province's medical College leadership, with whom they had tense relations.[1] By replacing Mindel and Cecil, Douglas perhaps hoped to send a signal that would placate organized medicine and keep the doctors onside in the future debate over publicly insured physician services—something it would ultimately take the CCF another eighteen years to achieve. In any event, pacifying physicians proved impossible, as the 1962 physicians' strike that attempted to block the creation of medicare attests. Mindel, always incisive, saw little benefit in Douglas's strategy. She would before too long become a quiet, but pointed critic. Writing to Sigerist in 1949 from her new home in Chapel Hill, North Carolina, where Cecil had found an academic position, she characterized the CCF's record as a "peculiar compound of recklessness and timidity."[2]

The Sheps's departure from the Saskatchewan government left some grieving their loss. Her Saskatchewan friend, Barbara Cadbury commented at Mindel's memorial service: "[Mindel and Cecil] were both the zest and the solid foundation of the whole experiment in the public good. For me at least it never recovered without them."[3] Known as assertive and radical in their support for socialized medicine, their brief Saskatchewan sojourn encapsulates the political dynamic that Gordon Lawson calls "the road not taken," the turning away from one health policy path (socialized medicine) and the choosing of another (public health insurance). Mindel's experience in particular, influenced as it was not only by her politics but also her gender and her Jewishness, complicates recent narratives about the openness and "cosmopolitanism" of the Douglas government.[4]

Embodying a political critique of the CCF's approach to health that simmered barely below the public surface, Mindel's short career evokes persistent limits to full equality in the culture of the western Canadian political left in the early postwar years.

At the time of her appointment to the Sigerist Commission, Mindel Cherniack Sheps was 31 years old. She was born in Winnipeg in 1913, the daughter of Joseph Alter and Fania (Goldin) Cherniack, immigrants to Winnipeg from southern Russia. Mindel was raised in the vibrant social and political atmosphere of Winnipeg's North End. Until after World War II, almost 90 percent of Winnipeg's Jewish community lived in the district.[5] The Jewish left was dominant in the area's social and cultural life, and its politics were diverse, ranging from the embrace of anarchism, communism, Labour Zionism and democratic socialism, to Jewish mutual aid organizations and trade union organizing.[6] Unsurprisingly, this diversity sometimes generated tensions and animosities.

Mindel grew up in a secular, left-leaning socialist—not communist—Jewish family. Her Labour Zionist father, Alter Cherniack, helped to found the I.L. Peretz Schul. He trained as a lawyer after immigrating to Canada, and was called to the bar in 1918. Alter formed a law practice with British Jewish immigrant Max Hyman, who lectured at the law school. Hyman was elected to the Manitoba Legislature in 1927 for the Independent Labour Party. Although Alter Cherniack was a member of the CCF during the last years of World War II, he worked alongside communists in the League Against Fascism and Anti-Semitism, despite the opposition of the Canadian Jewish Congress, which was opposed to united-front politics.[7] Alter was also "a Yiddhist, with a flair for theatre."[8] Political, social, and cultural life were dynamic in Winnipeg's relatively small and intertwined progressive Jewish community.

Mindel's mother, Fania, was born in Odessa, during Russia's late imperial era. Before immigrating to Winnipeg in 1908, she was jailed for her political activism in Socialist Territorialist causes. Neither

Fania (a seamstress) nor Alter (a watchmaker) had grown up in privileged circumstances in Odessa. After they married in Canada, Fania
supported the family while Alter went to law school. Their first two
children, a boy and a girl, died as infants. Fania Cherniack, like Alter,
was involved in several progressive Jewish organizations, including
the Peretz Schul. She was a member of the school's Muter Farein
(mother's club) and helped to establish a Jewish kindergarten in 1919.
Historian Ros Usiskin argues that Fania, like other Jewish women
on the left, valued modern early childhood education and believed
that "Jewish education should begin with the pre-school child."[9] Fania
appears to have supported her daughter in overcoming the sexism
and anti-Semitism Mindel faced as a young Jewish woman. Mindel's
younger brother, Saul Cherniack, described his mother as a "strong
person" and both of his parents as "gender conscious" and feminist.[10]

Teasing apart the multiple threads of Mindel's background
and identity poses certain interpretive challenges. While Canadian
scholars such as Ruth Frager and more recently Jodi Giesbrecht have
explored the relationship between gender, Jewish identity, and working-class activism, historians have paid less attention to women like
Mindel Cherniack Sheps, who came of age in the interwar political
left, but who were not working class.[11] Neither are there abundant
clues to be found in the history of medicine, as there are very few historical studies of Jewish physicians in Canada, male or female. Harry
Medovy's 1972 article, "The Early Jewish Physicians in Manitoba,"
mentions no women, which reflects perhaps the gendered perspective
of the author, but also indicates the barriers facing Jewish women
seeking to enter the profession at the turn of the twentieth century.[12]
Nevertheless, Canadian historian W.P.J. Millar notes that significant
numbers of Jews in North America entered faculties of medicine in
the first half of the twentieth century, despite the growth of quotas
limiting their enrollment. At the University of Manitoba, as many
as 28 percent of medical students came from Jewish backgrounds in
the early 1930s, before quotas would reduce that number to 9 percent

by the early 1940s.[13] These figures (particularly pre-quota) suggest that Jewish Winnipeggers entered medical school at rates disproportionate to their percentage of the population; in 1931, 7.7 percent of Winnipeg residents were Jewish.[14]

Why were medicine and science so appealing to modern Jews? Noah Efron's recent study, *A Chosen Calling: Jews in Science in the Twentieth Century*, examines the overrepresentation of Jews in science and medicine in three locales: the United States, the Soviet Union, and Jewish Palestine. Ephron argues that the linkage between Jewish identity and science and medicine was about more than professional advancement or social mobility; it reflected the twinning of "scientific spirit and democratic faith":

> In all three places, one finds similarly enthusiastic rhetoric about the role of science in fashioning a good society. In all three places, the "values" of science were said to comport with and bolster the most dearly held social values: democracy, equality, progress and more. In all three places, Jews held a generally uncritical attitude towards the sciences and technology, and toward government by scientific principles.[15]

Efron's study, however, includes no women and accepts the premise of a gendered male medical profession.

Feminist scholarship suggests that Jewish women, like Gentile women, were largely excluded from medicine before the nineteenth century.[16] Prior to migration from the Russian Pale of Settlement, life for Mindel's ancestors was characterized by oppression, poverty, and little social mobility. Poverty often meant Jewish women and girls played an essential economic role in family life. Paula Hyman has argued that "the strong, capable working woman [was a] dominant cultural ideal."[17] Jewish women took advantage of opportunities for medical education when the Russian state made them available. In 1889, after a brief period during which women had been encouraged to enter medicine, Jewish women represented 24 percent of all female physicians, while Jews made up only 4 percent of the total population of the Russian empire.[18] They often saw medicine as a calling, and were likely to be employed by the state in some form of community health, such as the rural regional (zemstvo) clinics and hospitals or urban clinics. In the words of one such physician, Mariya Rashkovich, their commitment was "to be useful to the people through specialized knowledge."[19] Many Jewish women studying medicine, like Rashkovich, came from the "New Russia," particularly from Odessa, the home city of Mindel Cherniack Sheps's parents. According to Carol Balin, Odessa "has become legendary in the historical literature for its huge Jewish enrolment of both boys and girls in gymnasia."[20]

After migration, progress towards gender equality in the Pale confronted powerful pressures for Jewish families to conform to Anglo-Canadian gender and social norms, including normative health practices. Migration may have shaken the boundaries between domestic and private spheres, and represented the possibility of education and more open access to work, politics, and leisure for women, as suggested by Paula Hyman for the US case. However, migrants from Eastern Europe confronted negative attitudes toward immigrant health practices among the dominant Anglo-Canadian majority. Jews and Slavic immigrants were often viewed as ignorant of modern health standards, and as carriers of disease, not as sources of medical knowledge. They were the targets of public health reformers in Winnipeg, like in other North American urban contexts. Immigrant mothers in particular were blamed for high rates of infant mortality and infectious disease.[21]

Despite the oppressive Anglo-Canadian context within which turn-of-the-twentieth-century Jewish migrants settled in Winnipeg, as well as their initial poverty, they successfully built institutions and cultural life in the city. These efforts helped insulate them from their vulnerability to an anti-Semitic host society, while promoting greater social mobility and accommodation. By the Great War, these institutions included schools, a Jewish Children's Aid Society, an orphanage, a home for the Jewish elderly, and Jewish charities.[22] The North End also nourished a vibrant labour culture. Militant female labour activism in the garment industry, for example, was an avenue for Jewish women to resist economic inequality and contest gender norms. As Jodi Giesbrecht has noted, labour organizing was also a vehicle through which Jewish women integrated into Canadian economic and political life.[23]

The Jewish left community, of which Mindel's family was a part, played a role in nurturing her ambitions. She was an exceptionally bright child, completing grades 10 and 11 in one year.[24] She received her medical degree from the University of Manitoba in 1936, aged 23, one of only five women in a graduating class of 53. One other woman in Mindel's graduating class, Gladys Nitikman, was Jewish.[25] As Mary Kinnear has shown, although there was initially no formal bar to women's admission to the Manitoba Medical College (founded in 1883), the first woman was not admitted until 1890. Between 1890 and the First World War, the College only graduated four women. By 1941, 86 women had graduated, but 40 percent of them never registered with the College of Physicians and Surgeons, either by personal choice or because of gendered barriers to practice.[26] Naomi Rogers has argued that by the 1950s, a gendered medical profession in the US had established a male inner fraternity that employed a variety of mechanisms to repel women through hostility, neglect, and disrespect.[27] There is no evidence to suggest the Canadian medical profession was any more egalitarian.

Like many other North American medical schools, including the US ivy league institutions, the Faculty of Medicine at the University of Manitoba developed a system of gender and ethnic quotas, stated and unstated. Beginning in 1932, Dean of Medicine Dr. A.T. Mathers reduced the number of annual admissions to the school and introduced a deliberate quota system in which applicants were sorted into four lists: Jews; women; Ukrainians, Poles,

Mennonites and others; and finally the preferred category—Anglo-Saxon, French-Canadian and male Icelandic applicants. This quota system operated quietly for a decade, until it was publicly revealed in 1944 through the efforts of the Avukah Zionist Society, a group of Jewish doctors, medical students, and supporters. It became the subject of legislative committee hearings, and a public embarrassment for the school.[28]

To be a Jewish female medical student in this era meant working in an environment characterized by sexual and racial discrimination. Dorothy Hollenberg, who graduated from the Faculty of Medicine in 1929 (seven years before Mindel), explained the situation she encountered at the school:

> In Medical School there certainly was definite planned anti-Semitism. The Jewish students were herded into a separate group, they were put at separate tables in the Anatomy Department, and I as a woman was not put with Jewish people. I was put with another woman who was a Methodist .... The Professor of Anatomy would have a party for the students and the Jewish students were never invited, and this was the sort of anti-Semitism. It shouldn't hurt, but it does. One becomes accustomed to it ... and when it came to getting internships, [there were] never more than two Jewish students appointed as interns in the General Hospital.[29]

Discrimination, however, did not prevent all Jewish women from succeeding in medicine. Miller's analysis of medical students at the University of Toronto suggests that Jewish women were as successful as Jewish men, once admitted, and did better academically than their non-Jewish female counterparts, suggesting they were "highly motivated to succeed."[30] Dorothy Hollenberg, for example, would go on to build a successful medical practice with her husband in the St. Vital neighbourhood in Winnipeg. Mindel completed her internship at the Saskatoon City Hospital in 1935. She was a resident at the Winnipeg Children's Hospital in 1937, which was at that time the only hospital in Winnipeg's working-class, immigrant North End neighbourhood, where she had grown up. She and her husband, Cecil, went to London, England in 1937 or 1938, and Mindel worked at the Marie Curie Hospital in Whitechapel, in east-end London. Her Winnipeg and London experiences both brought home to her the impact of poverty upon health. By 1939 Mindel was back in Winnipeg, working in general practice.

Early in her medical career, Mindel worked for a time with the Winnipeg Birth Control Society, which later became a part of Planned Parenthood. Although few archival records survive for the Society—and those extant do not mention Mindel—two sources (her husband and her brother) confirm her involvement in the organization. According to the recollections of Mindel's brother, Saul, she worked closely with Dr. Harry Martindale Speechly, a local physician and provincial coroner, the husband of Mary Speechly, the president of the Winnipeg Birth Control Society. Mindel went house-to-house, teaching women about birth control, at a time when the dissemination of birth control remained a criminal offence.[31] In an oral history, Cecil described his wife as "the physician for the Planned Parenthood organization" for several years, providing birth control advice to over three hundred women. Cecil described Mindel presenting a paper to the Winnipeg Medical Society on data she collected regarding birth control needs:

> I remember sitting in the audience before the meeting started with the doctors slapping their thighs and chuckling because they figured that this would be lascivious stuff, and they were flabbergasted when they saw those most of these patients had had three or four children. I remember that scene very well. That kind of work didn't get very much recognition then.[32]

Her belief in female reproductive freedom formed a long-lasting part of Mindel's political identity. In 1972, while accepting an honorary Doctorate of Science from the University of Manitoba, she defended access to birth control, arguing that it "would ameliorate some of the inequities with which we live, increase freedom of choice and enrich life." She called for "universal availability of contraceptive information, and even more important, true equality of opportunity and freedom for women."[33]

Mindel's involvement in the Winnipeg Birth Control Society is worth probing because of the Society's apparent embrace of eugenics, and because the Sigerist Commission report itself supported sterilization of the unfit. The history of North America's birth control advocacy from the early twentieth century through the 1940s is intertwined with that of eugenics. Stern refers to eugenics as having a "multi-dimensional presence" in government, professions, and social movements—including socialism, feminism, medicine, and public health.[34] However, there was a wide range and diversity of opinion about eugenics even among broadly sympathetic actors who accepted the fundamental premise of race betterment through reproductive controls. There was not always a unified view on what, if any, action was best. For example, many physicians opposed sterilization laws when proposed by legislators, even when they agreed that racial improvement was a desirable goal of medical science. Physicians had individual views, religious beliefs, personal ethics, and histories that did not always fall into line with those of eugenics' proponents.

Similarly, those who agreed on particulars (such as the provision of condoms to the poor) may have done so for very different reasons. When we shift the lens to focus on gender and sexuality, as recent scholarship has, the history of eugenics, sterilization, and birth control becomes even more complicated. Stern comments that "unfit," poor, and racialized women (frequently the targets of sterilization measures) might themselves seek out sterilization as a form of birth control, or at least not object to sterilization programs. This argument has been echoed recently in Erica Dyck's *Facing Eugenics*, a study of the issue in Canada.[35] Not all women were passive victims of sterilization laws and welfare state programs; at a time when birth control remained illegal and especially difficult for the poor to access, sterilization held different meanings than we might expect for women themselves. Yet, their ability to access sterilization remained caught within the broader rubric of a male-dominated eugenics, which as historians such as Linda Gordon have argued, appropriated the agenda of feminists and family planners.[36]

Birth controllers and eugenicists had a complex relationship, and while their respective interests may have overlapped, they were not identical. In the US case, not all eugenicists supported greater accessibility of birth control, and some (notably the male leaders of the American Eugenics Society) did not want to be seen as supporters of advocates such as Margaret Sanger. At the same time, "most birth controllers," historian Wendy Kline argues, "supported eugenic goals."[37] Eugenics provided birth control advocates with a scientific discourse, lent it credibility and legitimacy, and connected birth control with the larger project of "racial progress." By working within the eugenics framework, birth controllers were liberated from disreputable associations and disconnected from sex. In this way, the purpose of birth control was, as Sanger argued, "more children from the fit, less from the unfit."[38]

The Winnipeg Birth Control Society's publications certainly drew on eugenicist discourse. The Society's longtime chair was Mary Speechly, the wife of Harry Martindale Speechly. Speechly was the woman appointed to the University of Manitoba's Board of Governors, and she is recognized on the campus by a residence named in her honour. Speechly's organization was perpetually short of funds, and was supported by A.R. Kaufman, the Kitchener, Ontario-based businessman who was, from the 1930s through the mid-1970s, the driving force behind the Parents' Information Bureau, which manufactured and distributed various methods of birth control, including diaphragms and condoms. Linda Revie has argued that Kaufman was a eugenicist. He was a member of the executive of the Eugenics Society of Canada, sought to provide birth control

to the poor to limit their reproduction, and supported the sterilization of the unfit.[39]

It is impossible to say based on archival evidence what Mindel's
views were on the question of "improving the race." Later in her life,
when she became a biostatistician and demographer of fertility and
did consulting work for the Ford Foundation in India, she took a
critical approach to programs attempting to lower the birth rates of
developing countries, urging their proponents to carefully measure
the results and impact of such programs and to exercise caution considering the lack of available evidence. In 1972, she defended some
birth control policies not for their population-limiting effect, but
because they "would ameliorate some of the inequities with which
we live, increase freedom of choice and enrich life." Here, specifically,
she supported "universal availability of contraceptive information,
and even more important, true equality of opportunity and freedom for women."[40]

M indel seemed destined for electoral politics. The Cherniack
family has had a long history of involvement in Winnipeg's
political left. In 1919, Mindel's father's cousin, Rose (Cherniack)
Alcin was elected to the Winnipeg school board for the Independent
Labour Party. Mindel's younger brother, Saul, a lawyer, was a
school trustee, city councilor and then Finance Minister in the
Edward Schreyer government, the first NDP government elected
in Manitoba in 1969. Her cousin David Orlikow was also a CCF/
NDP politician, eventually replacing Stanley Knowles as the NDP
MP for Winnipeg North Centre. Before she had turned 30, Mindel
ran for public office for the CCF. She was elected to the Winnipeg
School Board in 1942, a position from which she resigned in order to
serve the Saskatchewan government as the secretary of the Sigerist
Commission. She chaired the Manitoba CCF's research committee on health in 1944, and also served on the party's national health
research committee.[41]

Mindel Cherniack Sheps (as her name appeared in CCF campaign literature, perhaps to emphasize her familial connections) was elected to the school board for Ward 3 in November 1942 with the highest number of votes among the four successful candidates.[42] The CCF ran two other female candidates for school trustee in the 1942 election. Mindel was the only one of the women elected. One of Mindel's allies on the school board was Joseph Zuken. Zuken, a lawyer and committed communist, was an extremely popular politician in his north end Winnipeg community. After serving as a school trustee for 20 years, he was elected to City Council in 1961, where he served until his retirement in 1983.[43] Despite the tensions and competition between democratic socialists and communists during the 1940s, Mindel appears to have been disinclined to drive a wedge between herself and Zuken for partisan reasons. The two often worked together on school board issues, not shying away from controversy.

In early January 1943, Cherniack Sheps and Zuken dove right in to their work as school trustees, calling for a review of the entire school curriculum. A week later, they were part of a group of trustees calling for the Province of Manitoba to amend the Manitoba Public Schools Act, which allowed religious instruction in schools between the hours of 3:30 and 4:00 pm at the request of 25 or more parents, to be carried out by "any Christian clergy" or his designate. The trustees wanted decisions over religious instruction to be made by the school board, and for the instruction to be provided by teachers authorized by the trustees. Long time Independent Labour Party school trustee Meyer Averbach, who had moved the motion, claimed that a Jewish student at Grosvenor School had become upset, "when during the religious period the crucifixion of Christ was discussed."[44] Zuken's position was clear:

> I am opposed to any form of religious teaching in any public school. There is a place for religion, but not in our schools.

> Religion is a matter between the child, the parents, and a spiritual advisor ... the more we try to make the school do the work of the church, the more controversy we'll have.[45]

Mindel spoke in favour of Averbach's motion. The controversy this motion unleashed is indicated by the school board's reversal a few weeks later, when Averbach's motion was rescinded. Trustee George Macleod made his opposition to any non-Christian religious instruction the centre of his argument against amending the law, which he saw as a safeguard for Christianity against demands for "instruction in the Jewish religion, the Mohammedan religion, or any other religion."[46]

Mindel gained public notoriety while on the school board by advocating two measures in support of female school teachers: the first to remove the ban on married women working as teachers; the second to introduce equal pay for male and female teachers.[47] When her motions to this effect were introduced to the school board in March 1943, they were "squelched in short order," prompting an outcry from Mindel's ally, Joe Zuken: "Hitler would just love you guys." Opponents to equal pay, rather than voting on the motion, tabled it until the end of the year, which put an immediate stop to debate on the motion at the meeting. On the question of the employment of married women, at least one school trustee argued that the appropriate place for married women was in the home. Mindel argued that merit should be the only criteria for hiring school teachers. Despite the fact that five Labour school trustees supported Mindel's motions, they were defeated.[48] Mindel's advocacy for women teachers was immediately applauded by local women's organizations. The Local Council of Women and the Women's International League, then meeting in Winnipeg for a conference on Canada's postwar challenges, issued a statement to the press that they would be writing a letter of thanks to Dr. Mindel Sheps "for her recent effort to obtain recognition of women's rights."[49]

In addition to her work as school trustee, Mindel and Cecil were becoming more involved in the Manitoba CCF. In 1940, Cecil sat on the Manitoba CCF Provincial Council.[50] In late 1942, Cecil was elected to the Provincial Executive of the Manitoba CCF, as Chair of the Finance Committee.[51] He remained active with the Executive and the Manitoba CCF Expansion Fund campaign until he joined the armed forces in 1943. That year, Mindel became Chair of the Manitoba CCF's Health Research Committee, and prepared the party's Provincial Health Program, which was presented to Provincial Convention and then Provincial Council, with the intent that it would go to the CCF National Conference on Provincial Policy to be held in January 1944 in Regina. Her views on the relationship between social equality and health had started to take shape:

> At present a person's chances of survival or health depend on his income and the place where he lives; a 14-year-old boy of a wealthy family is on the average four inches taller than a 14-year-old boy of a poor family. Farmers and waged workers do not get in living conditions, preventive work or treatment anything comparable to what a small portion of our population receives.

The position paper supported aspects of the health insurance bill proposed by the federal government arising out of the work of the Heagerty Committee (although this legislation would fail to materialize).[52] However, Cherniack Sheps also pointed out its limitations: "health insurance itself is no more than a way of financing medical care." While insurance might alleviate the worst of the fears and economic insecurities that resulted from lack of affordable care, insurance was insufficient on its own: "The causes of illness often lie in economic insecurity and cure is often impossible due to the same causes." Thus, health care insurance should be paired with improvements to social and economic conditions through a planned economy, including a housing program, programs providing economic security, industrial medicine, and coordination between health personnel and "industrial administration" in order to facilitate rehabilitation and special employment opportunities for the chronically ill.[53]

In March 1944, just months before being hired by Premier Douglas, Mindel, representing the CCF, gave a radio address on health, broadcast on the private Winnipeg radio station, CKY. It was a lecture on social medicine and marked out the distinctions between the CCF's health platform and the federal government's proposals for health insurance. Sheps described the federal proposals as "a plan to spread out the cost of illness ... partly [out] of contributions made by the government out of general revenues, and largely of special contributions made by each of us. These contributions will vary in size, but the poor man will pay much more in proportion to his income than will a wealthy man." Sheps also took on the Conservative Charlotte Whitton's proposal of two-tiered medical care—a minimum standard of care available publicly, with those able to afford it purchasing better care outside of the public system.

These ideas were inadequate to the problem of health inequality in Canada, Mindel Cherniack Sheps argued: "piecemeal concessions given the voters by the old political parties." Health "is not only a question of treating disease, of providing means to pay doctor and hospital bills." Rather:

> The problem of health and disease is a social problem. The best services in the world are to no avail if the people receiving them are working under poor conditions, are suffering hunger whether actual or hidden, are living in unsanitary homes, without sufficient rest or fresh air ... it's of little benefit to prescribe vitamins and milk to a child in a family of six, living on an income of 20 dollars a week. It's of little benefit to suggest a long vacation at the lake to the mother of this family, or lighter work to its father.
>
> Therefore an absolute essential to thinking about health is to plan for a life of plenty for all.

Mindel's radio address argued that the war effort revealed the capacity for society to afford the things it decides it must have, provided that the technical knowledge and human resources are available. Providing fair employment, good wages, better housing, food, and health care might be costly, but no more costly than could be managed through "cooperative, democratic planning" and utilizing resources for the common good. The health of rural people, which was poorer than that of those living in urban areas, would require special attention. Cherniack Sheps called for grants to municipalities for hospitals and diagnostic centres in rural areas, with ambulance service for those too remote to reach them. Where needed, travelling clinics could be used.

The key principles of CCF health policy, Mindel stated, were financial accessibility and cost borne according to ability to pay. Health services were to be democratically administered by providers and recipients of care. Prevention and health education must be emphasized, and health services must be coordinated with other areas of policy that affect health, such as income support.[54] These elements of a program for socialized medicine would find their way into the Sigerist Report, as would the focus on rural health needs.

The opportunity to work with Henry Sigerist must have been extraordinarily exciting for Mindel. She and her husband knew of Sigerist's work and reputation. In the early 1940s, Cecil had written Sigerist, requesting information about his courses in social medicine at Johns Hopkins University and about the *American Journal of Soviet Medicine*, which Sigerist founded and edited. Cecil (and perhaps Mindel with him) had seen Sigerist speak in Ann Arbor, Michigan in 1941.[55] Mindel and Henry became active correspondents. Mindel wrote her first letter to Sigerist on August 12, 1944, just before her departure for Regina to take up her new position. After introducing herself, she added that she and Cecil had been "very great admirers of yourself ever since we first read your book on

Soviet Medicine in 1937—an impression which has been fortified by everything of yours we've read since then."[56] Sigerist responded with the warmth and informality that characterized his letter-writing style, which gave the impression of picking up the thread of a conversation already in progress:

> I was delighted to receive your letter of August 12 and I apologize for answering it so late. It reached me with some delay in a cottage on the Delaware Bay where I tried to escape the terrific heat we had in Baltimore. … I am looking forward with greatest pleasure to working with you and I think that we have a unique opportunity of doing a truly constructive piece of work.
>
> I fully approve of the general procedure [for the Commission] that you outline. … I will need a few days to get the atmosphere of the local situation and I count on you and Mr. Douglas to give me some leaders. What counts and what makes me very optimistic is that we have the people of the Province with us. They have expressed their will unmistakably in the last election.[57]

Henry Sigerist and Mindel Cherniack Sheps developed a close personal bond during Sigerist's few weeks in Saskatchewan during the fall of 1944, when they spent an intense period of time together travelling the province for the Sigerist Commission.[58] Of the many letters they wrote to each other in the fall of 1944 and early 1945, most of them discussing the work of the Commission, one of the best indications of their friendship was the letter Sigerist wrote on October 9, 1944, just after his departure from Regina. Changing planes in Winnipeg on his journey home to Baltimore, Sigerist had phoned Mindel's father. She sent a note back a few days later to say that the phone call had given her father "very great pleasure, as I knew it would. And I am very grateful to you for it."[59]

After the finalization of the Sigerist Report, Mindel Cherniack Sheps remained in Regina, working directly with the Premier to move this agenda forward. "And Douglas now wants me to prepare some legislation," Mindel wrote to Sigerist. Ten days later she wrote to tell him about the excitement surrounding the CCF's first legislative session:

> I have pretty well cleaned up things in connection with the survey and am leaving for two weeks holiday at home on Friday night. On my return I expect to plunge into work on the Planning Commission and this is when I expect to start missing you most sorely. … the Legislature begins tomorrow and huge crowds are expected to be here for the opening of the first Socialist Parliament of North America. It should be a worthwhile occasion. [60]

Mindel and Thomas McLeod drafted the Douglas government's new legislation, the Health Services Act (1944), which provided comprehensive health care for those receiving provincial assistance payments, such as pensioners, women receiving mothers' allowances, and the blind. Planning these services, which would benefit some of the most economically vulnerable residents of the province, had started before Sigerist's arrival. In August 1944, Mindel began negotiating with a committee of the College of Physicians and Surgeons for public payment of physician services for those covered by the legislation, while hospital care was developed in discussions with the Saskatchewan Hospital Association. The Social Assistance Medical Care Plan was implemented January 1, 1945, when the CCF had been in power only six months. It immediately covered medical and hospital care and in-hospital drugs for nearly 25,000 people. The program grew to include dental and optical services, nursing, and physiotherapy and by 1950 had over 30,000 annual beneficiaries. [61]

The Health Services Act also created the Saskatchewan Health Services Planning Commission (HSPC), which had been recommended by the Sigerist Report. Mindel was Secretary between fall 1944 and February 1946, when her husband, Cecil, became Acting Chair of the HSPC. [62] The government also appointed a large (21-member) advisory committee to the HSPC. The work of the HSPC was critical to the development of health policy: it was responsible for implementing the health regions framework, deciding on crucial questions of how to organize services, and deciding how to finance them.[63] Working directly under the Premier, who was also Minister of Public Health, the HSPC faced intense political pressure to fulfill the CCF's health commitments, in a context of growing opposition from organized medicine. Transforming the ideals of the Sigerist Commission into reality was immediately contested.

In addition to health care coverage for public pensioners and single mothers, the HSPC began planning a regionalized health care scheme. In February 1945, the HSPC submitted to government its "Report on Regional Health Services: A Proposed Plan." The rural plan recommended the creation of fourteen health regions, in which salaried general practitioners would work out of fully equipped Local Health Centres. Physicians would also be offered pensions, paid holidays, and periodic leave for post-graduate training and development. Specialists would be located in larger regional centres. In its 1945 report, the HSPC stressed the importance of local autonomy, in balance with central "supervision and co-ordination."[64] Thus, the Health Services Act did not itself create health regions. The responsibility and authority to initiate health regions was vested at the local level. The Douglas government took this approach out of commitment to local lay governance, which was important to the CCF's political base and to advocates of socialized medicine. At the same time, however, the permissive nature of the legislation may have been intended to diffuse conflict with organized medicine.[65] If so, the strategy failed, as organized medicine opposed and attempted to block regionalization and lay governance from the outset, and local authorities lacked the firm central mandate of the Province for the regional health centre model.

In November 1945, the tentative health regions were mapped out, each to serve about 50,000 people; the regions were sub-divided into smaller districts of about 15,000. Local residents would control district services through a local health council. Regional boards would be created from representatives elected by the district councils. The establishment of health regions would depend on enthusiasm at the local level, and a very high bar was set for measuring this support. Municipalities were to petition the Minister of Public Health, and a majority of voters had to approve a public referendum.

Initially there was a high level of optimism about this regionalized system, designed along the Sigerist Report's model. As early as June 1945, Mindel Sheps and Tom McLeod travelled the province encouraging municipalities to form regional plans. In September 1945, Dr. Orville K. Hjertaas was appointed as Regional Organizer to help promote the establishment of fourteen health regions. Hjertaas was born in Saskatchewan and received his medical training at the University of Manitoba and the University of Edinburgh. Mindel saw citizen participation as essential to realizing the goals of the Sigerist Commission. As part of her strategy to engage the public behind the regional plan, Mindel organized a series of citizen forums in rural centres, with the help of the government's Adult Education Division. She wrote to Sigerist, "Our hope is that from these conferences there will grow communities who will take it on themselves to see that their local services are surveyed and that a health region is organized."[66] Called "Better Health Services for Our Community and District," citizen conferences were planned for Sturgis, Canora, Kamsack, and Saltcoats for October 1945.

Duane Mombourquette and Malcolm Taylor have argued that a major barrier to rural health regions with a health centre model of delivery was not lack of local support for the idea, but the lack of medical personnel in rural areas. Solving a rural physician shortage was one thing. But organized medical opposition to salaried doctors in rural health centres also undermined the implementation of the Sigerist model. The HSPC's health plan was condemned by the Saskatchewan College of Physicians and Surgeons (SCPS), which not only opposed salaried payment for rural doctors, but also saw that the plan would give local residents a great deal of control over public services and lessen the SCPS's influence over health policy. Mindel Sheps privately expressed frustration as she attempted to move the Sigerist Report recommendations forward. Her personal experience confirms the view of scholars Harley Dickinson and Renée Torgerson that "tension between professional autonomy and democratic control characterized the introduction of medicare."[67] Mindel commented with evident sarcasm in a letter to Henry Sigerist in March 1945: "The doctors on the Advisory Committee found that [the regions] did not agree with their perfectionist standards, and that what we needed were large hospitals and centres where the people could travel from sixty to a hundred miles, and have all their health needs looked after by city practitioners."[68]

While attempting to establish health regions, the Douglas government was also working to expand the number of municipal doctor schemes in the province. Its plan was to induce physicians to take up municipal positions through the promise of a stable salary, three weeks' vacation, and three weeks of post-graduate leave every other year. The HSPC developed a "model contract" for municipal doctors; those municipalities that had signed a contract would begin to receive provincial financial support beginning June 1945. The original model contract stipulated that municipal doctors would be paid salaries, without extra fees, perform preventive care (such as immunizations), and included prenatal care, child care, and mental health services. However, the SCPS insisted that fee-for-service contracts be allowed. Between 1946 and 1950, the number of municipal physician contracts more than doubled, from 58 to 117.[69]

The HSPC's regional framework was less successful. Although initial interest was expressed by as many as ten of the proposed regions, over the next five years only six were formally established. Douglas and the HSPC wanted to establish a viable "model" health region, with a full array of services. They considered focusing on the

Weyburn-Estevan area, where there were some keen local advocates, but according to Joan Feather, Weyburn was not the first choice of either the health planners nor of Douglas himself. Local physician opposition was a barrier, as was competition between Weyburn and nearby Estevan. Politically, any failure in Weyburn would be potentially embarrassing for Douglas because this was his home constituency. Mindel wrote to Douglas concluding, "Weyburn would not seem to be the best place to start."[70] Instead, Mindel and the HSPC proposed Moose Jaw, where work began on establishing a health region in May 1945.

The HSPC commissioned a US economist, Paul Dodd, to formulate a medical care insurance plan for the Moose Jaw health region. Since 1928, Dodd had taught labour economics at University of California Los Angeles (UCLA). He rose to public prominence as a labour arbitrator during a teamsters' union blockade of the Los Angeles Harbour in the 1930s.[71] In 1934 Dodd was appointed Director of the California Medical-Economic Survey, a project that originated with the California Medical Association (CMA) and was partially funded by the New Deal Works Progress Administration. Its work would eventually be known as the Dodd Report. At the same time, a resolution passed in the California Senate calling for a committee to investigate a health insurance act, which became known as the Senate Committee on the High Cost of Illness. The Committee listened to expert opinion and held public hearings. For a time, during the height of the Depression, a public health insurance scheme seemed viable. However, physicians in California were divided on the issue. As the possibility of state action became more likely, the leadership of the CMA grew more reluctant to entertain supporting public health insurance. As a stalling tactic, the CMA argued the Senate should wait for the Dodd Report before acting.

Dodd submitted a preliminary report to the CMA in January 1935. The draft made it obvious that "the CMA had received more than they bargained for."[72] Dodd presented statistical evidence of significant economic barriers to medical care among Californians, and also argued that many physicians were earning paltry incomes. Dodd concluded that compulsory health insurance was a reasonable solution to these inequities. The Dodd Report led to heated internal debates. Key members of the CMA Council condemned the report and held enough influence to have the project terminated. Over the next year and a half, Dodd spent $1000 of his own money and hired a research associate to help him finish the report, which was presented to the CMA in October 1936.

In March 1935, the CMA's House of Delegates passed a compromised resolution that advocated a health insurance system that was "mandatory as to certain population groups and voluntary as to certain population groups," and which would give the medical profession control over the "scope, extent, standards, quality, compensation paid for, and all other matters and things relation to, the medical and medical auxiliary services rendered under the system." Even this resolution, which was truly equivocal in its support for public measures, and some distance from supporting socialized medicine, defied the official stance of the American Medical Association, which was opposed to any significant state role in medical care. At the same time, efforts to pass a health insurance bill foundered in May 1935, and in the end the California legislators agreed only to study the issue further. The CMA published the Dodd Report in November 1937, but it suppressed all references to compulsory health insurance.

Like other American health planners who would make a contribution in Saskatchewan, Dodd was a survivor of the ideological war over health care in the US. With his valuable political experience, Dodd's advice could have become a lynchpin in the planning of medical coverage. But by the time Dodd submitted his report on medical insurance for the Moose Jaw region in November 1945, local organizers in Swift Current had moved ahead of the HSPC and become the first region to organize a health plan. The Dodd plan for Moose Jaw was never implemented.

While Swift Current's enthusiasm was welcome in many ways, from a planning perspective the HSPC had lost control over a fast-moving local situation. Energy now shifted to local organizers, who wanted hospital and medical care as part of their regional health services and were ready to proceed immediately. Joan Feather documented the creation and early evolution of the Swift Current health region in two articles published in the early 1990s.[73] As she points out, the southwest part of the province had a long history of government provision of health services, including a health district project in the Gravelbourg region during the late 1920s that was partially funded by the Rockefeller Foundation.[74] The project focused on public health measures such as infectious disease containment, school medical inspections, pre- and post-natal visits and education, and sanitation. According to the Rockefeller Foundation reports examined by Feather, this focus was not altogether popular with local people, who felt they had been promised free medical treatment, not just preventive measures (such as immunization) and advice. "It is hopeless to advise these people to have tonsillectomy performed on three of four children. Even the cost of vaccine and toxoid protection is utterly beyond many hundreds of people in our District," one report noted. An area woman noted "Most of us mothers know ... what is wrong with [our children], but, for want of money, can do nothing but watch them suffer ... We must have a little more than advice."[75] The project was terminated in 1932.

The community of Excelsior had one of the first municipal doctor schemes, created in the late 1920s. By 1945, the proposed Swift Current health region had four municipal doctor schemes operating within its boundaries. One of these, the RM of Pittville, led by the dynamic Bill Burak, who had presented to the Sigerist Commission (see chapter 3), had instituted medical and hospital coverage partially funded through taxes. The nearby RM of Webb introduced a similar plan in 1943, and in 1944 added dental care to its coverage. In many ways, the region was ideally placed to make a health region work, with experienced lay leadership. But according to Feather, the determining factor in the region's timing was the funding crisis and disrepair facing the Swift Current General Hospital. The hospital appealed to the province for help and met with Mindel Cherniack Sheps and the HSPC in August 1945. At that time, Mindel made a commitment to support building a new hospital, if a regional health centre was made part of the package, with the province agreeing to cover the extra building costs and paying for a full-time public health service.

Feather argues that Mindel did not see the immediate local push to organize the entire health region coming. Bill Burak seized the initiative and wanted to do more than address the hospital's needs. Burak, a "skilled lobbyist," also assertively promoted his own vision of what a health region should do, arguing that the region could provide "complete" medical and hospital services to residents for $9 per capita. Burak was insistent that hospital and medical coverage should be a priority. There certainly were skeptics among the municipal leaders, but Burak was able to convince nearly half of the municipalities in the region to send representatives to a meeting in September 1945. Tom McLeod and Orville Hjertaas attended on behalf of the HSPS. Local media reports of this meeting indicated there was "little discussion of the scope and financial implications of this ambitious program array."[76] Debate at the meeting was less about whether the proposed plan was the right one than it was about who should pay (that is, which levels of government should pay) and what form of taxation (land tax, personal tax, or business tax) was best. There was also debate about whether a referendum vote of ratepayers was required. Because local opinion in the area about the health region scheme was not uniform, the HSPC decided to hold a referendum in the Swift Current region on November 26, 1945; another vote was held the same day on establishing a health region in Weyburn-Estevan.

The HSPC sent out organizers Tom McLeod, Orville Hjertaas, and Mrs. A.M. Lydiard to promote the two health regions. The three spent several weeks travelling to small communities, speaking to members of the public. The HSPC prepared print advertisements, handbills, and radio broadcasts by McLeod, Mindel Cherniack Sheps, and Tommy Douglas. Douglas's broadcast suggested that the Province still considered federal health insurance legislation imminent. The CCF's first priority for regional health care was the establishment of public health services, to be followed by improved diagnostic and specialist services to rural people, and then by the provision of full hospital, medical, and dental coverage. This program, however, was not what Burak had in mind. Burak organized effectively for his own agenda, publishing opinion pieces in local weeklies, stressing medical and hospital insurance provision, and estimating that comprehensive services could be provided for less than $10 per capita.

On November 26, 1945 residents of both the Swift Current and Weyburn-Estevan areas voted about 70 percent in favour of establishing health regions. The government acted quickly and on December 11, 1945 Swift Current Health Region No. 1 was formally established by Order-in-Council. Hjertaas and Cherniack Sheps organized a meeting for January 17, 1946 with local representatives who would form the regional board; about 60 people attended. At this initial meeting, Burak's vision and ambition carried the day. A motion was passed that the Swift Current Health Region No. 1 should "provide complete health services," funded 25 percent through property tax and 75 percent through a personal tax. Hjertaas's account of the meeting was very positive: a "spirit of cooperation and unity of purpose ... prevailed," he wrote.[77] Nonetheless, Feather's observation that the HSPC had been placed in a reactive position seems fundamentally correct. Not only the pace but the direction of health reform and the regional plan were leaning very strongly in the direction not of public health and preventive services and the development of rural health centres, but rather health insurance that, while removing some of the economic barrier to health care access for individuals and families, nonetheless left conventional modes of health delivery intact.

Swift Current Health Region No. 1 became the first area in the province to provide hospital and medical coverage to residents covered by the plan, and as such became a model for other regions to follow, at least in theory. But the implementation of the Swift Current "model" had repercussions for health care organization that would affect future health planning in significant ways. The most important of these was the decision to allow physicians to charge fee-for-service, rather than place them in a salaried service.

The Swift Current case illustrates how, even in a well-informed population with high levels of support for the new CCF government, health planners had their work cut out for them. The CCF was firmly committed to local control and engagement in its early period, but quickly learned that local input could be a fast-moving train, impossible to steer. Citizens and lobby groups who had actively pressured government for health programs in the interwar years wanted a voice in shaping Douglas's policies, particularly in this crucial formative period. Mindel Cherniack Sheps was at the forefront of what could often be a quixotic exchange on both sides. In Swift Current, she and her fellow HSPC staff failed to contain the scope of local expectations or shift their focus toward the HSPC's priorities. Grassroots support could be heartening and gratifying, but there were many strong personalities involved who had years of investment in the issue, while she was a newcomer and an outsider—a "carpet bagger," as her husband Cecil would eventually call himself and other health planners hired by Douglas.

Mindel's experience with the main citizen lobby group, the State Hospital and Medical League was also mixed. She described the group, and particularly its publicist E.R. Powell, as politically supportive, but obstructionist. She expressed some cynicism toward the group in her correspondence with Sigerist, writing of Powell, "He tosses from one argument to another in an effort to find a) something to criticize and, b) something whereby he can get a job."[78] Always direct in her correspondence, her harsh words may have reflected the frustration of a public servant bearing the pressure of public expectations and unhappy with the uneven pace at which the Sigerist Report was being implemented. She was also overworked, exhausted, and in charge of a health agenda unfolding on multiple fronts, all of them bringing distinct challenges.

Mindel's formal status never quite matched her level of responsibility and behind-the-scenes influence. She was appointed Secretary of the Sigerist Commission and Secretary of the HSPC. She never acted formally as Chair. The most likely explanation was her gender. The CCF was not, in the mid-1940s, a feminist party, nor was Douglas's government. Women were marginally represented in key government positions, and in the Legislature itself, although they were not entirely absent. The first CCF government caucus did include one woman, Beatrice Janet Trew, elected in 1944 for one term as MLA for Maple Creek.[79] She was only the second woman ever elected to the Saskatchewan Legislature—the first was Sarah Ramsland (Liberal), who was elected in 1919 as the representative for Pelly, a seat vacated when her husband died in the influenza pandemic. Trew, a teacher originally from New Brunswick and married to a Saskatchewan farmer, was the president of the Swift Current Homemakers' Club leading up to the 1944 election. She was also a respected leader in the CCF, and would serve as a member of the national council for eleven years and as a vice-president of the Saskatchewan section of the party for eight years. In the early 1960s, she sat on the Thompson Advisory Planning Committee on Medical Care, which led to the introduction of universal physician-care coverage in Saskatchewan in 1962.[80] Nevertheless, throughout the Douglas and Woodrow Lloyd years, the CCF only ran three women for provincial office, electing two.

The gender politics of the CCF have come under close scrutiny by several scholars, including Joan Sangster and more recently David

McCrane. The Saskatchewan CCF, while in office, appeared to pay little attention to the gender implications of its policy measures, and formulated policy based on a traditional view of gender relations in family and society, emphasizing women's role in the household and the importance of supporting male breadwinners. From 1944 to 1964, CCF electoral platforms never explicitly mentioned women.[81] Women did key organizational work in the party and in activist groups (such as the Grain Growers), but they were seen as organizers, not part of the party's brain trust.

As McCrane has argued, "the dominance of males within both the CCF party organization and state institutions controlled by the party while it was in government did not create an atmosphere congenial to the advancement of women's issues."[82] Nor, quite evidently, did it create an atmosphere congenial to the advancement of women in the civil service or as political advisors. Recent historical works, such as *Tommy's Team: The People Behind the Douglas Years*, celebrate the "people behind the stage," virtually all of whom are men.[83] The government did pass a law requiring equal pay for equal work irrespective of sex for women working in the civil service; however, in 1946, when the Douglas administration amended the Public Service Act, it introduced restrictions on the employment of married women in the civil service. Under "emergency" situations, married women could be removed from their jobs, unless there was evidence of "special need, circumstances or particular skills." Joan Sangster observes, "CFF women were extremely disturbed that the government had bowed to public hostility to married working women."[84] Women in the party organized opposition to the measure, and were successful in having this aspect of the legislation later reversed.[85] However, a further blow was dealt to CCF women when, despite the urging of the drafter of the Bill of Rights, Morris Shumiatcher, and feminists in the party, the CCF's pioneering human rights legislation did not refer to sexual discrimination.[86] Mindel's response to Douglas's failure to prohibit sexual discrimination under the law has not surfaced in the archival record, but her past advocacy for women's equality makes it unlikely that she was neutral about it.

Mindel and her husband Cecil were two of several recruits to government from outside of the province. But for those who, like them (and later health advisors Leonard Rosenfeld and Milton Roemer), were Jewish, Saskatchewan's history of anti-Semitism also coloured their experience. During the interwar years, Saskatchewan's Anglo-Protestant majority had been a fertile recruiting ground for the Ku Klux Klan, which reached a membership of 25,000 by 1929, serving to polarize the politics of the province.[87] By the end of the Second World War, the CCF had taken a national position against discrimination based upon religious or racial difference. As historian Carmella Patrias has noted:

> Speaking out in Parliament against the deportation of Japanese Canadians, Alistair Stewart, CCF MP from Winnipeg, employed the language of rights: "Any citizen of this country, whether he be Jew or Gentile, Catholic or Protestant, black, white or yellow, believer or unbeliever," he argued, "has exactly the same rights as any other citizen."[88]

Taking up this equal rights and anti-discrimination discourse, Saskatchewan in 1946 became the first province in Canada to pass a Bill of Rights. Patrias has pointed out that there were pragmatic political reasons for this position which suggest it may not have been entirely a principled stand in support of civil rights. The CCF saw the defence of civil liberties against discrimination as key to electoral success among ethnic voters, especially during an era when the party faced active electoral competition from the Communist Party of Canada.[89]

Internally, the party still struggled with its own racism and anti-Semitism, which affected the Sheps's experience in the Saskatchewan civil service. In July 1946, Mindel wrote to the national leader of the CCF, David Lewis. Anticipating seeing Lewis at the

upcoming national CCF convention being held in Regina, Mindel
was direct in her observations about attitudes toward Jews within
the government and the party, and disagreed with Lewis on the best
way of dealing with the problem:

> Some time ago we agreed to disagree on whether it is good
> policy, particularly good socialist policy, to try to keep too
> many Jews out of the limelight. Well, I'm not going to argue
> that point again now. What I should like to suggest is that when
> you, David Lewis, mention those considerations to the aver-
> age, in-prejudice-weaned, non-Jew, you are helping to reinforce
> his prejudices and, more, to give them an aura of rightness and
> "respectability," that is, "socialist respectability." Specifically, I
> am referring at the moment to Don Black, whom I like ... Don,
> however, as you may know, is not quite among the vanguard of
> the socially enlightened. I think this is revealed in his attitude to
> women, possibly to his children, and definitely I felt to Tamaki.
> .... When he was introduced to David Schwartzman he said
> (I am told)—"Oh yes, ... say, how many Jews are there in this
> damn government anyway?" And when it was pointed out that
> the number was fairly small came out with a remark about how
> clever we all are. Later he explained to those who had introduced
> him to David Schwartzman that you had told him that D.S. had
> not been appointed to the National Office because he is a Jew.[90]

Mindel did not refer to her own experience, but it may well have
been why she raised the issue with Lewis. Lewis thought that the
way to deal with anti-Semitism in the CCF was for Jews to avoid
drawing attention to themselves: in her experience, this was not possible in any case in the Saskatchewan party. She challenged Lewis
to change tack.

Mindel was not interested in hiding or apologizing for her
Jewish identity. Indeed, her radical Yiddischist upbringing had
defined her world view and shaped her health politics, quite possibly

her feminism, and her commitment to social equality. Yet, as a woman, Mindel was also largely excluded from membership in a self-defined group of North American Jewish public health advocates who referred to themselves as "medical careniks"—a club in which Cecil would enjoy full membership throughout his long career as a health educator and administrator. In a tribute to Cecil after his death in 2004, Donald Madison, a professor of social medicine at the University of North Carolina School of Medicine who knew Cecil well, defined the medical careniks this way:

> The suffix, nik, is both Russian and Yiddish. It means something "associated with or characterized by" … Almost all in the group of whom I speak were physicians. Virtually all were male. Most were veterans of World War II. Most were Jews. In intellect they ranged from superior to brilliant. And they shared the same commitment to public health and social justice.[91]

Madison went on to name some of the US medical careniks: Sy Axelrod, Dick Weinerman, Milt Roemer, Les Falk, Milton Terris, Leonard Rosenfeld, Paul Cornely, George Silver, and Cecil Sheps. Sheps, Rosenfeld, Roemer, and Weinerman all had connections with the Douglas government. It was an all-male cohort. But Mindel is notably absent from Madison's list, as is Fred Mott who replaced Mindel and Cecil in Regina. A non-Jew, Mott, despite many overlapping professional and political relationships, was not defined as a carenik.

Perhaps coincidentally, Mindel left the Douglas government the same year the Public Service Act was amended to discourage the government employment of married women. She and her husband purchased a house in Regina and adopted a son, Sam.

Around the same time, Cecil was appointed a member of the Committee on Free Hospitalization, established in late October 1945, and Acting Chair of the HSPC, with an appointment as Assistant Deputy Minister in the Department of Public Health in February

1946. Cecil's time at the HSPC was short. Douglas planned to set up a Health Insurance Commission and recruited Dr. Frederick Mott from the US to begin building a hospitalization program. Mott's work in Saskatchewan is discussed in chapter 6.

It is notable how often historians of the period (several of whom worked in the Douglas Administration themselves) have felt the need to comment on the Sheps's characters, but even more interesting is how their individual personas have often been conflated. In *Dream No Little Dreams*, Al Johnson describes Mindel and Cecil as "a husband and wife team from Winnipeg," who had "strong personalities."[92] Thomas McLeod, in his political biography of Douglas, describes them as "experienced physicians, as well as socialists of outstanding ability and great energy."[93] David Naylor, in *Private Practice, Public Payment*, argues that Mindel had a poor relationship with the SCPS, who "made no secret of its disapproval of Dr. Mindel Sheps."[94] However, this claim is difficult to verify, since Naylor's sole historical source, the Presidential Address to the 1946 Annual General Meeting of the SCPS, criticized the appointment of Cecil Sheps as Acting Chair of the HSPC in February 1946, while making no mention of Mindel.[95] Untangling these perceptions is a bit of a guessing game, but given the gendered nature of the political culture, it is not terribly speculative to observe that Mindel's confidence and assertiveness may have been an issue for a male-dominated medical elite.

Whether Mindel or Cecil was the main offender in the eyes of the SCPS, or whether it was Cecil's appointment as Chair of the HSPC that was problematic for the SCPS is difficult to say for certain, but, the profession had in fact correctly identified both as a political barrier to their goals of physician control and fee-for-service remuneration. Mindel and her husband were committed to a fully socialized system. Although Naylor and Gordon Lawson see salaried payment as the main sticking point, there were multiple points of tension between the Sheps and organized medicine, including the regional health centre model (which integrated primary and preventive care), lay governance, and the role of the provincial government in directing health policy.

While Mindel was mobilizing popular support behind health regions, Douglas took action to mollify organized medicine in the province. According to David Naylor, "leaders of the college [SCPS] repeatedly bypassed the HSPC and members of his staff to negotiate with Douglas directly," which allowed the physicians to negotiate "a variety of concessions."[96] In a September 1945 letter to the SCPS Health Services Committee, Douglas attempted to reassure the College that it would have "unrestricted jurisdiction over all scientific, technical, and professional matters," and control over "the general character of the agreement and arrangements whereunder the profession will provide medical services."[97] Douglas had not set aside the regional model or lay governance, but neither did he make Mindel's task easier by giving physicians the impression that they had the Premier's ear. The SCPS, for its part, sought to manipulate the situation by claiming publicly in the *Canadian Medical Association Journal* that the Minister, that is, Douglas, had disavowed plans for fully socialized medicine in favour of a health insurance model.[98] It turns out that they were essentially correct. By 1946, efforts to secure lay governance in a regional health centre model were losing ground, and soon they would collapse altogether. Early in 1946, Douglas shifted health policy direction away from laying the groundwork for socialized primary and preventive care and toward prioritizing the creation of a universal hospitalization plan. It was hospitalization that came to dominate the health agenda for the remainder of Douglas's first mandate. By 1950, the HSPC itself was wound up, its role in planning socialized medicine at an end.

Mindel Cherniack Sheps's contribution to the founding of medicare in Canada is largely absent from the historical record. Her efforts to implement a socialized model of public health care were undoubtedly affected by the gendered context in which she was

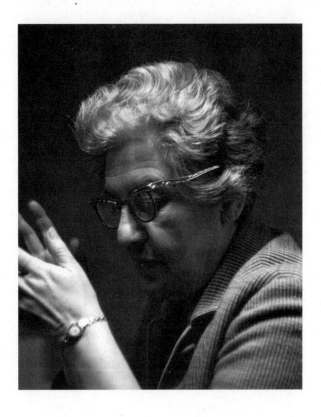

Mindel Cherniack Sheps
COURTESY SAUL CHERNIACK

asked to perform as a health policy advisor. Additionally, as a Jew she felt on the outside. She was handed the CCF's most politically sensitive file and had to resign herself to Douglas's active interventions. Ultimately, the vision for socialized medicine was rejected in favour of health care insurance paid by the taxpayer but controlled largely by health care professionals and hospital administrators—a far cry from the Sigerist Report's model.

Although Mindel's and Cecil's positions were never formally terminated by the Douglas Administration, they left Regina for the US in the fall of 1946 with their young son Sam and never returned. When the couple was informed about a year later by the new Chair of the HSPC, Frederick Mott, that the Government of Saskatchewan was not offering them re-appointments, Mindel and Cecil were caught off guard. They had believed they would be going back to continue their health planning work in Regina. Jobless and unhappy, they settled in Chapel Hill, North Carolina, where Cecil found a teaching position at University of North Carolina. They would never again live in Canada and left behind the western Canadian Jewish political culture in which they had been immersed.

Their friend and Winnipeg CCF comrade, Ann Rivkin, after a visit with Mindel and Cecil in Chicago, wrote to David Lewis to express her outrage at how the couple had been dismissed by the Douglas administration. Judging from Ann's letter, she had been allowed by the Sheps to read Mott's letter to them:

> As to the Sask situation, I have purposely delayed writing about it so that I might do so in retrospect and hence be somewhat more objective than while watching the Shepses going through their mental anguish. ... Fred's letter was, to put it mildly, a rude shock. Not the slightest concern was in the least bit evident as to the feelings or future of the recipients of that document. Evident only was the fact that the Shepses had done untold harm to Sask. (govt.) and they should never have the opportunity to doing so

again. If they had made even the slightest contribution to the
good, it couldn't be found with a magnifying glass, in Fred's letter.

Ann Rivkin went on to accuse Douglas of duplicity in his version of
events to other CCF supporters:

> while Min and Cecil were seeing their world in ruin and hadn't
> the slightest idea of what they were going to do next, T.C. was
> blandly and benignly telling the Lipsetts in Toronto, that the
> Shepses had had such wonderful offers that he couldn't dream
> of standing in the way of their future.[99]

Something of the difficulty of these events for Mindel can be gleaned
from her personal correspondence. She and Cecil remained in
touch with Henry Sigerist after he and his family had returned
to Switzerland from the US. In the short term, it was Cecil who
exchanged letters with Sigerist. It took some time for Mindel to find
her voice and a way to talk to Sigerist about the negative outcome
of the hopes and experiences they had shared in Saskatchewan. In
August 1949, Mindel wrote a long letter from Chapel Hill. Perhaps
Mindel felt she could finally write because she had found a new direction for her career, after three or four years of feeling "rudderless"
after their departure from Regina. She had decided to return to university, to earn a Master of Public Health from University of North
Carolina. "It is difficult to explain or justify a near-adolescent lack
of purpose, and a lack of (or rather loss of) faith," Mindel wrote to
Sigerist, before beginning her response to a question he had raised
in his recent letter:

> "What has happened to the CCF?" is a question which ties in
> well with my own feeling. They lost considerable ground in the
> Saskatchewan provincial election last year, and in the federal
> election this year they did very poorly everywhere and strikingly
> so in Saskatchewan. Our friends in Canada write glibly that a

fear of a Conservative victory drove the voters to the Liberal camp. While this is probably true to some extent it seems an inadequate explanation. It seems to me that there must be other factors of importance. One of these is surely the record of the Saskatchewan government. That record is a peculiar compound of recklessness and timidity, planlessness and compromise, with spots of determined courageous adherence to a well thought out plan. Also that these spots are so few and so small. ... Nor can they show any new techniques in democratic government, any signs of attempts to create a new way of life. In short—another reform government that accomplished a few good things in the old way.[100]

Mindel admitted to her friend a certain bitterness, and an under-lying pain that for a time deprived her of the single-mindedness she expected of herself. Although her criticism of Douglas was not personal, her disappointment is obvious. Her letter reflects her own "loss of faith" in her party.

In reference to herself as rudderless, Mindel was perhaps exaggerating. A letter from Cecil to Henry Sigerist a year before had stated that Mindel was running three baby clinics in the Chapel Hill area and working half days at the Rapid Treatment Centre in Durham, which treated sexually transmitted diseases.[101] After receiving her graduate degree in public health in 1950, she held positions at the University of North Carolina, Columbia University, the University of Pittsburgh, and Harvard University, where she taught in both the medical school and the school of public health. After 1963, she published almost exclusively in the field of population demography and biostatistics, a discipline she helped to create, researching patterns of female fertility. She did consulting work for the Ford Foundation, the Pan American Health Organizations, and the World Health Organization, linking her research on fertility patterns and birth control to what was then known as the "population problem" in developing countries. She received an honorary doctorate from the University of Manitoba in 1971, and died in 1973 of cancer, aged 59, at the peak of her career. According to her entry in *Jewish Women of America*, "a critical element of her work was her recognition of the links among poverty, fundamental social inequality, and population growth." For Cherniack Sheps, the entry continues, "demography became a science that could achieve social justice and clarify issues of women's rights and equality."[102]

In this description of Mindel are echoes of Noah Efron's interpretation of the twentieth-century Jewish relationship with science: "Jews looked to science to help refashion the societies in which they lived."[103] In Saskatchewan, though, Mindel had faced the challenges that came along with political engagement, which a scientific approach and reason could not alone resolve. Gender discrimination and the othering of her Jewishness within her own political party were daily realities. For all that, what appears to have loosened her connection to the political world into which she was born, was her inability to see the CCF as the embodiment of her ideals. A firm belief in socialized medicine and the health centre model had put her in opposition to powerful medical interests. Premier Douglas chose peace with the province's physicians over the early policy advice of the HSPC. Had Mindel returned to Saskatchewan after the couple's time in New Haven, she might have accommodated herself to the CCF's increasingly moderate health program. But she would have again faced the political culture of a male-dominated party and civil service, at times hostile to Jews, and would have remained an outsider.

ENDNOTES

1   "Sacrificed" is the term used by CCF activist Anne Rivkin. Library and Archives Canada (hereafter LAC), MG28 IV 1, CCF and NDP Fonds, Vol 60, Manitoba: General Correspondence 1938-1953, Anne Rivkin to David Lewis, 9 June 1947.

2   Yale University Library Manuscripts and Archives (hereafter YULMA), MS 788, Henry Ernest Sigerist Papers, Series 1 Correspondence, Box 22, Folder 794, Letter, Mindel Sheps to Henry Sigerist, August 20, 1949.

3   Transcript of "Memorial Service for Mindel Cherniack Sheps, January 18, 1973, University of North Carolina, Chapel Hill," courtesy of Saul Cherniack.

4   Erika Dyck refers to an "influx of cosmopolitanism" in her essay "Prairie Psychedelics: Mental Health Research in Saskatchewan, 1951-1967," in *Mental Health and Canadian Society*, ed. James E. Moran and David Wright (Montreal and Kingston: McGill-Queen's University Press, 2006), 226.

5   Daniel Stone, "Moving South: The Other Jewish Winnipeg Before the Second World War," *Manitoba History* 76 (2014): 2.

6   The most thorough examination of varieties of Jewish radicalism in Winnipeg is the essay collection Daniel Stone, ed., *Jewish Radicalism in Winnipeg, 1905-1960* (Winnipeg: Jewish Heritage Centre of Western Canada, 2002). See also Ester Reiter, *A Future Without Hate or Need: The Promise of the Jewish Left in Canada* (Toronto: Between the Lines, 2016), 32-33.

7   Henry Srebrnik, "Birobidzhan on the Prairies: Two Decades of Pro-Soviet Jewish Movements in Winnipeg," in *Jewish Radicalism in Winnipeg, 1905-1960*, ed. Daniel Stone (Winnipeg: Jewish Heritage Centre of Western Canada, 2002), 179.

8   Ava Block Super, "Preserving Winnipeg's Jewish History," *Canadian Jewish Studies* 23 (2015): 138-143.

9   Roz Usiskin, "Winnipeg's Jewish Women of the Left: Traditional and Radical," in *Jewish Radicalism in Winnipeg, 1905-1960*, ed. Daniel Stone (Winnipeg: Jewish Heritage Centre of Western Canada, 2002), 112.

10   Personal interview with Saul Cherniack, April 25, 2005.

11   Ruth Frager, *Sweatshop Strife: Class, Ethnicity, and Gender in the Jewish Labour Movement of Toronto, 1900-1939* (Toronto: University of Toronto Press, 1992); Jodi Giesbrecht, "Accommodating Resistance: Unionization, Gender, and Ethnicity in Winnipeg's Garment Industry, 1929-1945," *Urban History Review* 39, 1 (2010): 5–19.

12   Harry Medovy, "The Early Jewish Physicians in Manitoba," in *Jewish Life and Times" a Collection of Essays* (Winnipeg: Jewish Historical Society of Western Canada, 1983), 23–39.

13 Mary Kinnear, *In Subordination: Professional Women 1870-1970* (Montreal and Kingston: McGill-Queen's University Press, 1995), 63.

14 Stone, "Moving South," 3.

15 Noah J. Efron, *A Chosen Calling: Jews in Science in the Twentieth Century* (Baltimore: Johns Hopkins University Press, 2014), 8.

16 Harriet Pass Freidenreich, *Female, Jewish and Educated: The Lives of Central European University Women* (Bloomington: University of Indiana Press, 2002), 2–4.

17 Paula Hyman, *Gender and Assimilation in Modern Jewish History: The Roles and Representation of Women* (Seattle: University of Washington Press, 1995), 68.

18 Carole B. Balin, "The Call to Serve: Jewish Women Medical Students in Russia, 1872-1887," in *Jewish Women in Eastern Europe*, ed. Chaeran Freeze, Paula Hyman, and Antony Polonsky (Oxford and Portland, Oregon: The Littman Library of Jewish Civilization, 2005), 134.

19 Balin, "The Call to Serve," 151.

20 Balin, "The Call to Serve," 142.

21 Katherine Arnup, *Education for Motherhood: Advice for Mothers in Twentieth Century Canada* (Toronto: University of Toronto Press, 1993); Cynthia R. Comacchio, *Nations Are Built of Babies: Saving Ontario's Mothers and Children, 1900-1940* (Montreal and Kingston: McGill-Queen's University Press, 1998); Esyllt W. Jones, *Influenza 1918: Disease, Death and Struggle in Winnipeg* (Toronto: University of Toronto Press, 2007), 38–39; Marion McKay, "Region, Faith, and Health: The Development of Winnipeg's Visiting Nursing Agencies, 1897-1926," in *Place and Practice in Canadian Nursing History*, ed. Jane Elliott, Meryn Stuart, and Cynthia Toman (Vancouver: University of British Columbia Press, 2008), 70–90.

22 Harry Gutkin, *Journey Into Our Heritage: The Story of the Jewish People in the Canadian West* (Toronto: Lester and Orphen Dennys, 1980).

23 Jodi Giesbrecht, "Accommodating Resistance," 5-19.

24 Personal interview with Saul Cherniack, April 25, 2005.

25 Gladys Nitikman (married name Ellison) was born in Winkler, Manitoba. After graduation, she moved to Montreal and worked as an anesthetist at the Royal Victoria Hospital. She was a demonstrator in the Faculty of Medicine at McGill University from 1950 to 1958, and was awarded a position as Associate Professor Anesthesiology in 1959. *Jewish Post and News*, June 24, 1992. https://news.google.com/newspapers?nid=181 2&dat=19920624&id=-TghAAAAIBAJ&sjid=_mAEAAAAIBAJ&p-g=3079,3876300&hl=en Accessed January 14, 2016.

26 Kinnear, *In Subordination*, 56-59.

27 Naomi Rogers, "Feminists Fight the Culture of Exclusion in Medical
    Education, 1970-1990," in *Women Physicians and the Cultures of Medicine*,
    eds. Ellen S. More, Elizabeth Fee and Manon Perry (Baltimore: The Johns
    Hopkins University Press, 2008), 207.

28 Kinnear, *In Subordination*, 63-64.

29 Jewish Historical Society of Western Canada, "Jewish Life and Times
    Vol. VII. Women's Voices: Personal Recollections," (Winnipeg: Jewish
    Historical Society of Western Canada, 1998), 68.

30 W.P.J. Millar, "'We Wanted Our Children Should Have It Better': Jewish
    Medical Students at the University of Toronto, 1910-1951," *Journal of the
    Canadian Historical Association* 11, 1 (2000): 118–119.

31 Personal Conversation with Saul Cherniack, April 25, 2005.

32 John Lowe, "Hospital Administration Oral History Collection. Cecil G.
    Sheps In Person: An Oral History," Hospital Research and Educational
    Trust (1993), 8–9.

33 Mindel C. Sheps, "The Great Population Explosion as a Study in
    Dynamics," *University of Manitoba Alumni Journal* (Winter 1972): 19.

34 Alexandra Minna Stern, *Eugenic Nation: Faults and Frontier of Better
    Breeding in Modern America* (Berkeley: University of California Press,
    2005), 6.

35 Erika Dyck, *Facing Eugenics: Reproduction, Sterilization, and the Politics of
    Choice* (Toronto: University of Toronto Press, 2013).

36 Linda Gordon, *Woman's Body, Woman's Right: A Social History of Birth
    Control in America* (New York: Penguin Books, 1977); Wendy Kline,
    *Building a Better Race: Gender, Sexuality and Eugenics from the Turn of the
    Century to the Baby Boom* (Berkeley: University of California Press, 2001).

37 Kline, *Building a Better Race*, 64.

38 Kline, *Building a Better Race*, 65.

39 Linda Revie, "'More Than Just Boots!': The Eugenic and Commercial
    Concerns behind A. R. Kaufman's Birth Controlling Activities," *Canadian
    Bulletin of Medical History* 23, 1 (2006): 119–43.

40 Sheps, "The Great Population Explosion as a Study in Dynamics," 19.

41 Alan Mason Chesney Medical Archives of the Johns Hopkins Medical
    Institutions (hereafter AMCMA) Sigerist Collection, Box 153, Folder 12,
    Mindel Sheps to Henry Sigerist, August 12, 1944.

42 *Winnipeg Free Press*, November 26, 1942, p. 5; *Winnipeg Free Press*,
    November 28, 1.

43 Doug Smith, *Joe Zuken: Citizen and Socialist* (Toronto: James Lorimer &
    Company, 1990).

44 "Meyer Averbach, a lawyer and Hebrew Free School teacher and prin-
    cipal, also ran under the Independent Labour Party banner and was

elected a school trustee in 1933. He served in this capacity until 1949. Undoubtedly, his prominence within the Jewish community helped account for his success at the polls. He was active in the Poale Zion Club, the National Workers' Alliance, the Hebrew Free School, and the Canadian Jewish Congress, Western Division, of which he was secretary." Henry Trachtenberg, "The Winnipeg Jewish Community and Politics: The Inter-War Years, 1919–1939," *Manitoba Historical Society Transactions*, Series 3, Number 35 (1978-79), http://www.mhs.mb.ca/docs/transactions/3/jewish-politics.shtml.

45 "School Board to Ask Repeal of Religious Training Clause," *Winnipeg Free Press*, January 15, 1943, 13.

46 "Religious Instruction Motion Rescinded by School Board," *Winnipeg Free Press*, February 10, 1943, 13.

47 "Religious Instruction Motion Rescinded by School Board," *Winnipeg Free Press*, February 10, 1943, 13

48 "Same Pay for Same Work is Urged," *Winnipeg Free Press*, March 10, 1943, 3.

49 "Women Will Thank Dr. Mindel Sheps," *Winnipeg Free Press*, March 13, 1943, 11.

50 Archives of Manitoba (hereafter AM) MG14 D8, Cooperative Commonwealth Federation (CCF), Box 3, File 3, Provincial Convention 1940.

51 AM, MG14 D8, CCF, Box 1, File 1, Minutes of Meeting of Manitoba Provincial Council, December 2, 1942.

52 For discussion of the Heagerty proposals, see Heather Macdougall, "Into Thin Air: Making National Health Policy, 1939-1945," in Gregory P. Marchildon, ed., *Making Medicare: New Perspectives on the History of Medicare in Canada* (Toronto: University of Toronto Press, 2012): 41–70.

53 AM, MG14 D8, CCF, Box 3, File 6, Provincial Convention 1943.

54 AM, MG14 D8, CCF, Box 8, File 2, "Radio Broadcasts, 1944."

55 AMCMA, Sigerist Collection, Box 53, Folder 8; Box 138, Folder 8. Personal correspondence between Henry Sigerst and Cecil Sheps, Sept 18, 1941; c. October 1943.

56 AMCMA, Sigerist Collection, Box 153, Folder 12, Mindel Sheps to Henry Sigerist, August 12, 1944.

57 AMCMA, Sigerist Collection, Box 153, Folder 12, Mindel Sheps to Henry Sigerist, August 12, 1944.

58 Saskatchewan Archives Board, R-251, Health Services Survey Commission, "A Checklist of the Records of the Saskatchewan Health Services Survey Commission, 1944."

59 AMACA, Sigerist Collection, Box 153, Folder 12, Henry Sigerist to Mindel Sheps, October 9, 1944; Letter from Mindel Sheps to Henry Sigerist, October 12, 1944.

60 AMACA, Sigerist Collection, Box 153, Folder 12, Henry Sigerist to Mindel
    Sheps, October 9, 1944; Mindel Sheps to Henry Sigerist, October 18, 1944.
61 Duane Mombourquette, "An Inalienable Right: The CCF and Rapid
    Health Care Reform, 1944-1948," Saskatchewan History 43, 3 (1991): 104;
    Malcolm Taylor, Health Insurance and Canadian Public Policy: The Seven
    Decisions That Created the Health Insurance System and Their Outcomes
    (McGill-Queen's Press, 1987), 87–88.
62 Gordon S. Lawson, "The Road Not Taken: The 1945 Health Services
    Planning Commission Proposals and Physician Remuneration in
    Saskatchewan," in Making Medicare: New Perspectives on the History
    of Medicare in Canada, ed. Gregory P. Marchildon, vol. 26 (Toronto:
    University of Toronto Press, 2012), 181 note 40.
63 A.W. Johnson, Dream No Little Dreams: A Biography of the Douglas
    Government of Saskatchewan, 1944-1961 (Toronto: University of
    Toronto Press, 2004), 79–80; Lawson, "The Road Not Taken," 166–69;
    Mombourquette, "An Inalienable Right."
64 Quoted in A.W. Johnson, Dream No Little Dreams, 79.
65 Harley D. Dickinson and Renée Torgerson, "Medicare: Saskatchewan's
    Gift to the Nation?," in Perspectives of Saskatchewan, ed. Jene M. Porter
    (Winnipeg: University of Manitoba Press, 2009), 180.
66 AMCMA, Sigerist Collection, Box 153, Folder 12, Mindel Sheps to Henry
    Sigerist, August 16, 1945.
67 Dickinson and Torgerson, "Medicare: Saskatchewan's Gift to the Nation?,"
    176.
68 AMCMA, Sigerist Collection, Box 153, Folder 12, Mindel Sheps to Henry
    Sigerist, March 5, 1945.
69 Mombourquette, "An Inalienable Right," 105–6.
70 Quoted in Joan Feather, "From Concept to Reality: Formation of the Swift
    Current Health Region," Prairie Forum 16, 1 (1991): 69.
71 During World War II, Dodd served on the US National War Labor Board,
    charged with negotiating wage and price settlements, and as chairman of
    the President's Emergency Railway Labor Board. In 1946, Dodd would
    become a Dean of Letters and Science at UCLA, and he is credited with
    playing a key role in the growth and development of UCLA in the post-
    war years, including the creation of its medicine, nursing, and dentistry
    schools. Burt A. Folkart, "Paul A. Dodd; Former Dean at UCLA," Los
    Angeles Times, September 1, 1992 articles.latimes.com/1992-09-01/news/
    mn-6645_1_paul-dodd
72 Arthur J. Viseltear, "The California Medical-Economic Survey: Paul A.
    Dodd Versus the California Medical Association," Bulletin of the History of
    Medicine 44, 2 (1970): 146.

73 Feather, "From Concept to Reality;" Joan Feather, "Impact of the Swift Current Health Region: Experiment or Model?," *Prairie Forum* 16, 2 (1991): 225–48.

74 Feather, "From Concept to Reality," 61–62.

75 Quoted in Feather, "From Concept to Reality," 62.

76 Feather, "From Concept to Reality," 72–73.

77 Feather, "From Concept to Reality," 75.

78 AMCMA, Sigerist Collection, Box 153, Folder 12, Mindel Sheps to Henry Sigerist, March 8, 1945.

79 David McGrane, "A Mixed Record: Gender and Saskatchewan Social Democracy," *Journal of Canadian Studies/Revue d'études Canadiennes* 42, 1 (2008): 184. Although McGrane mentions that Trew was one of three women who ran for office during the CCF era in Saskatchewan, for some reason he does not mention that she was in fact elected.

80 "Beatrice Janet Trew," Saskatchewan Agriculture Hall of Fame https://www.sahf.ca/inductees/t/beatrice_trew.html accessed August 22, 2018.

81 David McGrane, "A Mixed Record," 184.

82 David McGrane, "A Mixed Record," 186.

83 Stuart Houston and Bill Waiser, *Tommy's Team: the People Behind the Douglas Years* (Markham, ON: Fifth House Ltd., 2010), vi.

84 The *Public Service Act* amendments are quoted in Joan Sangster, *Dreams of Equality: Women on the Canadian Left, 1920-1950* (Toronto: McClelland and Stewart, 1989), 214.

85 David McGrane, "A Mixed Record," 184 states that the legislation "forbid" the employment of married women in the civil service, but this was not exactly the case.

86 Carmella Patrias, "Socialists, Jews and the 1947 Saskatchewan Bill of Rights," *Canadian Historical Review* 87, 2 (2006): 280.

87 Bill Waiser, *Saskatchewan: A New History* (Calgary: Fifth House Publishers, 2005), 249–53.

88 Patrias, "Socialists, Jews and the 1947 Saskatchewan Bill of Rights," 270–71.

89 Patrias, "Socialists, Jews and the 1947 Saskatchewan Bill of Rights," 273.

90 LAC, MG28 IV 1, CCF and NDP Fonds, Vol 65, "Saskatchewan General Correspondence 1938-1958," Mindel Sheps to David Lewis, July 13, 1946. Don Black and George Tamaki were both key members of the staff of the General Finance Office, established by Douglas in 1947. Tamaki, a Canadian of Japanese ancestry, had been forcibly removed from British Columbia during World War II, and studied law at Dalhousie University and the University of Toronto before being recruited to Saskatchewan. Don Black was also a lawyer, educated at McGill University, who was recruited by George Cadbury, Douglas's key economic advisor. See A.W. Johnson, *Dream No Little Dreams*, 125.

91 Donald L. Madison, ed., *Cecil G. Sheps Memorial Volume* (University of North Carolina at Chapel Hill: Cecil G. Sheps Center for Health Services Research, 2005).

92 Johnson, *Dream No Little Dreams*, 79.

93 Thomas H. McLeod and Ian McLeod, *Tommy Douglas: The Road to Jerusalem*, 2nd ed. (Regina: Fifth House Publishers, 2004), 185.

94 David C. Naylor, *Private Practice, Public Payment: Canadian Medicine and the Politics of Health Insurance 1911-1966* (Montreal: McGill-Queen's University Press, 1986), 141.

95 "1946 Annual General Meeting," *Saskatchewan Medical Quarterly* 10 (December 1946): 11.

96 David Naylor, *Private Practice, Public Payment*, 140.

97 E.A. Tollefson, *Bitter Medicine: The Saskatchewan Medical Care Feud* (Saskatoon: Modern Press 1963), 36-38.

98 See David Naylor, *Private Practice, Public Payment*, 141.

99 LAC, MG28 IV 1, CCF and NDP Fonds, Vol 60, "Manitoba: General Correspondence 1938-1953," Anne Rivkin to David Lewis, 9 June 1947.

100 Yale University Library Manuscripts and Archives (hereafter YULMA), MS 788, Henry Ernest Sigerist Papers, Series 1 Correspondence, Box 22, Folder 794, Mindel Sheps to Henry Sigerist, August 20, 1949.

101 YULMA, MS 788, Henry Ernest Sigerist Papers, Series 1 Correspondence, Box 22, Folder 793, Cecil Sheps to Henry Sigerist, August 17, 1948.

102 Paula E. Hyman and Deborah Dash Moore, eds., *Jewish Women in America: An Historical Encyclopedia* (New York: Routledge, 1997), 1242-1243.

103 Efron, *A Chosen Calling*, 9.

CHAPTER 5

NEW DEAL MEDICINE MOVES NORTH

US Health Planners in Saskatchewan

The Soviet Union was not the only source of inspiration for radical health policy ideas in the 1930s. From our contemporary perspective it remains surprising, but in the US there was "a ferment at work in American medicine." Isidore Falk, a bacteriologist and health economist educated at Yale, described "a vast unrest [among] physicians, dentists, nurses, hospital administrators, pharmacists ... The times call for action and the problems for wise and judicious solutions."[1] New Deal era movements for health policy reform, while ultimately stillborn, provided key ideas and—crucially to the story of medicare—*people* to the medical left across the border in Canada.

In 1935, when Norman Bethune brought together the Montreal Group for the Security of the People's Health, he looked not only to Soviet medicine for inspiration, but also to the US, particularly the work of the Committee on the Costs of Medical Care (CCMC), of which Falk was the five-year project's associate director. In 1932, the CCMC released its benchmark final report, Medical Care for the American People. The document was not unanimous: two minority reports reflected polarization within the CCMC. The majority report recommended reforms such as group medical and dental practice, better public health services, some form of compulsory health insurance, improved coordination of medical services, and better education and training for all healthcare practitioners.[2]

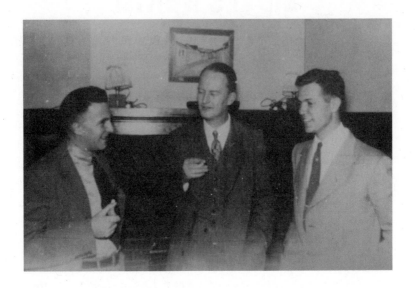

Milton Roemer, Fred Mott, and Leonard Rosenfeld, Regina, 1948

Although the proponent of what historian Alan Derickson has referred to as "mild liberalism," Falk was an elder statesman of health politics in the US because of his long-term advocacy of medical reform and state health insurance, in spite of the opposition it faced. Falk helped lead the charge of progressives into the US government during the 1930s, including two physicians, Fred Mott and Milton Roemer, who would later play important roles in Saskatchewan. In the US, Falk ultimately became the target of conservatives seeking to expose a communist plot behind "socialist medicine," as did many of his cohort.[3]

In 1945, an attempt to create a national health insurance plan in the US, the Wagner-Murray-Dingell Bill, failed to pass Congress. This defeat for the American health reform movement was to prove an unexpected opportunity for Saskatchewan. In 1946, on the advice of Cecil Sheps and Henry Sigerist, Douglas recruited Fred Mott to become the first permanent Chair of the Health Services Planning Commission (HSPC). Mott had a decade of experience, and a battle-hardened pragmatism gained trying to build government health programs in the highly polarized and complex world of US health politics. Mott, his New Deal colleague Milton Roemer, and a former student of Henry Sigerist, Leonard Rosenfeld, provide direct linkages between the Douglas Administration's early health program development, US health politics, and New Deal medicine, particularly the health programs of the Farm Security Administration (FSA). Rosenfeld had studied with Henry Sigerist at Johns Hopkins University. From 1942 to 1946, as part of US President Roosevelt's "good neighbour" policy, he helped to develop a public health program in Nicaragua, sponsored by the Institute of Inter-American Affairs. In 1946 he became the first director of the Saskatchewan Hospital Services Plan.[4]

While in charge of health planning in Saskatchewan, Fred Mott hired a third American, Milton Roemer, to prepare a crucial report advising the government on the provision of medical care to those in Saskatchewan receiving social assistance. Roemer had worked under Mott in the FSA. The two men co-authored a significant study of rural health, *Rural Health and Medical Care* (1948).[5] From 1953 to 1956, after Mott had left Saskatchewan, Roemer worked in the Saskatchewan Department of Public Health, implementing the hospital care program Mott had helped to establish. He and his wife, Ruth Roemer, arrived there to escape Cold War discrimination in the US, after the federal government had denied the necessary visas for him to continue in his position at the World Health Organization. For each of these New Dealers, Saskatchewan provided an opportunity to have an impact, unlike the US, where postwar anti-left sentiment in the government and within organized medicine had targeted their ideas and also them personally.

As Chair of the HSPC for five years, Fred Mott had the most influence of the three over Saskatchewan health policy. Mott was born in 1904 in Wooster, Ohio. He had a religious upbringing in an elite Methodist family; his father was John Raleigh Mott, the leader of the World YMCA, and a Nobel Prize winner (1946). John R. Mott had an international career, including several stints in Russia as a representative of the US government on diplomatic missions. During Mott's childhood, his father travelled extensively and was gone for long stretches at a time—for the first five years of his life, John Mott was abroad half of the time. While Fred, his brother, and his two sisters sometimes travelled with the family, considerable time was spent apart. Summers were spent together as often as possible at Lac des Iles, Quebec, sixty miles north of Montreal, where a cottage had been built after the Motts were invited to the area by Canadian YMCA friends in 1897. And so, canoe trips in the Laurentians, that quintessential experience for Canadians of a certain class in the early twentieth century, were part of Fred Mott's young life.[6]

Mott graduated from Montclair High School in Montclair, New Jersey in 1921, then attended the Mohonk School for a year. He did undergraduate studies at Princeton, where he graduated with an honours degree in history in 1927. Although then still a self-identified Republican, Mott was influenced by the teaching of progressive historian Clifton R. Hall. Between his junior and senior years at Princeton, he travelled in Asia and the South Pacific as his father's secretary. It was in the context of his father's missionary work, and visits to medical missions in what was then Sumatra and Java, that he became interested in a career in medicine.[7]

Mott went to medical school at McGill University, graduating in 1932 and winning the Thomas Wood Smith Gold Medal. In 1930, he married Marjorie Heeney, from Winnipeg, and the couple had three sons: Peter, Anthony, and Andrew. While at McGill, Mott became interested in social medicine and the problems of health organization. He was part of a group of students who "engineered an Osler Society session on health insurance," and in 1932 published his thoughts in the *McGill Journal of Medicine*—an article called "Some Aspects of the Case for State Medicine." The final report of the CCMC was released the same year. As Mott recalled toward the end of his career, upon receiving an award from the Group Health Association of America: "It's incredible that 43 years later most of what the CCMC stood for remains unaccomplished."[8]

Between 1932 and 1935, Mott returned to the US, interning at the Presbyterian Hospital in New York in internal medicine, then doing further specialized training in cardiology, gynecology, and dermatology. An influential mentor for Mott in New York was the surgeon Dr. James Peter Warbasse, the founder of the Cooperative League of the USA, who advocated for "organizing medical care along cooperative lines, in a professional-lay partnership."[9] In 1936, Mott helped to organized the Bureau of Cooperative Medicine with Warbasse, Esther Lucile Brown, a social anthropologist and expert in the health professions at the Russell Sage Foundation, and Dr. Kinglsey Roberts. Mott moved to Washington and began work on group pre-payment plans.

In January 1937 he became a medical consultant with the

Resettlement Administration in Washington, and later that year became Associate Medical Officer of the FSA. In February of 1942, he was promoted to Chief Medical Officer of the FSA, a position in which he served until leaving for Saskatchewan in summer of 1946. Simultaneously, from July 1943 through May 1945, he was Chief of the Health Services Branch of the War Food Administration. Mott was in Saskatchewan from August 1946 though the end of 1951. From Saskatchewan, Mott went on to work in health administration for the US labour movement. He returned to the US and became Senior Medical Consultant to the Welfare and Retirement Fund of the United Mine Workers of America, led by John L. Lewis, where he stayed for six and a half years. He acted as Medical Administrator of the Miners Memorial Hospital Association, which operated the union's health services in Kentucky, West Virginia, and Virginia. The Welfare and Retirement Fund created a regional network of ten hospitals with over 1000 beds and ten salaried group medical practices in the northern Appalachians; the hospitals opened in 1955 and 1956, during Mott's tenure, and cost $28 million dollars. The hospitals were meant for members of the Fund, but they were open to the general public.[10]

His next position was also with organized labour, this time as Executive Director of what would become in 1960 the Community Health Association (CHA) of Detroit, where Mott said "I learned the hard facts of negotiating, organizing and operating a membership based group health plan in an American city."[11] The United Automobile Workers, led by Walter Reuther, were looking to create a progressive, group-practice model health plan for union members. The union created a non-profit that provided to members comprehensive medical and hospital care. It purchased Detroit's Metropolitan Hospital, where the staff were put on salary, including physicians, and built five satellite health centres. The CHA emphasized prevention and health education. Despite considerable opposition from organized medicine, which sought to deny doctors in the plan admitting privileges, the CHA grew to 62,000 members from 1960 to 1966, only to be bought by Blue Cross/Blue Shield in 1972.[12]

The CHA was Mott's last big project. He consulted for the New York Academy of Medicine, then landed in Toronto in 1966, where he was Professor of Medical Care in the Department of Health Administration at the University of Toronto. During his time there, he participated in what was known as the Canada/World Health Organization Sault Ste. Marie Study. Steelworkers in Sault Ste. Marie had formed a Group Health Association, similar to the United Automobile, Aerospace and Agricultural Implement Workers of America (UAW) project in Detroit. He retired from his academic position in 1972.

Mott spent most of his professional life attempting to implement a health centre model of care delivery, which he sometimes referred to as a "network" model. His career unfolded in both government and private group health organizations. He remained committed to the progressive possibilities of private group insurance, in part because of his belief in the role of the health care recipient in the governance of prepaid health care organizations, and in part because of the pragmatics of the US situation, where the state's involvement in health care remained limited during the tenure of his professional life. And he concluded that state health insurance was not enough. "A program designed simply to finance health care, operating essentially through the fee-for-service system, does little or nothing to correct the maldistribution of services, to assure accessibility to needed care, to control costs, or to improve the quality of care," he argued. More critical from Mott's perspective were modalities of delivery that would guarantee accessibility, quality, parity (a world Mott like to use), and democratic control. As he said in 1975, late in his life, "it has never bothered me to switch back and forth in administering public programs of health care at one time and consumer-sponsored plans at another."[13] He had adapted to both socialized and consumer/co-operative models of health organization.

When Mott was recruited to Saskatchewan in 1946, he was an expert in rural health provision, and had significantly more experience as a health planner and administrator than his predecessor at the Health Services Commission, Cecil Sheps. Mott had been with the FSA Health Services Branch since its inception in 1937, when he was brought from the federal Public Health Service to serve as Assistant Chief Medical Officer to Dr. Ralph C. Williams.[14] Over the next nine years, Mott worked on several of the FSA's most creative health programs, particularly the migrant farm worker and experimental health programs of the early war years. He had four years of experience at the head of the New Deal's migrant health programs, which at their peak provided health care to as many as 200,000 of America's most impoverished migrant farm workers.

New Deal health care programs have received relatively little attention from historians. The only book-length study is Michael Grey's detailed and largely sympathetic history, *New Deal Medicine*, which provides significant grounding for this book, as does the chapter addressing the New Deal in Jennifer Klein's more recent *For All These Rights*.[15] As both scholars note, though in different ways, New Deal policies were situated within a broader context of health reform and advocacy, unfolding in multiple arenas (not only government) and influenced by multiple actors, including labour, women, African Americans, business, and organized medicine. Recent histories of the New Deal emphasize its antecedents in social reform movements of the Progressive Era, the Great War, and the 1920s: as Klein has noted, "we no longer talk about the New Deal as emerging full-blown from the forehead of Roosevelt and an inner-circle, male Brain Trust."[16] However, histories of 1930s and 1940s social policy and public health in the US tend not to address the significance of transnational networks, leaning towards American exceptionalism. Despite the transnationalism of many members of this cohort of health reform advocates, more remains to be done to demonstrate how knowledge and information circulated into, and out of, US health reform circles during the New Deal era.

As Klein has argued, the 1930s saw a great deal of "social experimentation" in health provision, especially at the local level.[17] The movement for "health security" in the 1930s and 1940s produced a wide array of prototypes for health organization, ranging from private health insurance, to group medical plans, to employment-related programs such as the Kaiser Permanente health plans, to health co-operatives and local health centres. To a significant extent, experimentation and innovation took place in the "voluntary" sector, as well as under the guise of state provision.

The interaction between "private" and "public" efforts to improve health security speaks to the movement qualities of the era, as the efforts of non-state sector groups and individuals influenced state policy, and New Deal policy itself facilitated debate and experimentation. Particularly during the popular-front era of the late 1930s and early 1940s, a broad coalition of progressive interests in the US— including labour, farmers, social workers, child welfare advocates, consumers' unions, health practitioners, and public health intellectuals—spoke of security against illness as "a matter of class justice," although the potential mechanisms identified for achieving health security were diverse.[18] Although under-resourced, the New Deal Office of Negro Health also provided improved health benefits to African Americans. Susan Smith demonstrates, however, that these efforts "rested on a foundation of black health programs put into place by middle-class black health activists long before the New Deal."[19]

New Deal era health advocates can be distinguished, Klein argues, from the earlier progressive-era health reformers. In part because of their involvement in the policy debates surrounding the CCMC and the failed attempt to include health care in the Social Security Act (1935), health reformers of the 1930s and 1940s were absorbed with questions around health financing and economics, delivery models for medical care, and governance issues. In one sense, this rendered health debates of the era highly technical, if not technocratic. Klein perceives a shift away from the progressive-era focus upon public health, occupational safety, and the social causes of ill health (such as poverty) toward demands for health in terms of equal access to good medical care. With the ascendancy of germ theory over sanitationism, and the availability of better (but more expensive) clinical care in hospitals, the stage was set for a shift in focus among health advocates, Klein argues.

This chapter questions the totality of any such shift in approach among health advocates who worked in the New Deal. While health care organization did increasingly take centre stage for Mott and his cohort, they did not reject earlier arguments about the links between income inequality, working and living conditions, and health. Neither did Mott underestimate the absolute necessity of public health and sanitation; on the contrary, he and others pointed to the inadequacy of rural infrastructure as a paramount consideration. Klein's focus is, to a significant extent, on urban movements for health security. When we look more closely at the social and economic analysis of rural health problems, a somewhat different picture emerges.

While segments of organized labour had always advocated for better medical care for workers and their families, the 1930s and 1940s witnessed an intensification of demand for affordable medical care to a broader segment of the public. Experimental projects were mounted by labour, employers, and private insurers such as the Blue Cross hospital service plan, which had four million subscribers in the US by 1939. Health reform discourse responded to these changing realities. As Dorothy Bellanca, Vice-President of the Amalgamated Clothing Workers of America argued in 1938:

> In the large cities as well as in the rural areas the low-income groups experience sickness and mortality today as if there had been no progress at all during these past fifty years. The results of medical science have reached those who could afford them.[20]

The era also witnessed a generational shift, as a new group of advocates such as Isidore Falk, Nathan Sinai, Rufus Rorem, and Henry Sigerist—men who often had PhDs in public health, medical sociology, or health economics—played a key role in public debate. Especially during the Roosevelt era, there was a fruitful relationship between universities, major foundations such as the Carnegie or Rockefeller foundations, the Millbank Memorial Fund or the Julius Rosenwald Fund, and the federal government, all of which nurtured a key group of scholars and public health experts and in some cases placed them in government positions where they could wield power, influence, and resources. The Roosevelt Foundation continued to support the education and development of experts in health organization.

An example of this context of public-private engagement was the background paper prepared on health insurance for the 1938 National Health Conference (convened by President Roosevelt) by the Technical Committee on Medical Care, entitled "The Need For a National Health Program." The National Health Conference was attended by a broad range of US health advocates, including labour representatives from both the American Federation of Labor and the Congress of Industrial Organizations, popular-front communists and socialists, and farm activists. The "emotional center" of debate at the conference was better access to medical care.[21] Labour women such as Florence Greenberg from the Council of Auxiliaries of the Steel Workers' Organizing Committee, Eve Stone of the UAW Women's Auxiliary, and Harriet Silverman of the People's National Health Committee called for community-based health care services—what Greenberg called "people's health centers." Eve Stone requested that the Works Progress Administration (WPA) provide funds to build and maintain health centers, which would first provide care to those receiving assistance from the WPA or other welfare programs, and then to everyone covered by the Social Security Act.[22]

The local community was often viewed as a site of innovation and citizen engagement in health care. Indeed, Klein argues, the future potential for a national health care system (a goal shared by the era's health advocates) was seen as intricately connected with the existence of local experiments in health provision.[23] Democratic control of health was also highly valued by most advocates, and community health plans "at their most ambitious" attempted to create frameworks for democratic (and implicitly local) control over health institutions, whether these be state-funded or non-state initiatives.[24]

Thus, health policy developed during the Roosevelt era in a milieu of debate about options for health provision, accompanied by concrete experimentation on how those options could work on the ground. This milieu often brought into direct contact grassroots advocates, labour, public health professionals including physicians and nurses, and government planners and program administrators, creating dialogue between "experts" and political activists. Boundaries between the two categories were at times blurred. In the context of meetings such as the National Conference on Health, such a dialogue could not be without its gaps and power imbalances. But the inclusion of consumer groups, as some referred to them, at the highest level of policy debate reflected the relationships between advocates forged in the broad push toward state provision of medical care.

Klein's overall argument in For All These Rights is that the focus upon medical care provision, and in particular the financing of medical care through some form of contributory social insurance, narrowed the perspective of health reform and limited the scope of its social critique. The leading minds of left-leaning health policy became focused on the admittedly thorny but nonetheless circumscribed question of how to best organize, pay for, and deliver medical services in the community and in hospitals. The challenge to capitalism as a root cause, built into the most radical of progressive-era critiques of health inequality, tended to get lost in the movement for

health security. Although not without its sharp critiques, the search
for mechanisms to deliver medical care equitably forced the movement into a box, Klein argues:

> the New Deal health insurance advocates comprehended that
> the politics of security was part of a comprehensive challenge to
> the control of economic resources and services by business cor-
> porations, insurance company executives, and physicians. Yet the
> remedy that these health security advocates would increasingly
> focus on, contributory social insurance, would circumscribe the
> expansive political potential of that challenge.[25]

US health reformers did put considerable energy into the passage of
health insurance legislation, especially the Wagner-Murray-Dingell
Bill. Their position on health insurance was complex, however. As
reformist as the movement for health insurance may have been, there
were radical elements to its discussion of health organization. Indeed,
as this chapter will reveal, for advocates like Mott there remained
more than one model of payment. More important was how services would be governed and delivered, and the guarantee of equal
access. As long as there was a viable way of financing care (through
co-operatives or through state subsidy, for example), the real issue of
concern was how to organize care in an equitable way: how to create
a system that allowed for local and consumer input, utilized funds
optimally with multidisciplinary staffing, and saw physician power
held in check. Above all, Mott, Roemer, and others came to believe
that systemic and structural inequalities, between the poor and the
wealthy, between the rural and the urban, could not be allowed to
stand in the way of health "parity." They saw contributory insurance
as a potentially achievable framework for financing. Regardless of
how it was financed, the goal was to organize care along what this
book refers to as the health centre model.

Mott and other members of the FSA health program staff attended the National Health Conference in 1938. By then, they had several years' experience of rural health work. The FSA was created in 1937, but health services to poor farmers had begun under the Resettlement Administration (RA). Nor was the FSA the only New Deal agency to provide health care. The Federal Emergency Relief Administration (FERA), Roosevelt's first Depression-relief aid program, mandated state and local relief agencies to provide emergency nursing, dental, and non-hospital care. In 1934, 46 states were providing medical care relief. Other New Deal programs in the mid-1930s such as the Works Progress Administration (WPA) provided support for public health initiatives including mass inoculations, school medical checkups, and health education.

It was the FSA health programs, however, that made the most impact upon rural health. By 1942, the FSA had developed a network of prepaid medical care co-operatives in more than one-third of all counties in the US, in which over 650,000 poor farmers had enrolled. The role of the FSA was to support the establishment of these co-operatives by encouraging farmers and their families to enroll and facilitating negotiations between the co-operatives and local medical practitioners. The FSA provided a workable model for the medical co-operatives, as well as financial support. The co-operatives functioned as medical group practices. Families, with the support of the FSA where necessary, would pay annual membership dues, which entitled them to general medical care and, in some cases, surgery, obstetrical care, and hospitalization. The mix of services was dependent upon local arrangements, into which co-operative members had considerable input.[26] The FSA also provided nursing services and other health supports, such as sanitary engineers and funds for building local health centres and hospitals. While the main emphasis of the program was on the provision of medical care to impoverished farmers, there was also close attention given to prevention and health education. As Michael Grey has noted, the rationale for the FSA's health programs explicitly acknowledged the economic need to improve the health of rural people.[27]

In addition to FSA's efforts to improve the health of poor farmers, the program focused greater attention on those whose lives were devastated by Depression-era agricultural conditions, such as migrant farm workers. The migrant labour programs provided health care to families who often could not access other public and private services, either because they could not afford to pay for health care, or because they failed to meet state or local residency requirements. And even though, as historians have pointed out, there was racial discrimination and inequality at the heart of New Deal initiatives, there were also attempts to improve the appalling lack of access to health care experienced by African Americans and Latinos.[28]

The FSA established a migrant health program that provided "acute care, hospitalization, and preventive services to a migrant population swollen by the combined effects of national drought, farm mechanization, and the near collapse of the nation's farm economy."[29] The FSA built health clinics in the government's migrant farm labour camps. In the Midwest, the program made use of mobile health clinics—"clinics on wheels"—which moved with migrants themselves. In California, the FSA established 23 mobile clinics and permanent clinics in 35 farm labour camps.[30]

The program was also, over eight years, able to establish seven regional or state-wide migrant health plans, under the auspices of semi-autonomous Agricultural Workers Health and Medical Associations (AWHMAs), organized similarly to the medical co-operatives. The AWHMAs ran their own health programs under the guidance and with the fiscal support of the FSA. The largest of the AWHMAs were in California and Arizona.[31] Others existed in Washington, Idaho, Oregon, Texas, and Florida; regional associations were formed in the Atlantic seaboard, the Midwest, and briefly on the Great Plains. In the most drought-affected states of North and South Dakota, the FSA supported the establishment of state-wide health insurance plans. The FSA migrant health programs were not all identical, varying according to local and regional needs, but as a whole they provided a comprehensive range of services including: hospitalization; medical, nursing and dental care; prescription drugs; and a higher level of preventive care, including immunizations and prenatal and postnatal care.

In a speech to the Wisconsin Welfare Council in 1942, Mott outlined a multidisciplinary model of care. Health care teams should include the public health worker, the nurse, the medical social worker, the health educator, and the physician.[32] Nurses played a key role in the work of the FSA health programs and continued to do so in the War Food Administration, which incorporated the FSA's health programs beginning in 1943. In the 1946 AWHMA Report of Activities, nursing occupied nearly one-quarter of the program's expenditures.[33] The report stated: "To many farm workers, the clinic or field nurse was their only contact with the farm labor health program. In peak seasons more than 300 nurses were employed in all associations ... Nurses alone, acting under standing order, handled 265,000 cases, 2.5 times as many cases as those seen by physicians."[34]

Nurses worked in a variety of settings, from migratory worker camps through local clinics and hospitals built by the FSA. The AWHMA handbook illustrates the full range of nursing work, which was documented for budgetary and statistical purposes. Nurses performed home visits to patients' residences or migratory farm labour camps. They provided treatment and prevention of contagious diseases—such as diphtheria, scarlet fever, measles, smallpox, and malaria—at clinics and during field nursing visits to patients. Nurses also provided monitoring and care for venereal diseases, and referrals to physician care where necessary. Testing and immunizations—for typhoid, smallpox, diphtheria, and tetanus—were done by either physicians or nurses. Nurses were responsible for tuberculosis control and treatment, or referral to sanitoria or other treatment centres.

Maternal and child health was an intellectually dynamic field, including "health conferences" described as meetings at which a "group of expectant mothers, mothers, and children are brought together to consider their maternal and child health problems." A conference session might include examinations and treatments. Nurses also delivered maternal and child health care "in the field" and visited nursery schools to "inspect" children.[35]

By 1942, the FSA had led some of the most innovative and revolutionary health programs ever seen in the US. Policy experts like Mott began to push more aggressively for an extension of the FSA's role in health provision. In part, this was motivated by the need to develop a broader base of involvement and support for medical co-operatives, which struggled financially due to the poverty of their members. By working towards the inclusion of more consumers who could afford health insurance premiums, the FSA staff hoped to make the co-operatives more fiscally sustainable while providing health care to more working- and middle-class Americans. Fiscal incentives were deepened by the conservative turn in politics during World War II, which saw lessening public support for New Deal initiatives. The FSA saw the need to insulate itself against criticisms that it provided expensive and unsustainable services.

Late in 1942, the agency established six new rural health services and two special demonstration projects, "administered locally through incorporated entities," along the lines of medical co-operatives. As Grey observes, "this approach gave them a strategically necessary distance from the federal government and enabled the FSA to claim that the experimental health plans held to the spirit of the AMA's policy on third-party involvement in financing medical care."[36] While most of the health plans paid physicians on a fee-for-service basis, one used a capitation model, and the model program in Taos County paid its three physicians annual salaries.

FSA health programs expanded significantly the reach of previous federal initiatives aimed at rural health and provided a model for health reform that challenged the status quo in several significant ways. First and foremost, they represented in the eyes of staff and health reform advocates an actually existing model that could service as a template for radical health organization and policy. Activists inside and outside the Roosevelt Administration were calling for the establishment of a national health insurance scheme, and legislation was being advanced toward that end. The FSA programs were intended to show how things might be done, should national legislation provide the financial base that rural health initiatives had thus far lacked.

Second, the FSA health programs were based in a socio-economic critique. FSA leaders emphasized that the economic hardships of rural America were inseparable from the high incidence of poor health. Rural incomes were inadequate, leading to poor health, and furthermore this problem circled back on itself in a vicious cycle. The FSA argued, for example, that nearly half of all farm-loan defaults were due to illness. Economic rehabilitation in rural communities, therefore, relied significantly upon improvements in the health of farmers, wage earners, and their families. In order to achieve better health, rural people needed health care, which they could not afford because of poor levels of income, either individually or in the aggregate. This recognition of the health impact of inequality, rather than a liberal humanitarian or individualist perspective, was key to the case for the FSA's rationale for its involvement in medical care delivery.[37]

Third, the philosophy underlying FSA health programs significantly challenged the power of organized medicine by supporting a multidisciplinary approach and "broad public health orientation."[38] FSA programs did not only remunerate the private rural physician, they also employed nurses, sanitarians, nutritionists, and health educators. The delivery of migrant health programs (the FSA's template for reform) achieved a high level of multidisciplinarity, giving extensive scope to nurses to deliver primary care, and incorporating other technical and health and social welfare professionals. FSA administrators were, however, careful to form positive, pragmatic relationships with rural physicians, and attempted (although ultimately unsuccessfully) to bring organized medicine on side. The program "promoted the social and professional status of allopathic physicians," economically supported struggling rural doctors, and made significant compromises on issues such as voluntary participation and patient choice of physician.[39] However, the multidisciplinary team model of health care organization, often accompanied by arguments for salaried remuneration, was radical and it was opposed by organized medicine.

In the 1930s and early 1940s, tensions among medical practitioners over issues such as physician payment and the organization and distribution of primary care, could be exploited successfully by skilled advocates of a health centre model. Organized medicine seldom wavered from its virulent opposition to group practice, let alone state control. But many physicians voted with their feet and worked with private and public sector health plans that used a group practice model. They were motivated in part by the economic challenges of the time, when many doctors earned low incomes and had difficulty getting paid for the care they delivered. But there were also those who supported greater equality of access to health care and saw little difficulty in working for group plans and co-operative schemes that improved their ability to provide patient care to those who needed it. This is not to say the FSA did not encounter physician opposition. Criticism always existed and it intensified as the wartime economic recovery took hold.

By the end of his FSA tenure, Mott had become a vocal advocate for a transformation in American health care delivery. His years at the FSA helped him to formulate an effective argument about the barriers to rural health parity, and this informed his speeches and publications. He viewed untrammeled physician power over state policy as contrary to the kind of change needed in order to achieve health equality. In his concluding remarks to a conference on medical care health services and facilities in rural Ohio in March 1946, Mott argued:

> [Rural people] ... need a sanitary and safe environment. They need an adequate number of well-trained health personnel of all kinds—physicians, dentists, nurses, and others. They need modern hospitals and diagnostic and health center facilities. They must have access to comprehensive medical services—preventive, diagnostic and therapeutic—services for the mind as well as the body. We must permit no barrier of dollars—no sheer lack of ability to pay—to stand between human needs and the health resources of the community.[40]

Mott and members of his FSA staff campaigned in favour of national legislation (the Wagner-Murray-Dingell Bill). This open political commitment left Mott open to personal attacks from the AMA. It perhaps had negative consequences for FSA programs already under attack in Congress.[41] With the defeat of Wagner-Murray-Dingell, optimism faded. As the New Deal encountered mounting political opposition and waning public support at the end of World War II, the FSA was disbanded. Within a short period, all of the programs Mott and his staff had built were gone—the co-operatives could not survive without state financial support. In this context of defeat Mott received an invitation from Saskatchewan that he ultimately could not refuse, although he felt regret at leaving behind the battles for health insurance in his own country, as well as his staff and colleagues.

Mott's support for Wagner-Murray-Dingell is a signal of his intellectual commitment to state intervention in health, and also, presumably, reflective of his own position as a state administrator. Grey's interpretation is that Mott (and his colleague Milton Roemer) were "driven by a streak of idealism."[42] However, Mott's health politics drew together several strands of health politics. With the exception of the paper he published as a medical student at McGill, Mott never directly endorsed "state medicine." He was clearly supportive of a role for government, including universal public health insurance. He had first-hand knowledge of how difficult it was to alter established patterns of health care delivery without a centralized government initiative. At the same time, Mott had a persistent affinity for co-operative-consumerist approaches, from his early period in the Bureau for Cooperative Medicine to his years building union health programs in the 1950s and 1960s. He remained committed to local input into government programs and felt there was a role for a private, but collective, sense of ownership and control.

Mott was a member of a technically skilled elite , and in some senses a technocrat. But he did not fully embrace technocracy, if by that we mean "the government or control of society or industry by an elite of technical experts."[43] As a health planner, Mott's job was to design and deliver an innovative government program and to utilize the power of the state toward the achievement of a broader social goal: the elimination of health inequality. He would have fit easily into what Philip Abbott described as the "public, collective, informal" democratized masculine culture of the New Deal planners.[44] Roosevelt himself spoke of "a pioneer spirit of cooperation and understanding of the need of building up, not a class, but a whole community."[45] Abbott reads public servants like Mott as emblems of a new masculinity forged in the New Deal era: "At no period in American history was the bureaucrat portrayed in the heroic terms that New Deal apparat presented themselves." The New Deal employee was a man of action, an empowered male figure "who helped plan and administer great projects."[46]

This ethos of empowered masculinity and great projects became "cluttered," as Alan Brinkley has noted, its central project out of focus. Being a Roosevelt New Dealer did not necessarily require rigidity or discipline to a central principle. Yet, by the time Mott left the US for Saskatchewan, the New Deal did appear to be a particular sort of project, with its own notion of the role of the state. The late New Deal, which followed the 1937 recession, saw a new group of "younger liberals" come to the fore, more skeptical than the earlier brain trust that the problems of capitalism could be solved through a regulatory impulse. While advancing the rights of the consumer, Brinkley argues, late New Deal economic policies came increasingly to rely upon the fiscal powers of the state—the power to tax and spend— to "stimulate economic growth and solve social problems."[47] While health spending itself benefitted very little if at all from this shift, the greater comfort with the role of the state had its parallel in the health politics of the FSA, whose experimental health care programs (introduced during the war) relied less upon contributory co-operative health insurance than they did upon government financing and control of a more deeply radical model of care.

Lessons learned during his FSA years allowed Mott to become a publicly recognized expert on the problem of rural health. In speeches and publications, Mott developed both a critique of rural health inequality, and a program to change it. Not long after Mott began his employment in Saskatchewan, he and co-author Milton Roemer published *Rural Health and Medical Care*. J.T.H Connor notes, "despite its mundane title, *Rural Health and Medical Care* was a lightning rod for debate as it was arguably a blueprint for major health policy reform in the United States."[48] The book became a widely used resource in medical, nursing, and public health circles in North America. Impeccably researched and weighted with statistical data and sociological analysis, the book drew heavily upon government data and reports, to which Mott had easy access during his years with the FSA, and analyses accumulated during his years of experience in rural health programming.

The main argument in *Rural Health and Medical Care* was that the health of rural Americans was lagging behind that of urban dwellers. Rural people, Mott and Roemer argued, had not benefitted equally from the health reforms of the early twentieth century, such as improved communicable disease control or even sanitation. In America in general, scientific advancement had moved more quickly than social adjustment; this gap between medical science and medical care "has been most extreme in the rural sections of our country," they stated in the book's preface. "The country dweller is the last to be served."[49] The reality was that progress made in US cities toward better sanitation and the provision of physician and hospital care to the poor had scarcely reached those outside of the city: rural health had failed to develop while urban dwellers were enjoying the fruits of modernization.

Threats to the health of rural people included: the political economy of agriculture, especially its increasing commercialization and industrialization; the impact of rural poverty on both health status and the accessibility of preventive care and medical treatment; and the health inequality facing African Americans. Mott referred to the need for "health parity" for rural people. His speeches argued that the health inequality of farm families was created in part by where they lived: "The fact that they live on farms seems to constitute almost as great a barrier in obtaining medical care as does the fact that they are poor."[50] Certainly, rural health inequality was related to rural poverty and inadequate farm incomes, but rather than purely a function of economic determinism, rural health was considered a complex and dialectical problem. Rural people faced multiple challenges: those posed by spatial and social isolation; a lack of access to physician and nursing care, hospitals, and diagnostic services; and the inadequacies of rural public health infrastructure and sanitary engineering. Mott's FSA experience had taught him that, while boosting farm incomes would help to solve rural health inequality, sick farm families needed access to medical care in order to labour and earn.

Unlike some of their contemporaries, and earlier generations of social commentators and reformers,[51] Mott and Roemer did not

assume the overall healthfulness of the rural environment, or accept
unequivocally the notion that "the rural landscape is the site of all
things good for the health of body and mind," as they ironically put
it.[52] While accepting that certain aspects of rural life, such as "fresh
air, sunshine, and the 'hardening' effects of physical work" might
have health benefits, they argued that the healthfulness of rural life
was exaggerated. In a talk given to the Minnesota State Conference
of Social Work in St. Paul, Minnesota in May 1943, Mott mocked
the myth of the healthful rural environment:

> In the cities people lived tense, crowded, pestilence-ridden lives;
> in the country they breathed the free air of mountain and prairie;
> their fruits and vegetables were fresh from the soil; they were not
> spoiled by the decadent luxuries of civilized life.[53]

To Mott, this was an outdated view. According to the Census Bureau,
in 1940 rural rates of infant and maternal mortality, typhoid, diphtheria, malaria, pellagra, and influenza/pneumonia were all higher
than those in cities. These data echoed the work of the CCMC.
Other factors including exposure to animals and insects were likely
to make a rural American less healthy. Mental health was no less an
issue in rural areas than among urbanites, Mott and Roemer argued.[54]

Despite this sympathetic analysis of the underlying causes of
rural health inequality, Mott did at times describe rural health
conditions with eugenics-inflected language, using terms like
"defective" to describe rural people. In 1941, delivering a speech to
the Population Association of America on behalf of the then-Chief
Medical Officer, R.C. Williams, Mott referred to "alarming" numbers of young men rejected for military service on medical grounds,
which he linked to the "physical condition of our low-income farm
people." Rural people suffered from "untreated diseases and unrem-
edied defects ... an average of 3.5 significant defects per person in a
large sample of the rural population examined by the Farm Security
Administration in 1940." Defects included poor vision (found to

affect 28 percent of white people and 17 percent of people of colour), hearing problems, poor teeth and tonsils, hernia, pelvic disrepair, hemorrhoids, varicose veins, hookworm, malaria, and syphilis. One child in twelve showed "evidence of malnutrition." Mott suggested the poor health of the rural dweller was insidious, as it was largely hidden from view. Aside from obvious defects, Mott opined, "much disability is not evident on physical inspection, but rather is functional and becomes apparent only on the performance of work. Easy fatigability, headache, malaise, attacks of indigestion, dizzy spells, weakness, lack of general vitality—these are important robbers of health that are not apparent on physical examination."[55]

Rural Health and Medical Care, too, paints a bleak portrait of rural life, and of farm life in particular. Although Mott and Roemer appreciate the efforts of the co-operative movement and other rural organizations to improve access to medical care, they have a view of the culture of farm life that is far from flattering. This portrait of "living habits and attitudes" is worth quoting at length:

> The demands of an agricultural existence tend to give the farmer a psychological make-up quite distinct from that of the city resident. Typically, his contacts with people tend to be fewer and he is thrown more completely on his own resources. All too frequently isolation prevents his exposure to new ideas. In general, he tends to be more individualistic and slower to accept novel viewpoints or unaccustomed ways of doing things. His closeness to nature and his relative helplessness against the ravages of drought or flood or windstorm make him somewhat fatalistic and, at the same time, rather stoical about the misfortunes of life.
>
> Obviously these attitudes have a bearing on the farm family's reaction to illness, injuries, or impairments and to the need for medical services. They tend to make the rural family less alert to the need for medical care and less demanding of medical attention than the city family. Thus the rural family, at least up to very

recent years, has tended to be more or less satisfied with—or at least tolerant of—the old country doctor or the old dug well. ... almost every rural health worker has found it necessary to hurdle the attitude bound up in the expression "what was good enough for my grandfather is good enough for me."[56]

Mott and Roemer's judgment of farm people veers towards distaste at times, and their commentary was frankly sexist. They thought farm wives had a "weary demeanor," and claimed a combination of poverty and lack of education "results in a loss of pride in their personal appearance ... a drab and meagerly furnished home within dilapidated, insanitary, and unsightly surroundings does little to encourage sound habits of mental or physical hygiene." The authors refer to the "vicious circle" that results as children and youth are raised in this context of low living standards and lowered expectations. Rural communities also have a closed, if not closed-minded tenor. The relative homogeneity of rural communities led to resistance against "foreign ideas." While strong family bonds and close relationships between neighbours dependent upon one another contribute strength, and while class differences in rural communities are less marked than in urban areas, Mott and Roemer conclude that "the sharpest caste system ever known to American life, slavery, was a rural institution."[57]

Thus, Mott and Roemer replaced an essentialist notion of rural healthfulness with an analysis that tended to pathologize the conditions, and the character, of rural life. They attributed rural health problems to socio-economic challenges, but also to "social psychology and other cultural characteristics." This came close to attributing responsibility for rural health inequality to rural people themselves.

Medical and public health practitioners needed to improve their awareness of both the rural health situation and the sorts of "corrective action" required.[58] In *Rural Health and Medical Care*, Mott and Roemer identified similar targets for reform as did urban activists in the early twentieth century—sanitation, housing, and education. Their analysis of housing was incisive. They pointed to a paradox in rural housing conditions: despite the availability of ample space, labour, and building materials (lumber), housing was often "crowded, of poor quality, and in a state of disrepair." Again, statistics were marshaled to demonstrate the disparity between urban and rural conditions: 16 percent of farmhouses were overcrowded, compared with six percent of urban housing units. Citing a 1945 US Department of Agriculture report on housing, Mott and Roemer argued that two-thirds of rural housing was either beyond repair or in need of major renovation. "Rural slum housing frequently fails to provide even basic shelter from the elements," they noted. [59] These conditions were magnified among tenant and migratory farm labour families and contributed to accidents and ill health.

The state of rural infrastructure presented further barriers to health. Water supplies, sewage disposal, electricity, or household amenities such as screens on windows, refrigeration, heating, or telephones were all lacking. As the authors noted, the health implications of these conditions hardly needed elaboration. Even mid-century, electricity was a luxury in rural America: in 1940, nearly 70 percent of farm families had no electricity in their homes. This did not only mean no electric lighting—it also meant no reliable refrigeration of food, either in homes or in locations such as schools. Mott and Roemer are well aware of the financial challenges facing rural communities and state governments in terms of education provision. Their analysis seems to suggest that the problem is not the lack of willingness to spend public funds on education, but rather relative lack of availability of public funds to begin with. Financing services, including health care, is a challenge in areas where the revenue base for public spending is small, due to low incomes.

Echoing the faith in scientific development and medical progress common to progressives of this era, Mott and Roemer nevertheless saw the basic underlying problem in rural health to be an economic one. In their view, America was increasingly characterized by urban-rural wealth inequality, with even the urban industrial worker having incomes far higher than the average farmer. According to Mott and Roemer, the average annual industrial wage in the US in 1940 was $1273, while the average annual net farm income was $531. "Although persons living on farms made upon 23 percent of the nation's population in 1940, they received only 10 percent of the national income."[60] Mott and Roemer approach this problem as an outcome of increased industrialization and marketization of agriculture. They link rising living standards to the increasing cash orientation of the market, and make the simple point that farmers must grow crops for cash in order to enjoy the standard of living enjoyed by urban dwellers. Thus, "farming for the market" displaced older forms of agricultural production and left farmers vulnerable to price changes. Unfortunately for the farmer, in a climate of fierce competition, productive capacity for the market far exceeded market demand for agricultural products. Competition placed the farmer in a similar position vis-à-vis the market as the artisanal worker confronting industrialization: to be unable to compete, because of inadequate land holdings or out-of-date machinery, was catastrophic. "To operate a dairy farm in Winsconsin with an inferior herd, or to cultivate wheat in North Dakota with a plow and a mule, is as much economic suicide as to weave cloth on a hand loom in price competition with a modern textile mill."[61]

Mott and Roemer observed that the realities of the agricultural marketplace meant many farms were not economically effective and produced inadequate incomes. They estimated that in the years leading up to World War II, only one in five farm families earned an income adequate to meet basic economic needs, and within agriculture itself there were stark disparities between the most and least productive farms. In 1939, the top two million farms in the US produced 84 percent of all agricultural goods on the market; the bottom two million only three percent. "The story is one of too little land, too poor soil, too little machinery, and farmers with too little training."[62] Working to counteract the myth of the American family-owned farm with some hard data, Mott and Roemer pointed out that only just over half of farmers were the sole owners of the land they farmed, and many of those "owners" were heavily indebted. As the "concentration of agricultural wealth" increased during this period (and not only due to the conditions of the Depression), tens of thousands of farmers lost their land every year to larger land-holders. By 1940, 4.3 percent of farms controlled almost half of all farm acreage in the country. Cash and share tenants farmed more and more of the land, a situation that was by no means restricted to the southern US—in Nebraska and South Dakota, 52 percent of farms were operated by tenants. The implications of this were viewed thus:

> tenancy usually means insecurity, frequent moves, lack of farm and home improvements, poor sanitation facilities, and chronic exploitation of land resources and dilapidation of buildings. It presents issues of deep social, political, and economic significance.[63]

The agricultural economy was also dependent upon the labour of hired farm hands—two to three million of them—between a quarter and a third of them migratory workers. Conditions were the worst for those in the south, especially for African Americans, where incomes were as low as $295 per year in 1939. Hired workers in the agricultural sector earned 37 percent of the average income of industrial workers. They were not covered by legislation meant to ameliorate other waged work, such as workers' compensation or health and safety laws, minimum wage or hours of work laws, unemployment benefits, or welfare or social security legislation, however modest. Although the plight of migratory farm workers during the Depression years was well documented by American writers and legislators alike, Mott and Roemer argue that there was little overall structural change in the agricultural economy.[64]

Mott and Roemer saw this structural inequality as more than a
short-term crisis. Although conditions improved slightly as a result
of wartime demand for goods, the wartime boom did not eliminate
rural poverty, nor the comparative gap in incomes between rural and
urban people. Even in the late 1940s when their study was published,
after the heightened awareness of poverty among farmers during the
Depression years, Mott and Roemer still felt that the plight of farm
families received inadequate societal response. Although there were
obvious parallels between the poor farmer and the urban unemployed, more had been done to develop social welfare supports for
the urban poor than for the rural poor. Rural underemployment was
"very largely concealed or overlooked," whereas urban poverty was
"apparent," and had elicited social responses varying from unemployment benefits to "free" medical care for the urban poor. Not only did
rural poverty contribute to higher rates of disease, it also prevented
rural people from accessing medical care: "The chief deterrent to
modern medical care in rural areas is low purchasing power and the
consequent economic barrier between patient and physician. Rural
deficiencies in health resources and in medical services stem almost
entirely from economic roots."[65]

Mott and Roemer struggled throughout the book to balance
bleak facts and analogies with a belief in the possibility of political
change. This is the classic reform dilemma. In their chapter, "The
Characteristics of Rural Life," they speak of the conservative culture
of rural America, but also "the awakening of the farm population,"
and its "mounting demand for improved rural medical facilities and
services."[66] In part, their work is meant to facilitate this demand,
to put the facts and evidence at its disposal. At the same time, the
main audience for *Rural Health and Medical Care* is public health
professionals, such as themselves, and potential legislators and policy
makers. It is not those farm people and rural residents about whom
the study was written.

The final section of *Rural Health and Medical Care* outlined Mott and Roemer's view of the future objectives of health policy and services. These objectives were summarized as: access to care according to need by rural people; construction of hospitals, health centres, and sanitation facilities, integrated along regional lines; recruitment of physicians and other health care providers to work in rural areas in greater numbers; an improvement in the "scientific quality" of medical care in rural areas; and enhanced preventive and educational public health, integrated with treatment services.[67] These health policy objectives were contextualized by the need to address what the authors refer to as the "maladjustments of American agriculture." Mott and Roemer advocated a wide range of economic and social measures that should be taken by government, from agricultural credit, to unemployment compensation for farm labourers, to investment in roads, electricity and telephones.[68]

The authors stressed that, in a context of limited economic resources, the problem of the high cost of medical care could not be solved by most individuals. A societal solution was required. Mott and Roemer argued that there was widespread acceptance in the US of the need for some sort of "prepayment" or "insurance" model of coverage for health care, although the method of organizing it was clearly a question of debate. By the late 1940s, Mott had rejected the notion that voluntary action would be sufficient to tackling rural health inequality. This was based on his own research, and his hands-on knowledge with the FSA. Although there were any number of local, voluntary health care schemes operating in the US, as well as various government programs that provided limited health coverage to targeted sectors of the population, their coverage was highly variable, patchwork, and often financially inaccessible to those who needed medical care the most. This was the basis for Mott's belief in the need for a universal public program.

Mott and Roemer viewed the critics of compulsory insurance or state-provided services as unable or unwilling to face the facts:

To claim that voluntary health insurance plans can solve the
overwhelming problem of medical costs, as is done by certain
articulate groups, is simply not to face economic facts or the lessons of world-wide as well as American experience. In assessing
this claim, we must not only face the cold facts regarding the
highly uneven levels of income in different parts of the nation, but
we must examine, in particular, how many farm families could
afford to join comprehensive voluntary medical service plans.[69]

The facts they marshaled did seem damning. Only five percent of
Americans were covered for health care by pre-payment plans and
less than three percent of rural people had Blue Cross coverage for
hospitalization. Mott and Roemer estimate that, in 1945, 0.5 or 1 percent of rural residents had insurance for medical care.

Thus, Mott's years in the FSA seem to have convinced him of
the impossibility of providing health care to rural people through
voluntary insurance plans. Much of what Mott attempted to do during those years was facilitate the establishment of voluntary health
co-operatives. By the end of the war, he evidently believed that this
had been a failed effort. Mott and Roemer give a clear analysis of
all of the challenges facing voluntary, locally based health pre-payment or insurance plans in communities where people are poor, sick,
and often both. In a voluntary pre-payment scheme, the healthy and
young tend not to buy in, making the actuarial realities of any plan
unworkable. Insurance is based on shared risk, and when the people
who bought into plans were older and sicker than average, their use
of the service drove costs beyond what the plan could sustain. They
also argued that voluntary plans could never cope with the sheer
lack of infrastructure confronting rural areas, for example, or solve
the problem of personnel shortages, especially shortages of specialist care. In the late 1930s, even the AMA had agreed with them on
this latter point. These were problems Mott and his colleagues at
the FSA faced again and again during the New Deal health program

era, and their familiarity with every potential way of tweaking private voluntary insurance was comprehensive.

Their frustration with liberal individualism and opposition to state involvement in health care provision motivated them to take an increasingly political stance. Mott and Roemer became passionate critics of the health and human toll of the status quo and what they called "economic law." Thus, *Rural Health and Medical Care* concludes with a call for national compulsory health insurance legislation:

> It is clear that a choice must be made today. The way of voluntary health insurance is an improvement over the past, but its toll is one which must be calculated honestly. It has its cost in almost certain failure to bring anything approaching maximum health opportunity to the majority of our 57 million rural citizens. There is a hidden cost in terms of delay that must be faced, a cost that can be measured in daily suffering and deaths that need not occur.[70]

Written during a period when reform possibilities seemed real, but not published until after the defeat of Wagner-Murry-Dingell, *Rural Health and Medical Care* continued to carry the banner for a reformed health system in the US.

Rural Health and Medical Care proposed re-organizing health services through regionalized planning for rural areas and the use of health centres and mobile units to make maximum use of coordinated resources. These ideas were consistent with a health centre model of care, and added an emphasis upon rural health. Mott and Roemer conceptualized regions as essentially concentric, organized around a hub of scientific knowledge, such as a university medical centre, and including a network of district hospitals, smaller rural hospitals, and health centres to serve outlying and isolated areas. This, of course, is very similar to the schema suggested for Saskatchewan in the 1944 Sigerist Report.

The health centre model here, and in general, emphasized the need to make medical care accessible to those who found it difficult to get it for financial or geographic reasons, and the integration of various components of health care, including curative and preventive care. In *Rural Health and Medical Care*, however, Mott and Roemer argued not that physician care should be brought under the auspices of state provision, but rather that private practice physicians could and should operate under the same health centre umbrella as preventive public health services. The issue was less about how physicians would be paid (fee-for-service versus salary) and more about the underlying question of the physician's relationship with the state. Mott and Roemer wished to avoid this thorny and highly politicized question by suggesting that private practice could happily co-exist with public facilities and programs—in other words, their model did not pose an explicit threat to the free-enterprise ethos of American medicine. They believed that rural physicians stood to gain under their model, with better access to supportive services and technology (such as diagnostic services) than they would be able to purchase individually, and by sharing the cost of secretarial, nursing and laboratory assistance with public health facilities.

Rural Health and Medical Care attempts to communicate solutions to detailed policy and organizational problems in health care delivery. Perhaps because of their own experience in delivering health care services in the FSA, however, the authors remained committed to putting "human needs above theory." This included the needs of the sick, but also of rural physicians and communities themselves. They believed local public control of facilities was necessary—their model would not work with a network of privately-run health care institutions, whether for profit or not. This requirement might mean that local governments would take over "proprietary hospitals" and bring them under community control.[71] Health centres were viewed as community institutions:

A true community health center has a contribution to make to
rural living. It goes beyond the provision of specific medical and
public health services. It serves to focus interest on health and,
along with the rural church and school, it can do much to build
a more complete and meaningful rural community life.[72]

Writing in the late 1940s, Mott and Roemer were fully aware that
the health centre concept was not entirely new, and situated it in an
international context, citing for example a League of Nations Health
Organization conference on rural hygiene in 1931, the report in support of health centres issued by the British Medical Association
in 1942, and then-current planning taking place in Saskatchewan
and Manitoba. Although US health reformer Hermann Biggs had
planned the use of rural health centres in New York State after
World War I, his plans had never come to fruition. Mott and Roemer
considered the US to be comparatively backward in this regard.

Countering the opposition to socialistic or communistic health
care, Mott and Roemer pointed to the experience of "the 30 or more
nations that have established programs of compulsory health insurance."[73] But if this was a kind of shorthand for the backwardness
of US social policy, theirs was not a particularly outward-looking
analysis, either. Mott's speeches suggest the influence of his transnational, cosmopolitan cohort, though he remained, more so than
some, rooted in the North American context. He was well informed
about health and the state internationally and conceptualized historical developments in the US in a context of a changing medical
care landscape in Europe, the UK, Canada, New Zealand, and elsewhere—most of which pointed to a growing state involvement in
health and social welfare provision, "in the midst of a struggle for the
preservation of the rights of the common man." Yet, in a 1943 speech
Mott described the FSA as "peculiar to America ... an inherently
American combination of governmentally sponsored and voluntary
health insurance."[74]

The Soviet Union, about which their mentor Henry Sigerist appeared to know so much, was mentioned only three times by Mott and Roemer in *Rural Health and Medical Care*. Other nations were not held up as models in any specific sense, and the borrowing of specific policy ideas appeared, at least on the surface, to be minimal. For Mott and Roemer, the solutions to American problems seemed to belong largely to Americans. Perhaps more than any other aspect of their book, this assumption illustrates the growing impact of Cold War tensions. Sigerist could write about Soviet medicine and make it to the front page of *Time* magazine in 1939; by 1945, the "paranoid style" of US health politics made such open admiration for Soviet society a distant memory.

By the end of World War II, America's medical Cold War was already well underway, spurred by the battle over the 1945 Wagner-Murray-Dingell Bill. Opponents to the legislation had referred to it as "the most socialistic measure that this Congress has ever had before it."[75] An anonymous article in *Medical Economics* suggested Truman's health legislation was a plot by the International Labor Organization (ILO) to socialize US health care.[76] Medical opponents framed national health insurance proposals as a foreign notion and a Soviet-communist wedge into American society. Some argued publicly that health reform advocates within the public health service, including Mott and Roemer, were controlled by the Soviet Union. Grey quotes a 1947 issue of *California and Western Medicine*: "In some instances, known Communists and fellow travelers with the Federal agencies are at work diligently with Federal funds in furtherance of the Moscow party line."[77]

J.T.H. Connor, in his study of the medical politics surrounding the publication of *Rural Health and Medical Care*, argues that "physicians could become political casualties during the early days of the Cold War."[78] Advocates of health reform, including key public figures such as Mott, who had spoken so firmly and publicly in favour of a universal state health insurance program, were put back on their heels. In the immediate postwar context, health reformers in the US were faced with increasingly hostile and personal attacks. FSA staff were accused of subversion and of being Communists or fellow travellers "in furtherance of the Moscow party line." According to Grey, this "led directly to purges of various federal agencies, including the FSA Health Services Branch."[79] Led by the relentless Marjorie Shearon, Isidore Falk and health economist Michael Davis, among others, were branded by their critics as the leaders of a communist health conspiracy. This was referred to in posters and diagrams as the "House of Falk," its web-like structure depicting an insidious network of colluders. Having worked for the FSA and spoken publicly in favour of the Wagner-Murray-Dingell Bill, Mott was publicly identified as a member of the "House of Falk."

This conspiracy theory was taken up by medical societies and members of the medical press opposed to health insurance. Mott's former boss at the United States Public Health Service (USPHS), Thomas Parran, was censured in an AMA resolution for activities "in opposition to American democratic processes."[80] Parran was accused by the AMA of misappropriating government funds when he sent a USPHS physician to New Zealand to study their health care system. Some of the physicians targeted by the AMA were called to testify to the House Un-American Activities Committee. By 1947, federal government employees were being investigated by both houses of Congress and by the FBI. The House of Representatives argued that federal employees' advocacy in favour of national health insurance was unlawful, and evidence of their involvement in a broader international campaign to achieve socialized medicine. While this might well have been an accurate assessment of the situation in some regards, support for state involvement was seen by the Republican Party, organized medicine, and others on the broader political right, as de facto evidence of disloyalty to the US, and even as part of a Soviet plot.

The heavy involvement of government employees in promoting Democratic Party-sponsored legislation left many public servants vulnerable to critique. Derickson has argued, however, that they also faced repercussions because of weak Democratic leadership and because two presidents did not adequately support the legislation. Derickson refers to the legislative campaign for national health insurance as "an army composed largely of lieutenants."[81] Public servants like Falk and Mott were left to rally the troops and mobilize public support, but they did so without a general leading the charge. Both Roosevelt and then Truman failed to champion health insurance. By 1948, the Democratic Party platform no longer endorsed a national health program. Derickson's assessment of the Wagner-Murray-Dingell Bill's legislative failure is that its supporters relied too much on technical arguments and insufficiently on a mass base of popular political support, which presumably might have been mobilized. Even organized labour (both the AFL and the CIO) "deferred to ... policy intellectuals" who had a "more reserved and elitist strategy."[82]

If that was the case, it was perhaps only part of the problem. Timing was against the Wagner-Murray-Dingell Bill. The end of World War II and its intensified Cold War context corresponded with a closing of the moment during which truly innovative and radical social policy might be possible. When the tide turned against health legislation in the US, many supporters of health reform lost their jobs, their status and authority, and their faith in the political process. The FSA itself was dismantled as of December 31, 1946: all of the programs Mott had built—the medical care co-operatives, the migrant health program, and the experimental health plans—were almost without exception terminated.[83] In this context, Saskatchewan's offer of a senior position gave Mott a way out of a bleak situation, though the opportunity was bittersweet.

ENDNOTES

1   I. S. Falk, "The Present and Future Organization of Medicine," Milbank
    Memorial Fund Quarterly 12, 2 (1934): 125.

2   J.T.H. Connor, "'One Simply Doesn't Arbitrate Authorship of Thoughts':
    Socialized Medicine, Medical McCarthyism, and the Publishing of Rural
    Health and Medical Care," Journal of the History of Medicine and Allied
    Sciences, 72, 3 (2017): 249.

3   See Alan Derickson, "The House of Falk: The Paranoid Style in American
    Health Politics," American Journal of Public Health 87, 11 (November 1997):
    1836–43. Mott is named in Marjorie Shearon's diagram "Nationalization of
    Medicine Dominated by THE HOUSE OF FALK. Spheres of Influence,
    Interlocking Directorates, Collaborationists," 1838.

4   Rosenfeld and his wife Irene were lifelong friends of Mindel and Cecil
    Sheps, and both men were associated from the 1970s on with what became
    known as the Cecil G. Sheps Center for Health Services Research at
    University of North Carolina Chapel Hill, still open today.

5   Frederick Dodge Mott and Milton I. Roemer, Rural Health and Medical
    Care (New York: McGraw-Hill, 1948).

6   Charles Howard Hopkins, John R. Mott, 1865-1955: A Biography (Grand
    Rapids: Eerdmans, 1979), 212, 680.

7   Biographical information in this section is drawn from Yale University
    Divinity School Library (hereafter YDSL), Special Collections, Record
    Group 45, John R. Mott Papers, Box 102 Folder 1795, "Group Health
    Institute, Chicago, June 24, 1975, Acceptance of Award by Frederick D.
    Mott"; and "Biographical Sketch of Frederick D. Mott, M.D."

8   YDSL, Special Collections, Record Group 45, John R. Mott Papers,
    Box 102 Folder 1795, "Group Health Institute, Chicago, June 24, 1975,
    Acceptance of Award by Frederick D. Mott."

9   YDSL, Special Collections, Record Group 45, John R. Mott Papers,
    Box 102 Folder 1795, "Group Health Institute, Chicago, June 24, 1975,
    Acceptance of Award by Frederick D. Mott."

10 YDSL, Special Collections, Record Group 45, John R. Mott Papers, Box
    102 Folder 1795, "Biographical Sketch of Frederick D. Mott, M.D."

11 YDSL, Special Collections, Record Group 45, John R. Mott Papers,
    Box 102 Folder 1795, "Group Health Institute, Chicago, June 24, 1975,
    Acceptance of Award by Frederick D. Mott."

12 YSDL, Special Collections, Record Group 45, John R. Mott Papers,
    Box 102 Folder 1795, "Biographical Sketch of Frederick D. Mott, M.D.";
    "History of HAP," https://www.hap.org/about/history, accessed August 24,
    2018.

13 YDSL, Special Collections, Record Group 45, John R. Mott Papers, Box 102 Folder 1795, "Group Health Institute, Chicago, June 24, 1975, Acceptance of Award by Frederick D. Mott."

14 Michael R. Grey, *New Deal Medicine: The Rural Health Programs of the Farm Security Administration* (Baltimore and London: Johns Hopkins University Press, 1999), 50.

15 Jennifer Klein, *For All These Rights: Business, Labor, and the Shaping of America's Public-Private Welfare State* (Princeton NJ: Princeton University Press, 2004), 11.

16 Jennifer Klein, "A New Deal Restoration: Individuals, Communities, and the Long Struggle for the Collective Good," *International Labor and Working-Class History* 74, 1 (2008): 42.

17 Klein, *For All These Rights*, 11.

18 Klein, *For All These Rights*, 116–117.

19 Susan Lynn Smith, *Sick and Tired of Being Sick and Tired: Black Women's Health Activism in America, 1890-1950* (Philadelphia: University of Pennsylvania Press, 1995), 59.

20 Quoted in Reginald Atwater, "National Health Conference—A Review," *American Journal of Public Health* 28, 9 (September 1938): 1103–1113.

21 Klein, *For All These Rights*, 143.

22 Klein, *For All These Rights*, 144.

23 Klein, *For All These Rights*, 11.

24 Klein, *For All These Rights*, 118.

25 Klein, *For All These Rights*, 141.

26 Klein, *For All These Rights*, 135.

27 Grey, *New Deal Medicine*, 5.

28 Smith, *Sick and Tired of Being Sick and Tired*, Chapter 3, "A New Deal for Black Health."

29 Grey, *New Deal Medicine*, 5.

30 Greg, *New Deal Medicine*, 85.

31 Grey, *New Deal Medicine*, 81–82.

32 Speech to Wisconsin Welfare Council, Oct. 9, 1942. Library and Archives Canada (hereafter LAC), MG 31 J15, Frederick Dodge Mott Papers, File 47-12. This point of view actually represented a considerable evolution in Mott's thinking from his days as a medical student at McGill University in the early 1930s, when he consistently rendered male doctors the key agents in socialized medicine. His professional experience broadened his understanding of who should be doing what work, so that ten years later his vision encompassed the contributions of other health workers, not only "the doctor and the public health man."

33 LAC, MG31 J15, Frederick Dodge Mott Papers, File 31-12.

34 LAC, MG31 J15, Frederick Dodge Mott Papers, File 31-12.

35 LAC, MG31 J15, Frederick Dodge Mott Papers, File 31-12, Agricultural
    Workers Health Association Handbook, 44-45.

36 Grey, *New Deal Medicine*, 113.

37 Grey, *New Deal Medicine*, 5.

38 Grey, *New Deal Medicine*, 9.

39 Grey, *New Deal Medicine*, 7.

40 LAC, MG 31 J15, Frederick Dodge Mott Papers, File 47-12.

41 Grey, *New Deal Medicine*. See Chapter 6.

42 Grey, *New Deal Medicine*, 155.

43 *Oxford New Dictionary*.

44 Philip Abbott, "Titans/Planners, Bohemians/Revolutionaries: Male
    Empowerment in the 1930s," *Journal of American Studies* 40, 3 (2006): 473.

45 Abbott, "Titans/Planners," 472.

46 Abbott, "Titans/Planners," 475, 476.

47 Alan Brinkley, "The New Deal and the Idea of the State," in *The Rise and
    Fall of the New Deal Order 1930-1980*, ed. Steve Fraser and Gary Gerstle
    (Princeton NJ: Princeton University Press, 1989), 94.

48 J.T.H. Connor, "'One Simply Doesn't Arbitrate Authorship of Thoughts'":
    246.

49 Frederick D. Mott and Milton Roemer, *Rural Health and Medical Care*
    (New York, Toronto, London: McGraw-Hill Book Company, 1948), v.

50 LAC, MG31 J15, Frederick Dodge Mott Papers, File 47-8, "Physical Status
    of Low-Income Farm Families."

51 Mott and Roemer refer specifically to Henry David Thoreau and Ralph
    Borsodi's *This Ugly Civilization*, published in 1929. See *Rural Health*, 31.

52 Mott and Roemer, *Rural Health*, 31

53 LAC, MG 31 J15, Frederick Dodge Mott Papers, File 47-9, "Medical Care
    for the Rural Population."

54 Mott and Roemer, *Rural Health and Medical Care*, 107, 140.

55 LAC, MG 31 J15, Frederick Dodge Mott Papers, File 47-9, "Medical Care
    for the Rural Population."

56 Mott and Roemer, *Rural Health*, 42.

57 Mott and Roemer, *Rural Health*, 43.

58 Mott and Roemer, *Rural Health*, 46, ix.

59 Mott and Roemer, *Rural Health*, 32–33.

60 Mott and Roemer, *Rural Health*, 15.

61 Mott and Roemer, *Rural Health*, 16

62 Mott and Roemer, *Rural Health*, 20.

63 Mott and Roemer, *Rural Health*, 24.

64 Mott and Roemer, *Rural Health*, 26.

65 Mott and Roemer, *Rural Health*, 470.
66 Mott and Roemer, *Rural Health*, 45.
67 Mott and Roemer, *Rural Health*, 473.
68 Mott and Roemer, *Rural Health*, 475–476.
69 Mott and Roemer, *Rural Health*, 481.
70 Mott and Roemer, *Rural Health*, 484.
71 Mott and Roemer, *Rural Health*, 501.
72 Mott and Roemer, *Rural Health*, 503.
73 Mott and Roemer, *Rural Health*, 483
74 LAC, MG31 J15, Frederick Dodge Mott Papers, File 47-22, "Medical Care in a Changing World—Speech to PTA, Arlington Virginia, April 1943."
75 Quoted in Grey, *New Deal Medicine*, 160.
76 Derickson, "The House of Falk," 1837.
77 Quoted in Grey, *New Deal Medicine*, 163.
78 J.T.H. Connor, "'One Simply Doesn't Arbitrate Authorship of Thoughts,'" 248.
79 Grey, *New Deal Medicine*, 163.
80 Grey, *New Deal Medicine*, 164.
81 Derickson, "The House of Falk," 1840.
82 Derickson, "The House of Falk," 1840.
83 Grey, *New Deal Medicine*, 165.

CHAPTER 6

UNINTENDED CONSEQUENCES

Hospitalization Insurance and the Eclipse of the Health Centre Model

The Saskatchewan College of Physicians and Surgeons (SCPS) leadership was apprehensive from the outset about the CCF's intentions to socialize health care, and "view[ed] with suspicion any so-called experts from outside the province."[1] The SCPS wasted little time before going on the ideological offensive against elements of the Sigerist plan for a regionally based health centre model of care, engaging in disputes with the Health Services Planning Commission (HSPC) on issues from physician payment to lay governance. By the spring of 1946, the SCPS was reporting to the Canadian Medical Association annual meeting that HSPC staff promoted an "unsound" model for health services, and that some of the HSPC's personnel were "entirely lacking the confidence of the medical profession." The SCPS's critiques sometimes became *ad hominem*, as when they offered to "actively assist" Douglas in appointing a "qualified" chairman of the HSPC to replace Cecil Sheps[2] even though, for the previous eighteen months, the doctors had not put forward any names for this position.

With the Sheps's departure (discussed in chapter 4) leadership at the HSPC changed. On August 30, 1946 Frederick Mott and Leonard Rosenfeld were appointed Chairman and Vice-Chairman of the HSPC.[3] In a study written 30 years ago, David Naylor suggested that Mott, who replaced Cecil Sheps and became the first permanent chairman of the HSCP, was hired to mollify the SCPS leadership. Naylor characterized Mott as a "formerly high-ranking official in the US Public Health Service ... well received by the [medical] profession."[4] This portrayal credits Mott's interpersonal skills and his reputation, but leaves out Mott's well-known support for health reform. The previous chapter demonstrated that Mott was a veteran of highly partisan US health politics and its medical Cold War, and a forthright advocate for health security and planning during the New Deal. During his time in Saskatchewan, Mott maintained connections with that world, communicating often with his US colleagues. Though a behind-the-scenes actor, Mott devoted his career to building co-operative and state alternatives in health care. Privately, his view of physicians' organizations was skeptical, at best.

Leonard Rosenfeld shared a similar, if slightly less distinguished, career trajectory to Mott's. His background was known to the Saskatchewan public. According to the Regina *Leader Post*, Rosenfeld "was chief of a health and sanitation field party assigned to Nicaragua by the Institute of Inter-American Affairs, a United States government agency set up by an agreement between the foreign minister of American countries to aid the war effort by raising the health and economic status of the Latin American countries."[5] Rosenfeld had returned to the US at the end of 1945, and took up a Rockefeller Foundation fellowship in public health, during which US health reformers Alan Gregg and John Grant mentored him. Henry Sigerist and John Grant both encouraged Rosenfeld to go to Saskatchewan. As early as January 1945, Sigerist was writing to Rosenfeld describing his time in Saskatchewan:

> The job in Saskatchewan was most interesting. It is a young
> Province with highly developed cooperatives. What pleased me

most was that they have even cooperative funeral parlors so that profits have been removed even from death. It is obvious that you cannot socialize medicine completely as long as there is a shortage of physicians and building materials but I drew up a plan that foresees a development by steps and a good deal has already been achieved.[6]

A year later, Sigerist wrote to Rosenfeld to congratulate him on his Rockefeller Fellowship, but at the same time to make the case that he should go with Fred Mott to Saskatchewan:

> Now, I just received a letter from Fred Mott from which I was very pleased to learn that he has accepted the position in Saskatchewan. He also mentions that there is a possibility of your going with him for a while and I think this could be worked into your other program without too much difficulty. I have to write to John Grant anyway and will mention the matter.[7]

The Rosenfelds stayed in Regina until 1948, when Leonard took a position with the Office of the Surgeon General of the Public Health Service in Washington, as Chief of the Health Profession Branch. Rosenfeld's archives are silent on why he made the decision to leave, but the strain of the position and his ill health may have played a part. In June 1948, Milton Roemer wrote to Leonard, expressing concern about Rosenfeld's recurring malaria, presumably contracted during years in Nicaragua. The letter makes it clear that Rosenfeld was considering leaving Saskatchewan at the time.[8] In the 1950s, Rosenfeld would teach at the Harvard School of Public Health, then later at the University of North Carolina. From 1957 to 1960, he worked as an administrator for the Community Health Association of Detroit—a prepaid medical coverage plan established by the United Auto Workers under Walter Reuther. In this group medical practice, doctors were paid a salary, and patients were treated at the Metropolitan Hospital. In 1960, Fred Mott became

Executive Director of the CHA, while Rosenfeld became General Director of its Metropolitan Hospital.[9]

When Mott and Rosenfeld arrived in Regina in fall 1946, Premier Douglas had already passed his Hospitalization Act (April 1946). The legislation committed to public hospitalization insurance coverage across the province and was to be implemented by January 1, 1947. This program was an important reason the Douglas Government needed someone with Mott's experience. They had less than six months to get the program off the ground. The HSPC created the Saskatchewan Hospital Services Plan (SHSP) to administer hospitalization insurance, and Rosenfeld became Executive Director. Rosenfeld, acting as Mott's deputy, had to dramatically expand upon existing hospital resources (some private, some taxpayer funded), and create effective mechanisms for record keeping, tax collection, and cost containment and efficiency.

Because of the program's ultimate success, hospitalization insurance is remembered as the CCF's first capstone health reform and is generally framed as a key precursor to the federal government's eventual support for a national hospital insurance program, introduced in 1957. Malcolm Taylor's 1987 study of Canadian health care, *Health Insurance and Canadian Public Policy*, referred to Saskatchewan's decision in 1946 to create a system of compulsory hospital care insurance as the "first decisive action in the long chain of events leading to our present system" (that is, Canadian medicare).[10] Taylor, an employee of the HSPC himself, was directly involved in the establishment of the SHSP. He wrote a doctoral dissertation on the subject, and his publications have been vital to the crafting of a historical narrative that privileges the importance of the SHSP over other elements of the HSPC's program. The decision to immediately provide universal hospital coverage through a combination of personal and family premiums and government revenues was indeed a hallmark development in the CCF's first mandate, but hospitalization was intended to be only one element of a socialized health system. The HSPC's aim to build an integrated regional network of care with the health centre model at its heart, by contrast, is a story less often told.

Canadian public policy history's focus on the issue of insurance for hospital, and then later physician, services is explained in part by the obscured historical traces left by a failed alternative. Over the course of the CCF's first two mandates, Saskatchewan's health care policies were drawn further and further away from the early health centre model captured in the Sigerist Report—a model, as we have seen, that had grown out of a transnational movement for health equality. Since Taylor and David Naylor published their defining studies of Saskatchewan medicare, historians Joan Feather and Gordon Lawson have discussed two specific ways in which the CCF diverted from its early intentions: the unclear role of lay governance in a regionalized system of health care post-SHSP; and the apparent capitulation to organized medicine through a fee-for-service model of physician payment in Health Region No. 1 (Swift Current), and in the medical program for social assistance recipients.[11] Both of these lines of argument are essential to understanding what CCF health services looked like on the ground. Both historians attribute intentionality to the CCF's actions. Yet, there is abundant evidence that the government and its health planners were overtaken by the magnitude of the project they had taken on, and by the limits of what was feasible.

Providing universally accessible hospital care to the people of the province was a vast project, but the SHSP did not build a hospital system from scratch. The Union Hospital Districts (UHD) program, established in 1916, had enabled municipalities to work together to build and operate hospitals, and gave municipalities power to tax property owners to finance them. In 1934, provincial legislation was amended to allow for a flat hospital tax on individuals. By 1944, when the CCF came to power, there were 23 UHDs in the province, but the number of beds was far from adequate.[12] Sigerist observed that there was little point in universally insuring hospital care if there were few accessible hospitals in which people could seek treatment. The Sigerist Report had suggested the need for 1000 new hospital beds, half of which would be provided in 50 rural health centres across the province, and the other 500 at a new university hospital. The HSPC prepared a "Report on Free Hospitalization" in June 1945, in which it argued, optimistically, that ongoing hospital construction plans should provide enough beds for the introduction of hospitalization insurance. A Committee on Free Hospitalization was established, which included Cecil Sheps, Thomas McLeod, a physician, and a hospital administrator. It began meeting in October 1945. Legislation for public hospitalization coverage was introduced in March 1946.[13]

Whatever the HSPC's early enthusiasm for hospitalization coverage, by the time of Mott's arrival in fall of 1946, staff were urging a more realistic time frame. Thomas McLeod's biography of Douglas provides a firsthand account of the early years of health program development; McLeod worked in the HSPC and, as previously discussed, was part of the team led by Mindel Sheps that attempted to get the first health regions established. In McLeod's analysis, Douglas made universal hospitalization insurance a priority during his first mandate over the advice of Sigerist (who had suggested the gradual introduction of free hospitalization) and that of his planners at the HSPC, who viewed it as premature. As McLeod wrote:

> In embarking on the hospital insurance gamble, Douglas over-ruled the advice of his own planning commission. The planners reported that the province faced a huge hospital construction bill over the next few years. In addition, they pointed out that Saskatchewan lacked the technical, professional, and administrative staff to put a hospital insurance program into effect. Douglas ... judged that the risks of not proceeding outweighed any obstacles.[14]

Douglas hoped the federal government would begin to insure hospital care in the immediate future. The King Government had certainly made significant gestures in this direction, but in the end failed to carry through. Federal support for hospitalization was not introduced until 1957, a decade after Douglas's Hospitalization Act. Enormous fiscal pressures were created by the federal government's failure to deliver, and they had long-term repercussions on health policy. Had the federal government insured hospital care sooner, perhaps the pattern of development in health services in Saskatchewan would have been different, and greater attention to public health and the regional health centre model more achievable. Nonetheless, as Aleck Ostry has argued, the "major health reform initiated in the early years of the CCF government," hospitalization quickly tilted health services heavily towards the institutional, tertiary end of the care spectrum.[15]

The decision to focus on hospitalization insurance was consequential for health policy, but the political stakes were just as high. Douglas was by this point two years into his first mandate and needed to show meaningful progress on his party's signature issue. Hospitalization coverage offered the possibility of a high-profile accomplishment. This is not to say Douglas took the easy way out. To the contrary, as McLeod has noted, the strategy represented an enormous gamble. If public hospitalization insurance turned out to be a shambles, the CCF risked losing the next election, and the damage would extend far beyond the province's borders. Repeatedly heralded as the first universal public hospitalization program in North America, and watched carefully by health advocates across the continent, the HSPC could not afford to have the program break down. By McLeod's account, shortly after the arrival of Mott and Rosenfeld in fall 1946, "a delegation of planners came to the premier's office to ask for a one-year extension to January 1, 1948. Douglas rejected this appeal on the spot."[16] The Premier wanted the plan up and running well before the 1948 election.

The HSPC and the new SHSP got to work planning and constructing new hospitals, expanding and improving existing ones, creating an administrative mechanism for hospital care financing, and developing a bureaucracy capable of effective oversight. "Fred Mott's people worked under battlefield conditions," McLeod recalled. "Their office was an old retail store, their desks were plywood panels on trestles, and their filing cabinets were cardboard boxes on the floor."[17] Mott drew regular support during this hectic time from his correspondence with E. Richard (Dick) Weinerman. Weinerman had worked under Mott as Assistant Chief Medical Officer, Health Services Division during the last months of the US Farm Security Administration (FSA) health programs, planning rural medical care (the program was terminated in 1947). After the demise of the FSA programs, Weinerman worked with Milton Roemer and Sy Axelrod in the US Public Health Service, Division of Public Health Methods, on research and planning in rural health and medical care, including health care for migratory farm workers. Close personal relationships developed during this period in Weinerman's life that lasted throughout his career, including with Milton Roemer, Cecil Sheps, Sy Axelrod, and Fred Mott.

Weinerman, like others in this network, had a distinguished career in social medicine and health politics. Born in Hartford, Connecticut, Dick Weinerman was a brilliant student with a scientific bent. He excelled as a pre-med student at Yale University, and tutored in both chemistry and mathematics but was nonetheless denied admission to Yale Medical School, probably because he was Jewish.[18] His friend Milton Roemer believed that Weinerman was deeply affected by Yale Medical School's rejection. Weinerman studied at Georgetown University instead and, according to his obituary in the *Yale Journal of Biology and Medicine*, "had the highest national rank of anyone taking the basic sciences test of the National Board of Medical Examiners in 1940."[19] Weinerman's "medical intellectual hero" was Henry Sigerist, although he never studied with him. In 1950–51, Weinerman became a medical director of the Kaiser Foundation Health Plan, an alternative health care model in Oakland, California. The early influence of Kaiser Health on Saskatchewan's State Hospital and Medical League was discussed in chapter 3. In 1970, Weinerman and his wife Shirley Basch were killed on a flight to Israel when a bomb exploded on the airplane. Weinerman was 52 years old.

In August 1946, before Mott arrived in Regina, he wrote to Weinerman from his family's summer property in Entrélac, Québec. At the time, Mott anticipated that he would be "bound to be plunging into health centre planning," when he arrived in Regina.[20] He asked Weinerman to send him the architectural plans for the proposed San Luis Health Center in Costilla County, Colorado, a co-operative project between a local consumer health association, the Colorado State Health Officer, and the FSA Health Services and Engineering Divisions. This was one of the last major projects Mott had worked on while at the FSA. The original plans show an examination and treatment room, nurse's and doctor's offices, eight hospital beds, and labour and delivery rooms, as well as a nursery and a dentist office. Negotiations were underway with the state to have a public health officer and/or public health nurses located in the building. The San Luis Health Center was to be the home of the local health association's medical and hospital plan, which, according to notes taken by Weinerman in a meeting in Colorado attended by FSA staff in April 1946, would cover 500 families in six counties for an annual fee of $38. The plan would include medical care in the home and at the health center, obstetrics services, emergency care, public health services, basic drugs, and ambulance service. Physicians who worked for the plan would be guaranteed $6000 per year, and a portion of any fees paid to the health center for services to non-plan members.[21] Weinerman's return letter to Mott, in which he included documents on the San Luis Health Centre, offered enthusiasm and support to developments in Saskatchewan: "We are anxious for all

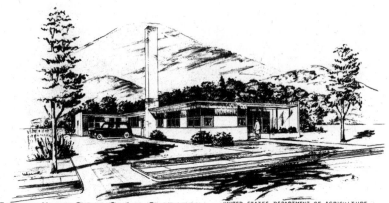

PROPOSED HEALTH CENTER · SAN LUIS · COLORADO · UNITED STATES DEPARTMENT OF AGRICULTURE
FARM SECURITY ADMINISTRATION · HEALTH SERVICE & ENGINEERING DIVISION

San Luis Health Centre Plans

the details of your program. The progress already made in health center and hospital construction is amazing."[22]

Weinerman's archives from his time working for Mott at the FSA include an undated typescript he authored, "Health Centres for the People." It was perhaps intended for a radio broadcast or mass publication to publicize the value of the Costilla health centre model:

> Farmer Brown works his land in a back-road rural area. ... He knows what a doctor looks like, because one day last spring, with Mrs. Brown in real agony, he had to drive the old farm truck 30 miles to the trade area center where the nearest physician practices.
>
> He can tell a hospital building when he sees one for his son, Jim, age 21, spent a long six months in a body cast on the ward of the city hospital, two hours' drive to the North.
>
> But Farmer Brown has seen no physician in his home county since the funeral of old Doctor Withers (died 1938, age 81). And the thought of a hospital building in his gas-station-general-store-and-post-office village never crosses his mind. ...
>
> It is a vicious circle. Folks know that a hospital is meaning-less without doctors to staff it. And the MDs shake their heads at the prospect of settling in a county where no proper clinic and laboratory facilities exist ...
>
> Yet, with community determination and cooperation, solu-tions can be found. One such is the Health Center.
>
> A health center takes its place alongside the town hall and the public school and the community social center. No two are exactly alike, but the recently organized health association in Costilla County, Colorado, is building a center that can be used as a working model. A simple, one-story structure on commun-ity-donated land is to be erected and equipped for about $30,000. Provisions are made for managerial, doctor, dentist, and nurses' offices. Headquarters for a unit of the district Public Health Department are included. A small laboratory and X-ray unit

adjoin a combination treatment room and clinic. In the "hospital" wing a kitchen and modern operating room serve eight to ten beds, set up for obstetrical and emergency cases. ...

The health center is the outlying link that feeds the central hospital system of the more urban areas. In the center the day-to-day ambulatory illnesses and accidents can be handled. Here the community preventive health program can be centered and coordinated with the curative services of the private practitioners whose offices are also in the center. Here, too, a few beds can be located to provide for the medical and surgical emergencies and to handle the ordinary child birth cases—reducing the need for undesirable home deliveries. The cases requiring specialty consultation, the hospitalized illnesses, the more complex diagnostic and curative work can be referred—without the need for made haste—to the nearest medical center facility.

Farmer Brown could, thus, see his "own" doctor and have a share in a local community health center.[23]

Weinerman was describing a health system virtually identical to the health regions model proposed by the Sigerist Report, although in the political context of the US, this model was to be implemented through a voluntary individual/family pre-payment health plan, not a compulsory government insurance scheme. Mott reiterated the general principles of this rural health centre approach in his address to the FSA Planning and Policy Conference on June 6, 1946, barely two months before his departure to Regina:

Hospitals and health centers must be constructed in an integrated network, with functional relationships between rural hospitals and larger urban institutions. More physicians, dentists, nurses and other health workers must be trained and attracted to rural sections. ... Well-financed and well-staffed local public health departments must extend into every rural district, and

there must be coordination of preventive and therapeutic programs under common administrative direction.[24]

In Regina, Mott could draw not only upon a model for rural health
centres, but also upon the FSA's concrete experience with health centre planning. Early in August 1946 he wrote to Weinerman:

> I plan to write to Sy Axelrod, asking for the floor plans of the
> health centers which have turned out to be best in the farm labor
> program from the point of view of practical experience—possibly
> the best each for Florida, Texas, California and the Northwest.
> ... I'm certainly sorry I never followed up ... the idea of bringing
> several of our best plans together in a little publication on health
> centers.[25]

Several of the western FSA rural health centres were designed
by modernist architect Vernon DeMars, with landscaping by
Garrett Eckbo.[26] The two worked under Burton Cairns, who was
the FSA's Chief Architect for the western region until his death
in 1939. DeMars received his architecture degree from University
of California Berkeley in 1931. He designed innovative housing for
migrant farmers and a series of hospitals and clinics for the FSA
health program. DeMars became a professor of architecture at
Berkeley in 1952, and worked there for the remainder of his career.
After wartime service, he taught at the Massachusetts Institute of
Technology (MIT) with the Finnish architect Alvar Aalto, among
others. Garret Eckbo had also studied architecture at Berkeley, but
he learned modernism at the Harvard Graduate School of Design
under professors like the Bauhaus designer Walter Gropius.[27]

Some of DeMars's health work was highlighted in the December
1942 issue of the modernist architectural journal, *The New Pencil
Points*. The article, "Farm Labor: After Shelter Comes Health" was
illustrated with photographs taken by Dorothea Lange for the FSA.
Three designs by De Mars and Eckbo were profiled: the Clinic

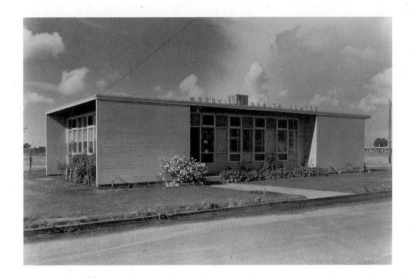

Woodville Health Centre, California

PHOTO BY DOROTHEA LANGE. VERNON DEMARS COLLECTION, 2005-13,
ENVIRONMENTAL DESIGN ARCHIVES, UNIVERSITY OF CALIFORNIA, BERKELEY.

Building in Woodville, California; the 100-bed FSA rural hospital in Fresno, California; and the Burton Cairns General Hospital and Convalescent Center in 11 Mile Corner, Arizona, which had started out as a clinic building and grew into a 60-bed hospital. The Woodville clinic was described as the "architectural expression of the social need which FSA is trying to satisfy."[28]

Mott thus arrived in Saskatchewan a firm adherent of the health centre model. He had relevant experience in line with Sigerist's recommendations and was excited about creating a regionalized network of rural health centres and hospitals. He also knew, however, that Douglas had an ambitious set of health care plans. Early in September, while settling into his role as Chair of the HSPC, Mott wrote again to Weinerman:

> Len Rosenfeld and I have plunged into a multitude of complex problems and more actual action than I have seen in a long time ... Len and I have secured approval for slowing things down and getting a master plan drawn up over the next six or seven months. Meanwhile, very small hospitals and health centres are going up all over the place. I don't doubt that most of them are needed in this very sparsely settled territory, but certain inevitable mistakes are probably being made. This is just a hint of one of the many problems facing us.[29]

This account differs slightly from McLeod's, which depicts Douglas as a rigid adherent to his aggressive timeframe. Mott may have convinced Douglas to give him more time to develop an overall plan for health reform, but the implementation date for hospital coverage remained unchanged. Thus, the SHSP entered a period of "feverish activity."[30]

Conveying his feeling to Weinerman that instituting compulsory hospitalization insurance was "far from a cinch," Mott touched on his ongoing attempts to maintain cordial relationships with organized medicine, while remaining cautious about their fundamental political orientation:

They are all being very decent to me during this "honeymoon" period, but I have no illusions about the future. The profession here does not differ in any fundamental respect from the profession south of the border. The chief difference—and I recognize that it is a big one—is that they have accepted the principle of compulsory health insurance.[31]

With hindsight, Mott might have conceded that physicians had accepted, more narrowly, *hospitalization* insurance. On other elements of the government's health platform, and ultimately on public insurance for medical care, their support could not be assumed.

One of the HSPC's first tasks was to register every eligible resident of the province for the hospitalization plan. Those living in cities were enumerated, while in rural areas, everyone was urged to register at the municipal office. The personal tax was collected by local municipalities. At the end of October 1946, Mott issued a public plea for registration in advance of the January 1, 1947 implementation date.[32] At the same time, Rosenfeld was working on the unglamorous task of developing standardized forms and procedures. In a letter to Weinerman written barely six weeks before Douglas's January 1, 1947 implementation deadline, Mott observed, "Len Rosenfeld is practically killing himself in temporarily heading up the [hospital insurance] plan, and the rest of the staff are not far behind him."[33] Rosenfeld's team put together the hospitalization program in five months. Launching the plan, Premier Douglas deployed his usual flair for the potent symbol. A ceremony was held at the Regina City Hall in late December 1939, at which City Assessor Arthur Robins presented Premier Douglas with SHSP card No. 1, entitling Douglas to receive hospitalization benefits after January 1, 1947. Douglas commented, "the eyes of Canada are on this province. We are establishing a pattern for socially minded people everywhere to follow."[34]

Like their Premier, each registrant was given a unique hospitalization plan number, and a card that was required to receive insured care. Patients were to use their hospitalization cards when admitted for treatment, and the hospital was required to keep a fairly detailed record of patient hospitalizations. From the outset, the HSPC emphasized the importance of gathering data on hospital utilization to support informed and knowledgeable debate about Saskatchewan's experiment in hospitalization coverage. As health planners and administrators Mott, Rosenfeld, and their cohort stressed the need to develop technical abilities that would put scientific knowledge to the service of humanity. To determine how best to gather information and monitor the performance of the hospitalization plan, Mott consulted American biostatistician Anthony Ciocco, who provided "help in sizing up our personnel requirements in the field of studies and statistics."[35] In 1947, Ciocco, employed at the time by the US Public Health Service, wrote a joint report with Frances Weekes of Canada's Dominion Bureau of Statistics (a precursor to Statistics Canada) on statistical procedures for the hospitalization plan. The report made recommendations on how to collect two needed sets of data for the purposes of health planning: routine data on everyday usage of insured hospital services; and data on the Saskatchewan population for the purposes of calculating rates. Data on patients and hospital usage would be gathered through the standard hospitalization card and based on hospital discharge information. This information would be used by the HSPC to assess the operation of the hospitalization plan in its early years.[36]

Data was also critical if Mott and the CCF were to successfully defend the government's health program—especially the hospitalization plan. In January 1947 Mott wrote to Weinerman for information he could use to shore up support:

> The 1947 session of our Legislative Assembly is due to start before the end of January. Our whole program will be subject to scrutiny during the session, both by our friends and by the Opposition. One criticism which is being heard here and there throughout the

province is that this program is going to be far more costly than small local programs such as those scattered here and there in the province in the past. One point of attack will undoubtedly be the overhead expenses of this provide wide program which we hope to keep below 10 percent, even this first year.

Mott thought friends at the US Social Security Board staff might have gathered data on administrative costs in countries with health insurance, as part of its own support for the Wagner-Murray-Dingell Bill: "I recall tossing off a few figures in my own testimony of the Wagner-Murray-Dingell Bill but I cannot recall their source at the moment." A few weeks later, Weinerman sent Mott a package of material suggested by Mott's former colleagues: Margaret Klem of the Social Security Administration, with whom Mott worked in the US Department of Agriculture Interbureau Committee on Postwar Problems; Jess Yaukey (who suggested Mott look at the report "Activities of an Experimental Rural Health Program,") and Louis Reed, who had prepared a table on "foreign administrative expenses in comparison with those of Blue Cross and medical society plans." Weinerman suggested Mott also draw upon the British experience through the reports of the British Ministry of Health.[37]

Mott was especially anxious in his letters to Weinerman to hear about the fates of his other former staff in Washington, asking after them by name. Mott's ongoing connection and concern was both personal and professional. For his part, Weinerman expressed to Mott his increasing anxiety about the future of the rural health programs they had built. With the disbanding of the remnants of the FSA rural health programs in early 1947, Weinerman spoke to Mott of the "witch hunt atmosphere around town these days." Like so many others, he left the US public service, entering the Harvard School of Public Health, with a recommendation from Mott. In February 1947, Mott responded to his friend with thanks, encouragement, and a handwritten note below typed correspondence.

It was a subtle apology for not being able to offer Weinerman a place in Saskatchewan: "Don't get too damned discouraged these days—FHA atmosphere must be awful. Wish you were here but I'm having to feel my way pretty carefully and use a Canadian where one can fill the bill."[38] Even in Mott's earliest days in the province, he obviously experienced some animus to his presence as an outsider to Saskatchewan. He would articulate this feeling again in a 1951 letter to Sigerist when he had decided to leave the province for Washington.

Scholars such as Seymour Lipset and Aleck Ostry have argued that hospitalization coverage was politically astute in the sense that everyone approved of it. Most critically, unlike other aspects of CCF health policy (lay governance, regionalized services, multidisciplinary health centres, alternatives to fee-for-service payment) it did not encounter sustained physician opposition. "It was practically the only reform in the period which was not opposed by organized medicine," Ostry argued, because it improved physicians' financial position and enhanced the services they could provide to patients.[39] However, implementation was certainly not entirely free of tension. In Douglas's telling, both physicians and hospitals initially resisted:

> Doctors were very much opposed, not because they objected to the idea of hospital insurance, but because they felt this was the beginning of socialized medicine. The hospital people weren't too happy about it, and about three weeks before the plan was to go into effect the entire executive of the Saskatchewan Hospital Association marched into my office and said, they were not prepared to co-operate with our legislation dated to become valid in January 1947. Their objections were on the grounds that the government would virtually take over the hospitals. Since we were going to pay all the bills, it was only natural that we would control the hospitals. We would be appointing auditors and managers,

and we would take control of municipal hospitals, and what was
even worse, we would take control of the private hospitals, particularly those run by the churches. I explained that our intention
was to centralize finance and de-centralize administration. We
would collect the money and then pay the hospitals for the care
given to the people protected under our plan. As far as we were
concerned, the running of the hospital would continue to be in
the hands of hospital administrators. But I told them that if they
couldn't run the hospitals under this plan then on 1 January, we
would take over the hospitals. I suggested that they think it over
and return later to give me their decision. They decided to go
along but they were most reluctant; they were quite prepared to
begin protesting the moment we took over the hospitals.[40]

In the end, hospitalization coverage proved double-edged for
Douglas. It stymied the move toward a health centre model of socialized care and laid the groundwork for future battles by enhancing
the power of key institutional actors, especially physicians and hospital administrators.[41]

Nevertheless, public use of insured hospital care was immediately high, which made the program politically valuable. It was also
expensive. According to a presentation given by Fred Mott to the
American Public Health Association in October 1947, the program
paid out more than $3 million to hospitals in its first six months
of operation, for an average of 10,000 patient accounts per month.
Saskatchewan's early hospital utilization rates were 1600 days per
1000 covered population per annum. From Mott's perspective, this
frequent use of the system was an outcome of previously unmet
health care demand and was "surely a far truer measure of real need
than the lower ratios characteristic of voluntary plans, with their
limited benefits and selective coverage."[42]

The SHSP broadened the revenue base for hospital care dramatically, through both the direct hospitalization tax and provincial

grants to hospitals and UHDs. The CCF funded hospital construction to the tune of $827,000 between 1945 and 1949.[43] By 1949, there were 78 UHDs, which together operated 40 percent of all hospital beds in Saskatchewan.

From the outset, funds raised through the tax were supplemented by provincial general revenue. In late 1947, 60 percent of the cost of the program was funded through the personal tax; 40 percent was funded from general revenue.[44] Prior to the plan's introduction, the taxation base of municipal governments was too small to adequately provide universal hospital services. The SHSP provided a more stable and reliable financial basis for hospital care, which is one reason municipal governments and emergent health districts and regions supported it.

Mott and Rosenfeld, as the HSPC's two most senior planners, promoted the hospitalization program, especially to elite health care stakeholders, writing articles and delivering speeches across the country. Mott spoke to the June 1947 meeting of the Canadian Medical Association (CMA) in Winnipeg, in which he outlined the Saskatchewan government's program for health reform. Mott pointed out this was the first universal hospitalization program in North America, and an historic achievement. Publicly insured and administered hospital care was not, however, the main focus of Mott's speech to the CMA. Speaking to "the social application of medical knowledge, in all its broad connotations," Mott emphasized the need for a comprehensive health program, in which hospitalization was "an integral part of a broad system of health services organized in relation to the fundamental social and economic characteristics of the province," which was predominantly rural and in the midst of significant population loss.[45] The main elements of this program were to be delivered through regional health units, in which treatment and preventive services would be melded. Regional boards were to be elected by district health councils, themselves made up of municipal representatives. That same year, writing in *Physicians'*

Forum, Mott referred to this "network" of health care, built upon district hospitals and regional health centres where specialist care and recent technologies would be accessible to local practitioners and their patients. The network would rely upon the principles of co-operative group physician practice, and capitation for physician payment, to ensure affordability in a public system.[46]

Mott again reminded his audience that Saskatchewan's "program of prepaid hospital care" was the only one of its kind in North America, an important step in an "overall program to provide adequate health services for every person in the province regardless of financial capacity." Its key principles were to achieve high standards of individual and community health through "removal of the economic barrier" to hospital care and to distribute the costs of hospitalization across the population. At the June CMA meeting, Mott emphasized the government's aim to provide "the opportunity for full participation in the benefit of scientific progress in the field of medicine ... Working out methods for using scientific and technical knowledge in the cause of humanity is the great central problem of our time." In this, Mott placed Saskatchewan in an international context, working towards reform alongside the UK, Sweden, France, the Netherlands, Australia, and South America—as well as the US. Mott's speech to the CMA emphasized community and social context, signaling the intent to create an integrated health care system in which hospitalization would play its role alongside efforts in community health, including public health and prevention.

It should not be surprising that senior health planners began to believe in the indispensability of their own program, and invest in its image of success. In June 1947, Len Rosenfeld argued in the pages of the quarterly *Public Affairs*, "hospitalization insurance has become established as a significant factor in the health security of the people of North America."[47] A universal, compulsory government-administered plan, such as Saskatchewan had introduced, was necessary to deal with the gaps in provision experienced in voluntary schemes in which rural people and those less economically secure were unlikely to be able to access or afford hospital insurance coverage. Rosenfeld highlighted the high level of popular support enjoyed by the SHSP: 800,000 individuals in 315,000 families had registered and paid their taxes to the program within the first six months of its operation, virtually every resident in the eligible population of 825,000.[48] Rosenfeld also defended the Province's decision to provide financial support for hospitalization in advance of necessary human and institutional resources, arguing that the SHSP allowed for the development of health care capacity. This was a reversed "if you build it they will come" justification (as in, "they will come and it will be built"), which may in fact have been accurate. Despite the apparent shortage of hospital beds, physicians, and nurses, the plan funded 35,000 hospital admissions in the first three months.[49]

Learning largely through trial and error, the plan had to develop three different methods of calculating payments to hospitals over its first five years of existence. The first payment method was a points and mill-rate system based on a 1943 proposal by Dr. Harry Agnew of the Canadian Hospital Council. The SHSP established a committee of physicians, nurses, and hospital administrators to work out how to apply this formula in Saskatchewan. A schedule was established that gave all hospitals a basic number of points, with higher points up to a maximum, given for hospitals according to "physical facilities and procedures available, but also [taking] into account the qualifications of personnel." Hospitals were paid an amount per patient day of stay based upon a negotiated mill rate multiplied by the number of points, with the mill rate declining after the first ten days of stay. For example, "if a hospital received 800 points, it would be paid at a rate of 800 x 6.5 mills, or $5.20 per day for the first 10 days of the patient's stay, $4.80 for the second 10 days, and $4.40 per day beyond 20 days. These rates were intended to cover all benefits provided under the plan." This method of payment was intended to encourage hospitals to provide complete, high-quality hospital services with qualified staff. By giving hospitals with greater amenities higher points (and therefore payments), the SHSP hoped to provide incentives for facility improvements. It was quickly discovered, however, that the payment plan caused a lot of financial difficulties for some hospitals, while others made a significant profit, which was not a desired outcome in a taxpayer-funded system. According to an analysis written by HSPC staff and published in the *American Journal of Public Health* in 1953, "The point rating system was revealed as arbitrary, failing to take into account legitimate differences in operating costs as between individual hospitals."[50]

Upward cost pressures caused difficulties from the start. The SHSP informed hospitals that 80 percent of their deficits would be covered by the plan if hospitals provided evidence to prove they were making efforts to contain costs and improve efficiency. In 1948, the points system was discarded in favour of a per-diem rate per patient day, based on estimated costs of efficient hospital operations, with daily rates again varying by length of hospital stay. General hospitals with more than fifteen beds were required to submit annual budgets, based on a standardized accounting procedure introduced the previous year. The government established a Rate Board that met with the administration of any hospital that requested a meeting. At the same time, the SHSP attempted to tighten hospital spending by agreeing to fund only 50 percent of any deficits incurred by hospitals with more than 50 beds, and 80 percent of deficits in hospitals with 15–49 beds. The smallest hospitals would have their deficits covered entirely if necessary, but also had to agree to administrative oversight from the Province should deficits recur.

But the per-diem system came with its own distortions. As the government quickly learned, making payments based entirely on the number of inpatient days encouraged some hospitals to keep patients longer than necessary: higher occupancy meant higher hospital revenues. Occupancy rates were seasonal, resulting in uneven cash flow from the SHSP. Further discussions between the health department and hospitals took place in 1950, and in 1951 the SHSP introduced yet another payment model: a stable semi-monthly lump-sum payment to hospitals, with an additional per-diem rate paid on patient days. Overall funding was determined by a hospital's annual budget. The lump-sum portion of funding was calculated at slightly above estimated fixed costs (such as physical plant, heating, and salaries); a now-reduced per-diem payment was calculated at slightly below the patient costs that fluctuated with occupancy (such as food, laundry, and drugs). The advantage to hospitals of this formula was that they would receive stable financial transfers from the SHSP twice a month, alleviating the problem of cash flow. The SHSP health planners argued that this formula would "reverse the financial incentives to hospital management in regard to occupancy."[51] Because hospitals would lose money for variable per-diem costs above budget, there was no longer a financial incentive to let patient stays lengthen or admit a high number of patients. According to the SHSP, this strategy resulted in a leveling off of costs in facilities where admissions and lengths of stay were higher than the provincial average.

The SHSP experienced a steep learning curve in its first five years of operation. This was not surprising, given the pace of implementation, and the shortage of comparable systems in North America from which to learn. Whatever the glitches, its popularity was demonstrated by the public's eagerness to use the new health benefits. High utilization served to intensify the pressures on the HSPC to focus more and more on the tertiary, acute-care end of health services, regardless of Mott and Rosenfeld's early intentions. Hospitalization did eat up resources. In 1947–48, the Province was spending over $10 million dollars a year on health services, 20 percent of its budget, up from six percent of the provincial budget in the year before the CCF came to power.[52] Nearly $7 million of this spending was on the SHSP.[53] Hospitalization costs increased significantly every year during the program's first decade. Hospitalization funding formula adjustments slowed the increases from 1952 on, but by then per-capita costs had doubled. Aleck Ostry argues that "explosive" growth in Saskatchewan's hospital infrastructure significantly surpassed the national average, and claims that by the mid-1950s Saskatchewan residents were the "most hospitalized" in Canada.[54] This has to be put in proper context, however, since Ostry is comparing the growth rate of hospital services and utilization in Saskatchewan to those in provinces without universal public hospitalization insurance. Expansion in the SHSP was driven by patient demand, some of it pent up from pre-insurance days when hospital care was prohibitively expensive for many people, and there were too few hospital beds to meet the need. Demand for hospitalization might also have been driven by the fact that, while hospital care was insured, physician care (outside of hospital) was not. Many residents likely sought out hospital care as a way to get basic primary care needs met, in the absence of universal coverage for medical care.

The SHSP was not free from criticism—including from its own architects and supporters. Rosenfeld recognized legitimate criticism of the $5 flat personal tax rate for each member of a household up to the $30 maximum, and early on considered a graduated tax for families as potentially more equitable.[55] Douglas also said later he had reservations about the per-capita tax:

> all of it ought not to be financed on a per capita basis. This means each family pays the same tax irrespective of whether their income is two thousand or a hundred thousand dollars a year, which to me is retrogression of the worst sort. Someday I would like to see a nominal per capita tax of five or ten dollars a family, five for the husband, five for the wife, and ten dollars maximum for the family.[56]

The CCF could have introduced a hospital system that was free at the point of access, as New Zealand Labour had done, for example. Surprisingly, Douglas believed that some fee was desirable and did not consider "free" services to be a point of principle:

I think people appreciate something if they've paid for it. If you give people a card from Santa Claus entitling them to free hospital services, it is not good psychology. But the amount should be sufficiently small that it doesn't impose financial burdens on anybody.[57]

Many advocates of socialized medicine in Saskatchewan would not have agreed with Douglas on this point.

The plan's greatest structural inequity, however, was its failure to ensure that Indigenous peoples benefited equally. Indigenous peoples sought access to medical care, but in the 1940s the Canadian health system provided them with utterly inadequate medical care. Even if hospital care was accessible to Indigenous people, Maureen Lux demonstrates that in western Canada and in the north, segregation was frequent: "The Indian annexes, Indian wings, and basement wards, demanded by community prejudice and inadequately funded by the state, actively shaped inequality and constructed an image of Aboriginal people as less worthy of care."[58]

For several reasons, the CCF's health policy did little to address the problem of differential access to care. In 1947, the HSPC discussed the inclusion of treaty peoples in the SHSP plan, but decided against it because the federal government refused to cover the cost of SHSP coverage for treaty Indians.[59] For its part, the federal government consistently denied the treaty right to health care in this period. The HSPC bemoaned this reality but chose not to waive the personal tax and provide coverage to the same care available to non-Indigenous peoples. Small modifications did broaden access in a piecemeal way. By the early 1950s, SHSP coverage was extended to status Indians who paid voluntarily into the plan, but only if they had been living off reserve for a minimum of eighteen months.[60] Discussions between federal and provincial officials about the full inclusion of status Indian peoples in the provincial plan continued into the 1950s without resolution.

The situation of non-status and Métis peoples is harder to trace. Little health data was collected on northern Saskatchewan Indigenous peoples before the 1960s.[61] While in theory Métis peoples should have gained access to improved health services equal to the white population, in reality this was not the case. For example, the SHSP did not extend to the north (that is, the region of the province north of the 55th parallel) until January 1, 1959. The majority of the population in the northern half of the province was Indigenous (status, non-status, and Métis). Non-compulsory hospitalization coverage was introduced in the north in 1948, but according to David Quiring it was mostly non-Indigenous peoples who opted in to the provincial plan. This may have been due to the poverty of Indigenous northerners, who may have found the premiums onerous. Beginning in 1945, the Medical Services Branch provided medical and hospital care for "indigents" in the north, but it still left the majority without SHSP coverage. By 1953, there were 1355 insured people in the region, only 17 percent of the non-status northern population.[62]

In the early years of its mandate, the CCF made some efforts to improve northern health care through the expansion of the existing outpost hospitals, more properly understood as nursing stations, at Buffalo Narrows (originally built by the Red Cross) and Cumberland House (a small log hospital built by local residents), and the creation of three new outpost facilities at Snake Lake (Pinehouse), Sandy Bay, and Stony Rapids.[63] In 1945, the CCF sent two nurses to New York to train as midwives, who then served northern women in Cumberland House and Buffalo Narrows. The outpost system, however, provided inferior health care coverage. In the late 1940s outpost facilities lacked modern diagnostic equipment, such as x-rays or laboratories. They were sparsely staffed by public health nurses: between 1944 and 1957 there were "only eight in the north at any given time."[64] Nursing care in the north was not free at the point of access; it operated on a fee-for-service basis. Outpost nurses were expected to try to collect some form of payment from patients, whether cash or in-kind services, such as providing wood. Living and working in poor northern communities, nurses resisted this role as fee collectors and "requested that they not be put in a position of having to badger people for payment."[65] Nurses struggled to meet increasing patient demand. In 1952 Buffalo Narrows alone handled 1550 outpatient visits.[66]

As nursing historian Lesley McBain has noted, the nurses who lived and worked in northern communities not only provided primary medical care, they promoted ways of living and western medicine within a colonialist paradigm that sought to displace Indigenous forms of knowledge and healing. This dynamic created an uneasy tension, what she calls an "ambiguity," in nurses' relationships with Indigenous patients. State policies of medicalization and modernization necessarily evolved on the ground. Not all northern public health nurses (who were white) responded in the same way to working in Indigenous communities. Some were more empathetic and respectful of Indigenous ways of life than others. The shortage of resources also meant nurses had to be flexible and innovative. There was a limit to how interventionist they could be in the lives of their patients given the daily realities of northern nursing, in communities where nurses were also reliant on the broader community for support.

Having said this, public health nurses did undertake work beyond physical care that revealed an underlying assumption about the inferiority of Indigenous traditions and ways of life. Nurses established a variety of organizations and clubs intended to assimilate Indigenous peoples into "modern" modes of living, such as women's auxiliaries, clubs for mothers with new babies, or craft clubs. Some of these clubs raised money to improve access to services such as dentists. Nurses promoted the message of assimilation into mainstream health norms and the "right" ways of living through presentations, films, slides, posters, and leaflets on topics such as handwashing, dental care, sanitation, child rearing, and how to prevent tuberculosis and venereal diseases. Health information was not translated into Indigenous languages, and white nurses who spoke only English had to rely on Indigenous translators in their daily work. Some felt they had more success with children than adults. One nurse encouraged the community's children to visit her home "hoping they may gain some knowledge of cleanliness and the ways of living properly."[67] Nurses also attempted to instruct northern women on changing their families' diets in accordance with the new Canada Food Guide, with its emphasis on fresh fruit and vegetables, as well as dairy products. Some nurses recognized these guidelines as unrealistic in the northern context, where many people continued to eat a traditional diet based upon wild meat, fish, and local plants. Other nurses "did not see the nutritional value of country food."[68]

After an early phase of expansion in the outpost network, the CCF "rested on its laurels."[69] For example, calls to upgrade Cumberland House were rejected. Until the mid-1950s, when an office was opened in Prince Albert, northern outpost hospitals were overseen by distant health officials in Regina. The Department of Public Health employed a part-time medical officer of health, who visited the north only four times a year. In addition to the nursing outposts, the CCF government also built new hospitals in LaRonge and Uranium City, which were predominantly non-Indigenous communities, while the Catholic church operated facilities at Ile-a-la-Crosse and La Loche, which served Indigenous peoples in the western part of the north, supported by the provincial and federal governments. In the early 1950s, Ile-a-la-Crosse had 22 beds, four nurses, and one doctor, while the La Loche hospital had ten beds and was operated by two nurses, with occasional visits from the Ile-a-la-Crosse physician. The province provided some operating costs, and a patient per diem. Thus, as late as the mid-1950s, health care for the entire north was provided by three physicians (two of whom were located in the white mining town of Uranium City) and a total of twelve nurses.[70] Indigenous patients in the central and western regions of northern Saskatchewan were especially poorly served.

Until the early 1950s, the leading cause of death among the Indigenous population was tuberculosis. Non-status Indigenous peoples also suffered a very high incidence of the disease. In the decade after the Second World War, rates of Indigenous tuberculosis did decline as a result of better screening programs and the impact of treatment with streptomycin. In the early 1950s, the rate of tuberculosis in northern Saskatchewan was still alarming: 400 cases per 100,000 population—over 20 times the provincial rate of 18.5 per 100,000.[71] Rather than formulate an independent policy or programs to combat Indigenous tuberculosis, the CCF relied on and supported the Saskatchewan Anti-Tuberculosis League (SATL) for tuberculosis treatment. The SATL funded its efforts through private donations, user fees, and money from all levels of government. Key figures in the SATL, such as Dr. R.G. Ferguson, held racist views of Indigenous peoples as "primitive" and a biologically inferior race to whites. The SATL also saw Indigenous people as a menace to the white population because of their high tuberculosis rates, a view shared by anti-tuberculosis advocates across Canada. There is no indication that the CCF, once in power, took issue with these views, which underpinned the SATL's approach to tuberculosis care for Indigenous peoples.

The SATL's interest in Indigenous tuberculosis had intensified in the 1920s. Ferguson was medical superintendent of the Qu'Appelle sanatorium from 1917 to 1948. Qu'Appelle did not accept Indigenous patients until the 1920s, when demand for the institutional care of whites had declined, and anxieties about tuberculosis shifted towards the putative risk of infection posed by diseased Indigenous peoples. "Tuberculosis associations had increased public awareness of tuberculosis prevention and treatment, and exerted steady pressure on the federal government to control the tuberculosis 'menace' on reserves."[72] Ferguson proposed an investigation into Indigenous tuberculosis, and a trial of the controversial BCG vaccine on Indigenous children. This project was supported by the National Research Council and the federal Department of Indian Affairs.

As Mary-Ellen Kelm has shown in the case of British Columbia, health research studies in Indigenous communities during this period were "key to a society that sought control through knowledge and the creation of a colonizing archive of data, rather than overt displays of force." Studies resulted in increased medical surveillance, but also delayed action and treatment. As "thousands of Aboriginal bodies came under the gaze of medical researchers," little was done to address the underlying social and economic causes of high tuberculosis rates.[73] Colonialist views of Indigenous bodies were articulated openly. In his 1928 BCG-trial preliminary report, Ferguson concluded that Indigenous peoples were more susceptible to tuberculosis because they lacked "white blood"—the same cause of their primitiveness.

Yet intervention, however paternalistic and inadequate, showed that improved health was possible with greater resources. Ferguson and the SATL established the Qu'Appelle Indian Demonstration Health Unit in 1930, with federal financial aid. The project did not focus only on vaccine testing, but also upon marginally improving living conditions and segregating active cases of tuberculosis. New homes were built, wells dug, families provided with chickens and garden seeds, and extra nourishment given to pregnant women and children. The project had a full-time public health nurse, who treated children suffering from infectious disease, and a medical officer, Dr. A.B. Simes. Members of the community with active tuberculosis were admitted to hospital. Within two years, even before the start of the BCG trial, the tuberculosis rate in the Qu'Appelle agency had been cut in half. The comparatively generous resources linked to Ferguson's BCG trial, however, certainly were not the norm. Nor did the study result in the expanded supports that would have improved Indigenous health.

Ferguson's vaccine trials began in March 1933 and ran until 1945. BCG vaccines were administered to 306 children; 303 control subjects were not vaccinated. Six vaccinated children developed tuberculosis and two died; 29 unvaccinated children developed the disease, and nine died. The trial was considered a success. What became clear during the trials, however, was that poverty and poor health conditions on reserves contributed to high mortality rates from diseases other than tuberculosis. Seventy-seven of the trial's participants died before their first birthdays—an astonishing infant mortality rate of 12 percent. After seven years, 105 children had died—17 percent of the trial group—mostly from gastroenteritis or pneumonia. "The most obvious result of the BCG vaccine trials was that poverty, not tuberculosis, was the greatest threat to Native infants," Lux concludes.[74] Knowledge about the persistence of very preventable and deadly health problems failed to translate into reformed policy at the federal or provincial levels.

The BCG trials marked an increased SATL focus on combating tuberculosis in Indigenous communities, extending beyond status and reserve peoples. But this campaign was slow to reach the north. According to David Quiring, the SATL's efforts in the north began in earnest only in the early 1950s, first through undertaking more aggressive diagnosis. The federal government provided funds for x-ray equipment at provincial outpost hospitals at Sandy Bay, Cumberland House, and Buffalo Narrows. Throughout the decade, outpost nurses employed by the province administered the BCG vaccine, although sporadically. Prevention and treatment measures did, however, have an impact. By 1960, the rate of tuberculosis in northern Saskatchewan had fallen to 40 per 100,000 population.[75]

This improvement came at a price. Northerners were sent south in significant numbers for treatment at sanatoria in Fort Qu'Appelle, Saskatoon, or Prince Albert, far from their home communities. In 1956, the province paid the SATL for over 25,000 inpatient days of sanatoria care for northern patients. Stays were often long—months or years—were disruptive to family and community life, and caused fear and suffering for some patients. Family could rarely visit distant sanatoria. Patients, especially children, experienced terrible loneliness.[76] The isolation from family sometimes meant people tried to avoid tuberculosis hospitals, but pressure was put on Indigenous people to accept treatment and institutionalization. Some resisted sanatorium care by leaving the institution. Doing so came with risks, however. Although provincial health regulations allowed for less coercion than did federal laws applying to status Indians, the RCMP in Saskatchewan were deployed to return patients to hospital; according to Quiring, some resisters were confined to locked psychiatric wards.[77]

Jurisdictional confusion and disputes over responsibility for Indigenous health between the federal and provincial governments made any reform more difficult, but it cannot entirely explain the CCF's record on Indigenous health. Neither do the admittedly significant challenges to improving care in a small northern population spread over vast distances with poor or non-existent transportation. Rather than integrate Indigenous northerners into the process of health reform, the CCF denied them an equal voice in developing their own health care. Services were overseen by southern experts in the Department of Public Health's Medical Services Branch and the Department of Natural Resources. The north was also excluded from HSPC planning, whether from the SHSP or the health regions framework. Indigenous health in the north was outside the HSPC's remit and this, in effect, rendered Indigenous health needs invisible in the CCF's health care planning process. Quiring argues, "the primary reason for having separate policies for the north and the south appeared to be that government, knowing that most northerners could not afford the plan, did not want the administrative and policy difficulties of creating a workable plan for the north." Acknowledging the CCF's "humanitarian" motivations, Quiring concludes that it had a colonialist mentality towards the north, which surely cannot be denied.[78]

With Mott and Rosenfeld investing most of their energy setting up the hospitalization insurance program, the establishment of health regions received less attention than it should have. Senior health planners did try to rectify this. In April 1948, Rosenfeld wrote to his former US colleague Mildred Walker, Health Consultant with the US Children's Bureau, that his role was shifting away from hospitalization towards struggling regional health services.[79] But Rosenfeld left Saskatchewan a few months later. He was replaced as secretary of the HSPC by Malcolm Taylor. After 1948, expansion of health regions essentially stopped. The Swift Current "model" (discussed in chapter 4) did not grow to other regions. It stalled.

As a result, integrating the new hospitalization plan (which was centrally administered) with the regionalized scheme suggested by the Sigerist Commission became that much more difficult. Hospitalization was moving ahead more quickly than other elements. In 1945, the HSPC had proposed a holistic model that emphasized integration, coordination, and innovative medical and preventive care delivery through health institutions from health centres on up. The health regions constituted the key link in this proposed system, the structure that connected the parts. The success of the health regions was therefore a lynchpin, if the model was to be realized.

Scholars such as Joan Feather have suggested that the centralized nature of the hospital insurance plan may have sealed the fate of the health regions. From an historical perspective, it is easy to conclude that health planners failed to find a successful method with which to integrate a hospitalization insurance plan, funded and overseen by a provincial body, into the Sigerist plan for a model that was intentionally decentralized and overseen by lay regional boards. At least in the first few years after hospitalization was introduced, the HSPC continued to try to find ways to make the health-regions framework work. Mott continued to struggle with the challenge of coordination and the integration of preventive and therapeutic capacity, which was a key principle of the health centre model. Why did their efforts not pay off?

The complexity of the existing system was part of the problem. In 1946 Saskatchewan's health program had two distinct institutional branches: the HSPC and the Department of Public Health. Mott was Chair of the HSPC, but became Deputy Minister of the Department of Public Health only in 1950. The Department oversaw not only services such as infectious disease control, but also many of the health programs that Saskatchewan had developed prior to the CCF's election, most notably mental health services and cancer care, as well as northern health care as we have seen. The Department also ran the CCF's new air ambulance service. The HSPC was responsible for developing a provincial plan for hospital and medical services, including oversight of future health care services administered by health regions and municipalities. It also administered medical care for groups receiving public assistance. Mott could see that close coordination of the Department and the HSPC was essential. In reality, co-operation between the two bodies may not have been easy.

Mott intended the health region to be an "important point of coordination"—not least between the HSPC and the Department of Public Health.[80] The boundaries of health regions were carefully shaped to correspond to what Mott called natural trading areas, within which trading centers were chosen as sites for district hospitals and preventive services. Public health districts and UHDs were to have common boundaries, to make coordination between prevention and cure possible. Specialist and advanced diagnostic services, as well as public health administration, were all to be located at the health region's major centre, where a division of regional health services would be located. The health officer for each region would work closely with a regional health board, "elected on the basis of population by district health councils, which consist of representatives from all municipalities in the area." The HSPC intended that primary medical care provision and hospital care would work together, and where possible occupy shared space. Mott suggested that health centres could either be incorporated into hospital buildings or be located nearby. Physicians' offices might also be housed in district or "outpost" hospitals. "District hospitals can provide a base for supplying local practitioners with facilities and equipment," Mott argued in 1947. In the regional centers, Mott advocated the creation of group-practice units of specialists, who were to serve their entire region, or refer their patients to the highest level of tertiary care, the large urban medical centres.[81]

Implementing such a regional model might have been more straightforward if all hospitals in the province had been "socialized" and centrally administered by the SHSP. In reality, the HSPC provided oversight and funding to hospitals that were variously run by voluntary organizations, UHDs, municipalities, and religious orders. HSPC planners resisted from the outset the charge that they sought to centralize the administration of hospital care. The UHDs and local hospitals retained their administrative roles, even as they became increasingly powerful institutional actors. This, in fact, created a dilemma for the HSPC, since the hospitals had their own governance structures and, from 1947 onward, a significant and growing resource base through SHPS transfers. While the HSPC was committed to the larger integrated model framed by the Sigerist Report, even after the passage of the Hospitalization Act some municipalities (especially urban centres), UHDs, and private hospitals were less committed. Hospitalization insurance was enormously and immediately popular with the public, and in fairly short order became a pathway for municipalities and districts to provide services that were in high public demand, and in the process secure valued resources for their communities. By contrast, proposed health regions were complex structures, promising much less tangible or immediate benefits—especially in the absence of insured physician services.

Ultimately, the intent was to include programs of general

medical care in the health regions. Without financial support from
the federal government for any element of its program, however, in
the late 1940s and early 1950s Saskatchewan could not afford further
expansion of services. Without a crystal ball, health planners did not
know that the federal government would delay the establishment of
health insurance for a number of years. Mott, fresh out of the US
context where national health insurance bills had emerged and failed,
would have had reason for pessimism. Without a broader program
for medical care province-wide, which would enable more regions to
provide medical coverage, Mott and Rosenfeld were trying to solve
the health regions puzzle with a critical piece missing.

The one break-out exception was the Swift Current Health
Region No.1. Chapter 4 argued that the creation of the province's
first health region in the Swift Current area was a mixed blessing
for HSPC health planners. Publicly, the government lauded Swift
Current as a model. Inside the government, views on Swift Current
were somewhat complicated. HSPC planners had lost control in
Swift Current. Their input into how and when the region developed
its health services was limited as local advocates moved ahead on
their own. In certain key ways, the region diverged from the plan
for regional health services put forward by the HSPC in 1945, especially in its formula for physician payment. In Health Region No. 1
physicians were paid on a fee-for-service basis. There was no attempt
to institute group practice or salaried payment—the original recommendation of the HSPC. Its dental care program, from the
HSPC's point of view, was too focused on restorative treatment
with not enough attention paid to prevention. In a province with a
serious dentist shortage, the Swift Current dental model could not
be broadly applied. Despite these concerns, once it was established,
the HSPC could not afford to let Swift Current fail. It had become
too closely identified with the CCF's health program. But problems
remained. Feather notes "there were continual struggles between
regions and province over the program's orientation."[82]

Under the terms of the Act, the establishment of health regions required public support and agreement and coordination among multiple local actors. The HSPC could not legally compel any community to participate in the regional framework. The hope that the impetus to form health regions would come from the bottom up, which had animated the HSPC in the first few years of its existence, began to fade in the late 1940s. The HSPC had few means to leverage physician buy-in to health regions, or to models like group practice. Opposition to the health regions was especially strong in larger urban centres where private practice was more economically viable than in rural areas, and where private medical insurance schemes continued to grow after the election of the CCF.

By 1951, seven health regions had been formed, out of the fourteen originally planned. These were Swift Current (1945), Assiniboia-Gravelbourg (1947), Weyburn-Estevan (1945), Moose Jaw (1946), North Battleford (1947), Meadow Lake (1946), and Prince Albert (1951).[83] The province also operated the Northern Administration District. Early advocacy by the HSPC had led to the quick establishment of several health regions, but after Rosenfeld's departure in 1948 only one region was organized. Notably, neither Regina nor Saskatoon had established health regions by 1951. As the most important locations of specialist and tertiary health services in the province, their absence challenged the overall goal of coordination of care, and the workability of the model.

Before his departure, Rosenfeld had tried to establish regional services in North Battleford and Saskatoon. The North Battleford campaign was successful; Saskatoon's was not. Planning documents for Saskatoon suggest the HSPC attempted to persuade the City of Saskatoon that there were benefits to a health region that encompassed the city and the outlying rural area. The concept of the trading area, based on existing interaction between rural and urban settings, was fundamental to the HSPC's planning model, but this appears to have been a hard sell to an urban municipality.

Saskatoon had operated its own health department for over 30 years and had little incentive to relinquish its authority to a regional board and regional health staff. To counter potential urban ambivalence, the HSPC argued "the health status of an urban community is very closely inter-related with the health of the surrounding rural areas," and used the fear of infectious disease as a point of persuasion. Typhoid, diphtheria, scarlet fever, and other diseases could spread from rural to urban areas through "food, water and contact," it cautioned. "Any deterioration of the health status in the surrounding rural areas … is reflected in the urban community." The HSPC also asserted that rural and urban communities had a mutually beneficial health care relationship, albeit one that could be improved. Rural residents in the Saskatoon area naturally turned to the city for medical specialists and advanced diagnostics; at the same time, rural use of urban facilities contributed to urban growth and development. The proposed Saskatoon Health Region would constitute a conscious effort to pool urban and rural resources, to create a "complete and adequate unit of public health service."[84]

It is important to note that, in these conversations, the term "public health" was not limited to the provision of sanitation or communicable disease prevention. The CCF used the term in a capacious manner, consistent with their overall emphasis on the integration of prevention and cure. This was signaled by the fact that Premier Douglas was the Minister of Public Health, overseeing the Department of Public Health. In other words, the term "public health" had potentially broad connotations. The HSPC's regional planning documents referred to three major factors that shaped the health of the community: the standard of living, "including standards of nutrition, housing, clothing, recreation, cultural development and adequacy of medical care"; educational standards, "which will determine the rapidity with which the community can grasp principles of hygiene … and methods and responsibilities in promoting individual and community health standards;" and a public health service with "good coordination between preventive and treatment services and effective participation of trained health personnel in determining standards of community development."[85]

Both the Saskatoon and North Battleford health region plans listed the following minimum services that should be provided by local health units within the region: maternal and child hygiene; communicable disease control; school hygiene; mental hygiene; sanitation, including supervision of the water, milk, and food supplies; health education; and vital-statistics records maintenance. Full-time public health personnel would be assigned to the region by the Department of Public Health, who would develop services in consultation with the elected district health councils and regional board. Their efforts would be overseen by a regional health officer.

When it came to the curative framework, however, the two plans diverged. The HSPC's regional plan for Saskatoon placed a priority on a broad public health mandate, but proposed that "no provision be made for the development of general medical care." The Saskatoon health region plan referred to the benefit of group medical practices at regional and district centres, "in keeping with modern trends in medical care," but the main purpose of the health region was stated to be the establishment of adequate public health services. In other words, the HSPC did not advance the Swift Current model (comprehensive health care provision, including physician services, hospitalization, and dental care) in the case of the proposed Saskatoon Health Region. The Province would only pay for 50 percent of the cost of public health services in urban parts of the region, and two-thirds of costs in rural portions, in addition to providing any buildings or furnishings needed to operate the program.

The HSPC's caution against proceeding to develop a general medical care program in the Saskatoon region was not a blanket policy. Documents for the proposed North Battleford Health Region, developed during the same time period (1946–48), did not oppose medical care coverage by the health region. In a very similarly

worded plan to the one proposed for Saskatoon, which prioritized
the provision of public health services, the HSPC's plan for North
Battleford stated, "additional services such as general medical care,
dental care, special diagnostic service be developed at the discre-
tion of the Regional Board, subject to the approval of the Minister
of Public Health." Subject to approval, the Province would pay 50
percent of the cost of specialist consultations and diagnostics, 50 percent of dental care, and 25 cents per capita for all persons covered by
a general medical services scheme introduced by the region. In this
event, the North Battleford Health Region did not opt for medical
or dental care provision.[86]

There were several potential reasons why the HSPC enter-
tained a medical care program for North Battleford, but not for the
Saskatoon region. One was the expense to the provincial government of introducing a general medical program in a large urban area.
Smaller rural plans, especially in areas that had already established
municipal doctor schemes, could be assisted without a huge fiscal
commitment, but a large urban program would need support beyond
what the Province could afford. The second issue was the problem
of securing public support. Any taxpayer-funded medical program
in Saskatoon would have to compete with two voluntary pre-payment plans that had already been established in the city: Saskatoon
Mutual, a co-operative plan that had 16,000 members by 1946; and
the rapidly expanding physician-controlled Medical Service Inc.,
which had 35,000 enrolled members by 1950. Medical Service Inc.
and its Regina counterpart, Group Medical Services (which had
taken over the co-operative Regina Mutual in 1949) together insured
47,000 people in 1950; this had ballooned to 185,000 by 1955.[87] The
growth of private medical insurance plans acted as a significant barrier to the formation of urban health regions, especially if regions
proposed medical care provision.

Malcolm Taylor argued in his 1987 book *Health Insurance and
Canadian Public Policy* that medical opposition to medical care

provision by health regions hardened in the early 1950s. Some physicians had accommodated themselves to the Swift Current model,
especially after salaried payment was taken off the table. Swift Current
paid physicians on a fee-for-service basis, and most were generally
pleased with this arrangement. For example, Dr. Howden, a physician
practicing in the region, told the annual meeting of the SCPS in 1949:

> Aside from the economic aspects there is fundamentally little
> difference in doctor-patient relationships, type of practice and so
> on. As there is free choice of doctor and patient, and as the work
> is done on a "fee-for-service" basis, there has been almost no dis-
> ruption of the present personalized system of private practice.[88]

A review of the Swift Current medical program by the CMA in
1948 concluded that it was "a successful experiment ... courageously
applied, efficiently managed, and remarkably free from attempts to
make the facts fit preconceived ideas, financial or otherwise."[89] Even
the Chairman of the SCPS's Health Services Committee, Dr. J.
Lloyd Brown, praised Swift Current in 1949 as a "rather sound system." He went on to say, "every encouragement should be given to
the people of this Region in continuing the excellent experimental
efforts they are so courageously undertaking."[90] It was, perhaps,
increasingly easy even for the SCPS to be magnanimous. They had
defeated the HSPC on salaried service. Co-operative mutual benefit
plans, such as Regina Mutual, lost the battle over salaried payment
early. The Regina Medical Society steadfastly refused to negotiate
a salaried contract, and successfully resisted the establishment of
health centres with salaried physicians in Regina.[91] The hospitalization service had given all physicians in the province open access to
a hospital system in which the CCF invested a lot of resources. The
success of hospitalization coverage had gone some way to convincing
Saskatchewan physicians that public health services could be recon-
ciled with physician self-interest, but only if physicians were able to
contain less-desirable elements of the health centre model of delivery.

Nationally, the end of the 1940s marked a shift in organized medicine's public position on public health insurance. Retreating from its supportive 1943 statement, in 1949 the CMA council voted to support private health insurance over public options. This result was reflective of nationally ascendant anti-public-insurance perspectives, bolstered by the nation-wide growth in private insurance plans, many of them physician controlled. Lack of government initiative at the federal and provincial levels left a vacuum into which private plans moved. In Saskatchewan, the SCPS publicly re-affirmed its support for "state-aided" health insurance in 1942, 1943, 1948, and again in 1949 after the CMA had reversed course. In 1951, however, the SCPS stepped back into line with the CMA, and passed a resolution endorsing the CMA's 1949 statement in favour of private insurance models.[92]

The HSPC, under Mott's leadership, continued to seek compromises with the province's physicians, but the context was growing less favourable. He spent the remainder of his time in Saskatchewan, until his 1951 departure, improving insured hospital services and developing a work-around on the key principles of a regional health structure, in the absence of progress establishing new health regions. The latter effort can be seen in the recommendations of the Saskatchewan Health Survey Report, released in 1951. Mott and his team worked on this report for more than two years. The Health Survey program was instituted by the federal government in summer 1948. It provided financial support to the provinces through the General Health Grant for surveys of health services and facilities, and to conduct research for recommendations to improve them. Mott was Chair of the Saskatchewan Health Survey Committee, and Malcolm Taylor was Research Director. The Committee included representation from rural and urban municipalities, labour, the SCPS, dentists, registered nurses, hospitals, and the Women's Section of the Saskatchewan Farmers' Union. Swift Current Health Region No. 1 also had a representative. The Survey's Sub-Committee on Hospitals included a representative of the Catholic Hospital Conference, and SHML activist Joseph Thain, who sat as a representative of the Trades and Labour Congress of Canada.

The Saskatchewan Health Survey (SHS) had a very broad research agenda, and it reviewed every health program the province offered (including those of the Cancer Commission, and tuberculosis and mental health care provision) as well as the needs of the health professions. While the Saskatchewan Health Survey Committee lauded the progress made on health services provision in the province, the SHS discussed ongoing problems, such as shortages of personnel, especially dentists, laboratory technicians, physiotherapists, and social workers. The development of public health services remained incomplete, and health services were not equally available in all areas of the province. The SHS estimated that about one-third of Saskatchewan's residents received general medical care through a variety of mechanisms: municipal doctor schemes, regional medical care plans, voluntary medical insurance plans, and the provincial medical care plan for social assistance recipients. The SHS Report's first recommendation was for the broadening of this coverage and the provision of complete health insurance benefits:

> A comprehensive health insurance program should be undertaken in Saskatchewan at the earliest possible date. This health insurance program should be integrated with and built upon existing health programs which should be extended, modified, and coordinated as required, to the end that adequate health care of high quality shall be available to all residents of the province on the basis of need and without regard to individual ability to pay.[93]

The committee called upon the federal government to adopt immediately a national health insurance program. According to the new Saskatchewan Minister of Health, T. J. Bentley, a comprehensive program should be based upon guiding principles of "universal coverage, comprehensive services, and the preservation of ministerial responsibility."[94] The SHS Report argued that universal coverage should include "treaty Indians," and that "health services for treaty Indians should be integrated with the provincial health services, with the required special financial arrangements being agreed upon between the Federal Government and the Provincial Government."

The second volume of the SHS Report was the 1951 "Hospital Survey and Master Plan." It included a set of 45 recommendations, the first 37 of which applied to hospitals. The Sigerist principles remained influential in these recommendations, but in this instance, they were applied to the sector of the health care system over which the government had been able to establish control through the introduction of public insurance—that is, hospitals. In the absence of a government medical care plan, physician services delivered outside of hospitals remained beyond the master plan's remit. The report recommended there be four types of hospitals: community hospitals or health centres; district hospitals; regional hospitals; and base hospitals. It also recommended that space be provided for physicians, dentists, and public health personnel in or adjacent to hospitals, in keeping with HSPC's consistent emphasis on integration, both between hospitals, and between hospitals and medical and public health practitioners. Integration between hospitals, especially between smaller facilities and regional hospitals, would be accomplished through the creation of new health service areas, in a fully regionalized hospital system.

The twenty-year master plan for health service areas appears intended to accomplish what previous regional plans had failed to achieve: a coordinated approach that allowed a mutually interdependent set of health services to grow within and between regions. Mott emphasized that hospital services must be available to all residents within a "reasonable distance" from where they lived; and that duplication and waste of resources should be avoided.[95] The proposal operated in some senses as a sort of parallel to the health regions mandated in the Health Services Act of 1944; or, as a regional system within a (failed) regional system. Again, though, the lack of medical care coverage left a huge gap in services.

Mott attempted to instill the principles of the health centre modelsuch as lay involvement and integrated preventive and curative services—within the hospital sector, but a truly integrated model was a pipe dream under the circumstances. The SHS Report once again emphasized the importance of prevention and health promotion, as well as "citizen participation," which the report described as "the most striking characteristic of the development of health services in Saskatchewan."[96] Co-operative action had proven effective in the development of health programs from tuberculosis care to health region boards, the report claimed. This commitment to lay engagement was a principle that Mott, in particular, articulated throughout his health service career, before and after his time in Saskatchewan. But the originally intended vehicle for this vision of health organization—the health region, built from the health centre up, with elected leadership helping to oversee a comprehensive range of health services—was further away than at any time since Mott had arrived in the province in 1946.

The seven existing health regions were referred to in the SHS Report as "public health regions" only. These were not health care regions that provided a full range of medical, hospital, and public health services (with the exception, as always, of Swift Current). The shift reflected the narrowed scope of responsibility for the regions compared with the original Sigerist blueprint. The term "public health regions" reflected more accurately the work the seven existing health regions performed; it was a practical descriptor. Even at that, the organizational chart for the Department of Public Health, after its 1950 consolidation with the HSPC, shows both a Regional Health Services Branch and a Preventive Services Branch, which included divisions from sanitation to nursing services. In fact, public health was overseen by both the department and by regional boards. Regional medical health officers had to answer to (at least) two masters.

The main recommendations in the report in regard to public health administration centred on the need to organize health regions, adequately staffed with full-time qualified public health personnel, in the areas of the province that had yet to buy in. But in 1951 there were few new tactics available to the HSPC with which to achieve this goal. Judging by the recommendations of the SHS, the government remained unwilling to compel municipalities to form regions. Health regions were to be democratically and locally determined. As was discussed earlier, urban areas were a particularly challenging problem. Recognizing the difficulty of persuading large urban centres to form regions with their surrounding rural counterparts, the report recommended an alternative—that a rural health region could be organized in place of a combined urban-rural region. Thus originated the idea to form regions known as Regina Rural and Saskatoon Rural, within which urban municipal health departments would continue to exist. In 1955, proposals for Regina Rural failed in a plebiscite.

Fred Mott resigned from his position in Saskatchewan effective the end of December 1951. In a letter to Henry Sigerist just before departing Regina for Washington, D.C., Mott suggested that he had done what could be done in Saskatchewan, and that the health program was being "left in good hands":

> After five extremely interesting and worthwhile years in Saskatchewan I am going to be associated with the progressive and expanding health program of the United Mine Workers of America Welfare and Retirement Fund. ... My position will be that of Medical Administrator of [the Memorial Hospital Associations of Kentucky, West Virginia, and Virginia] ... It might be premature to attempt to describe at this time the kind of health program which we hope to see developed in areas where there are concentrations of soft coal miners and their families,

but I might say that the possibilities in the way of constructive developments appear to be almost limitless. ... The decision to leave Saskatchewan has been made with a great deal of reluctance, for Saskatchewan is in the lead or is pioneering in North America in so many aspects of health services that one hesitates very much to sever connections here.[97]

In January 1952, Sigerist wrote to Mott from Pura, Ticino, in southern Switzerland, where he and his wife then lived. He thanked Fred for keeping him in touch with developments in Saskatchewan over the years. Always a skilled builder of professional and personal networks, Sigerist mentioned that that he had seen Milton Roemer and his family in Geneva, where Roemer was then working at the World Health Organization:

They have a very nice apartment and he is doing a splendid job with WHO. I attended a meeting of the Expert Committee on Social Medicine that he had called to advise the ILO (International Labor Organization) in their drafting of minimum and advanced requirements for a social security program.

Dick Weinerman had visited Sigerist in 1950. "And of course I see a lot of René Sand and the other Europeans who are working in our field," Sigerist wrote. "If you ever come to Europe, I very much hope that you will look us up in Pura."[98]

Fred responded to Sigerist's letter a few days after receiving it. His careful but honest assessment of his years in Saskatchewan provides a glimpse into Mott's measured personality as well as his ability to take the long view. It also illustrates in a subtle way the impact of growing Canadian nationalism and anti-American sentiment upon Mott's sense of his place in Saskatchewan.

Thank you very much indeed for your good letter of January 11. I can assure you that it was most difficult to leave Saskatchewan, for many personal ties were built up over the more than five years there and the program is still the most challenging one of its kind in North America. However, it seemed to us that the time had come to return to the United States and to have the program in Saskatchewan taken over entirely by Canadians.

The Saskatchewan Program is really in good shape, although it is still extremely difficult to get the support of the physicians for measures which would lead to a better quality of medical care in the various programs. The Saskatchewan Hospital Services Plan is stable, and despite some admitted abuses, is considered on the whole to be generally satisfactory to all groups concerned. The program of quite complete health service for social assistance beneficiaries is going on reasonably well except for a periodic crisis due to the desire of the physicians for more money. The program in the Swift Current Health Region is still generally popular with the doctors as well as the residents of the area, its chief weakness being that the local physicians resist any effort to build up a group of consulting specialists on a salary basis who might be located at Swift Current. ...

The development of basic public health services on a regional basis has been rather slow, chiefly because of the shortage of competent public health personnel. However, the new Prince Albert Health Region was established this past year and, when I left, steps had been taken to establish the Regina Rural Health Region. Moreover, there are plans for developing at least one if not two more regions during the coming year....

The opportunity to work in Saskatchewan for over five years was a most unusual one which I shall always consider to have been a privilege, and I want to express my appreciation to you for the part you played in getting me into that position.[99]

Mott's years in Saskatchewan gave him invaluable experience planning government health services, especially hospital care, which he would put to use as a hospital planner and administrator for the United Mine Workers and the United Auto Workers. He kept careful track of developments in Saskatchewan after he left, as his archives reveal.

In the end, the CCF's first flagship health program was not a regional network of health services built on the health centre model. It was the Saskatchewan Hospital Services Plan. The SHSP's success contributed to the national introduction of hospitalization coverage in 1957. In that aspect, Mott and Rosenfeld, two Americans who cut their political teeth in the US New Deal era, played a role in the creation of Canadian medicare that has never really been publicly appreciated. Canadians have been schooled in a quasi-nationalist notion that they have had nothing to learn from the US on health care. We've built an identity around our health care superiority, believing that we have a homegrown health system that transparently illustrates innate Canadian (especially Prairie) values. Saskatchewan's role in the introduction of universal health care has often been portrayed as singularly rooted in rural co-operative traditions.

As much as there is some truth to such interpretations, they are also lacking in historical depth. Mott, Rosenfeld, the Sheps, Henry Sigerist, and the activists of the State Hospital and Medical League, among others, shared a commitment to a model of health care that circulated outside nation-state boundaries. This shared framework for engagement, the health centre movement, had its roots in the idealized promise of Soviet socialized medicine, British health centres, New Deal medicine and a myriad of other experiments this book has only very partially traced. During the health centre model's moment from the mid-1930s to the early 1950s, there was a political opening for something more than what David Naylor decades ago termed "private practice, public payment." The model these health advocates shared was rooted in a social interpretation of health, an antipathy to the private medical marketplace, and a belief in scientific progress and the entitlement of the average person to benefit fully and equally in its preventive and curative capacity. Its moment reached into a small prairie province, with a political culture that created space for a broader transformation in health equity.

ENDNOTES

1   Malcolm Taylor, *Health Insurance and Canadian Public Policy: The Seven Decisions That Created the Health Insurance System and Their Outcomes* (McGill-Queen's Press, 1987), 243.

2   David Naylor, *Private Practice, Public Payment: Canadian Medicine and the Politics of Health Insurance, 1911-1966* (McGill-Queen's Press - MQUP, 1986), 142.

3   *The Saskatchewan Gazette*, September 16, 1946.

4   Naylor, *Private Practice*, Public Payment, 142.

5   Yale University Library Manuscripts and Archives (hereafer YULMA), MS 1360, Leonard Rosenfeld Papers, Acc 1996 Box 2 "American Gets Post— Health Services," *Regina Leader Post*, nd .

6   YULMA, MS 1360, Leonard Rosenfeld Papers, Acc 1996 Box 1, Henry Sigerist to Leonard Rosenfeld, January 14, 1945.

7   YULMA, MS 1360, Leonard Rosenfeld Papers, Acc 1996 Box 1, Henry Sigerist to Leonard Rosenfeld, May 18, 1946.

8   YULMA, MS 1360, Leonard Rosenfeld Papers, Acc 1996 Box 1, Milton Roemer to Leonard Rosenfeld, June 9, 1948.

9   YULMA, MS 1360, Leonard Rosenfeld Papers, Acc 1996, Box 2. For historical timeline of the Community Health Association see https://www.hap.org/about/history accessed Sept 21, 2017.

10 Taylor, *Health Insurance and Canadian Public Policy*, 69.

11 Joan Feather, "From Concept to Reality: Formation of the Swift Current Health Region," *Prairie Forum* 16, 1 (1991): 59–80; Joan Feather, "Impact of the Swift Current Health Region: Experiment or Model?," *Prairie Forum* 16, 2 (1991): 225–48; Gordon S. Lawson, "The Road Not Taken: The 1945 Health Services Planning Commission Proposals and Physician Remuneration in Saskatchewan," *Canadian Bulletin of Medical History* 26, 2 (December 2009): 395–427.

12 Aleck Ostry, "Prelude to Medicare: Institutional Change and Continuity in Saskatchewan, 1944-1962," *Prairie Forum* 20, 1 (1995): 92.

13 Duane Mombourquette, "An Inalienable Right: The CCF and Rapid Health Care Reform, 1944-1948," *Saskatchewan History* 43, 3 (1991): 107.

14 Thomas H. McLeod and Ian McLeod, *Tommy Douglas: The Road to Jerusalem*, 2nd ed. (Regina: Fifth House Publishers, 2004), 190.

15 Ostry, "Prelude to Medicare," 88.

16 McLeod and McLeod, *Tommy Douglas*, 190.

17 McLeod and McLeod, *Tommy Douglas*, 191.

18 Richard Weinerman's father, Charles, wrote to Yale University requesting that they re-consider his son's rejection, which he believed was based

upon their Jewish identity. L. A. Falk, "E. Richard Weinerman, M.D., M.P.H. (July 17, 1917—February 21, 1970)," The Yale Journal of Biology and Medicine 44, 1 (August 1971): 5. Physician and historian of medicine Barron Lerner has noted that Yale marked the admission applications of Jews with 'H' for Hebrew. "In a Time of Quotas, A Quiet Pose in Defiance," New York Times, May 25, 2009, accessed June 17, 2015 http://www.nytimes.com/2009/05/26/health/26quot.html?_r=0

19 Falk, "E. Richard Weinerman," 7.

20 YULMA, MS 692, Edwin Richard Weinerman Papers, Box 13, Folder 559, Mott to Weinerman, August 1, 1946.

21 YULMA, MS 692, Edwin Richard Weinerman Papers, Box 22, Folder 2.

22 YULMA, MS 692, Edwin Richard Weinerman Papers, Box 13, Folder 559, Weinerman to Mott, September 19, 1946.

23 YULMA, MS 692, Edwin Richard Weinerman Papers, Box 23, Folder 15.

24 YULMA, MS 692, Edwin Richard Weinerman Papers, Box 23, Folder 15.

25 YULMA, MS 692, Edwin Richard Weinerman Papers, Box 13, Folder 559, Mott to Weinerman, August 1, 1946.

26 University of California, Berkeley, College of Environmental Design, Environmental Design Archives, Vernon DeMars Collection, Finding Aid. http://www.oac.dclib.org/findaid/ark:/13030/c81j9gh8/entire_text/ Accessed October 10, 2017.

27 Martin Filler, "Landscape Visionary for a New American Dream," New York Times February 2, 1997. http://www.nytimes.com/1997/02/02/arts/landscape-visionary-for-a-new-american-dream.html Accessed November 28, 2017.

28 "Farm Labor: After Shelter Comes Health," The New Pencil Points (December, 1942): 32-41.

29 YULMA, MS 692, Edwin Richard Weinerman Papers, Series 1, Box 13 Folder 559, Mott to Weinerman, September 5, 1946.

30 Gordon Leslie Barnhart, ed., Saskatchewan Premiers of the Twentieth Century (Regina: University of Regina, Canadian Plains Research Center, 2004), 190.

31 YULMA, MS 692, Edwin Richard Weinerman Papers, Box 13, Folder 559, Frederick Mott to Dick Weinerman, September 25, 1946.

32 "Mott Urges Registration," Regina Leader Post, October 31, 1946.

33 YULMA, MS 692, Edwin Richard Weinerman Papers, Box 13, Folder 559, Mott to Weinerman, November 27, 1946.

34 "Hospitalization Card No. 1 Given to Premier," Regina Leader-Post, December 20, 1946.

35 YULMA, MS 692, Edwin Richard Weinerman Papers, Box 13, Folder 559, Mott to Weinerman, April 3, 1947.

36 YULMA, MS 1360, Leonard Sidney Rosenfeld Papers, Box 3, Folder 2.

37 YULMA, MS 692, Edwin Richard Weinerman Papers, Box 13, Folder 559, Weinerman to Mott, January 17, 1947.

38 YULMA, MS 692, Edwin Richard Weinerman Papers, Box 13, Folder 559, Mott to Weinerman, February 11, 1947. He reiterated this apology in his March 6, 1947 letter to Weinerman.

39 Ostry, "Prelude to Medicare," 88–89.

40 Lewis H. Thomas, ed., *The Making of a Socialist : The Recollections of T.C. Douglas* (Edmonton: University of Alberta Press, 1984), 229.

41 Ostry, "Prelude to Medicare," 88.

42 Frederick Mott, "Hospital Relations: Hospital Services in Saskatchewan," *American Journal of Public Health* 37 (December 1947): 1543.

43 Mombourquette, "An Inalienable Right," 106.

44 Mott, "Hospital Relations," 1542.

45 Library and Archives Canada, MG 13 Series J15, Frederick Mott Fonds, Vol. 47, File 13, "Recent Developments in the Provision of Medical Services in Saskatchewan," Address by Dr. F.D. Mott at the Session on Medical Economics, Canadian Medical Association, Winnipeg, June 26, 1947, p. 1.

46 Frederic Mott, "The Saskatchewan Hospital Services Plan," *Physicians Forum Bulletin* (Jan-Feb 1947).

47 Leonard Rosenfeld, "Province-Wide Hospitalization in Saskatchewan," *Public Affairs* 10, 3 (June 1947): 157.

48 Rosenfeld, "Province-Wide Hospitalization," 162.

49 Rosenfeld, "Province-Wide Hospitalization," 162.

50 Frederick Mott et al., "The Saskatchewan Experience in Payment for Hospital Care," *American Journal of Public Health* 88, 6 (1953): 753–54.

51 Mott et al., "The Saskatchewan Experience," 755.

52 Ostry, "Prelude to Medicare," 89.

53 Rosenfeld, "Province-Wide Hospitalization," 162. Rosenfeld estimated that hospitalization benefits would cost $6 million in 1947, with an additional $600,000 going to administrative costs.

54 Ostry, "Prelude to Medicare," 100.

55 Rosenfeld, "Province-Wide Hospitalization," 163.

56 Thomas, *The Making of a Socialist*, 227–28.

57 Thomas, *The Making of a Socialist*, 228.

58 Maureen K. Lux, *Separate Beds: A History of Indian Hospitals in Canada, 1920s-1980s* (Toronto: University of Toronto Press, 2016), 21.

59 Mombourquette, "An Inalienable Right," 112.

60 G.W. Myers, "Hospitalization Experience of a Government Hospital Care Insurance Plan," *Canadian Journal of Public Health* (September-October 1954): 2.

61 Lesley McBain, "Caring, Curing and Socialization: The Ambiguities of Nursing in Northern Saskatchewan, 1944-57," in *Caregiving on the Periphery: Historical Perspectives on Nursing and Midwifery in Canada*, ed. Myra Rutherdale (Montreal and Kingston: McGill-Queen's University Press, 2010), 288.

62 David M. Quiring, *CCF Colonialism in Northern Saskatchewan: Battling Parish Priests, Bootleggers, and Fur Sharks* (Vancouver: University of British Columbia Press, 2004), 223.

63 McBain, "Caring, Curing and Socialization," 285.

64 McBain, "Caring, Curing and Socialization," 280.

65 McBain, "Caring, Curing and Socialization," 298.

66 Quiring, *CCF Colonialism in Northern Saskatchewan*, 226.

67 McBain, "Caring, Curing and Socialization," 289.

68 McBain, "Caring, Curing and Socialization," 291.

69 Quiring, *CCF Colonialism in Northern Saskatchewan*, 225.

70 Quiring, *CCF Colonialism in Northern Saskatchewan*, 227.

71 Quiring, *CCF Colonialism in Northern Saskatchewan*, 232.

72 Maureen K. Lux, "Perfect Subjects: Race, Tuberculosis and the Qu'Appell BCG Vaccine Trial," *Canadian Bulletin of Medical History* 15,2 (1998): 282.

73 Mary-Ellen Kelm, *Colonizing Bodies: Aboriginal Health and Healing in British Columbia, 1900-1950* (UBC Press, 1999), 120.

74 Lux, "Perfect Subjects," 289.

75 Quiring, *CCF Colonialism in Northern Saskatchewan*, 233.

76 Kelm, *Colonizing Bodies*, 124–25.

77 Quiring, *CCF Colonialism in Northern Saskatchewan*, 234.

78 Quiring, *CCF Colonialism in Northern Saskatchewan*, 219.

79 YULMA, MS 1360 , Leonard Rosenfeld Papers, Acc 1996, Box 3, Folder 3, Letter to Mildred Walker, April 27, 1948.

80 Mott, "Hospital Relations," 1540.

81 Mott, "Hospital Relations,"1541.

82 Feather, "Impact of the Swift Current Health Region," 226.

83 Saskatchewan Health Survey Report (Regina: Queen's Printer, 1951), 35.

84 YULMA, MS 1360, Leonard Rosenfeld Papers, Acc 1996, Box 3, Folder 3, "Proposed Organization of Saskatoon Health Region."

85 YULMA, MS 1360, Leonard Rosenfeld Papers, Acc1996, Box 3, Folder 3, "Proposed Organization of Saskatoon Health Region."

86 YULMA, MS 1360, Leonard Rosenfeld Papers, Acc1996, Box 3, Folder 3, "Proposed Organization of North Battleford Health Region."

87 Taylor, *Health Insurance and Canadian Public Policy*, 258–61.

88 Taylor, *Health Insurance and Canadian Public Policy*, 251.

89 Taylor, *Health Insurance and Canadian Public Policy*, 251.

90 Taylor, *Health Insurance and Canadian Public Policy*, 252.

91 Taylor, *Health Insurance and Canadian Public Policy*, 253, 258.

92 Taylor, *Health Insurance and Canadian Public Policy*, 254, 256.

93 Saskatchewan Health Survey Report, 225.

94 Saskatchewan Health Survey Report, vii.

95 Saskatchewan Health Survey Report, 63.

96 Saskatchewan Health Survey Report, xxvii.

97 YULMA, MSS 788, Henry E. Sigerist Papers, Box 18, File 665, Mott to Sigerist, December 17, 1951.

98 YULMA, MSS 788, Henry E. Sigerist Papers, Box 18, File 665, Sigerist to Mott, January 11, 1952.

99 YULMA, MSS 788, Henry E. Sigerist Papers, Box 18, File 665, Mott to Sigerist, January 21, 1952.

CONCLUSION

DISAPPEARING FROM VIEW

The Health Centre Model's Dénouement

The last chapter detailed the process by which the health centre model was superceded in Saskatchewan by the introduction of publicly insured hospital care. That process was effectively over by the time of Frederick Mott's departure in 1951, although he still held out hope for the future establishment of health regions along the lines of the health centre model proposed in the Sigerist Report.

For certain, the demise of the health centre ideal was obvious by 1955, when the CCF government lost two public plebiscites on the establishment of two new health regions: Regina Rural and Assiniboia-Gravelbourg. In both cases, the full plan for publicly administered medical care services was put before the electorate. The proposal was for prepaid, comprehensive medical care coverage for all residents of the region, overseen by the regional board. The proposal sought to integrate preventive with curative care. Physician payment was to be a form of capitation, in which an overall budget for physician services would be established for the region, with each physician paid on a pro-rated basis according to volume of services provided. There had been a similar physician payment scheme in the Swift Current Health Region in the past, but it had been abandoned due to physician opposition. According to Joan Feather, "that abandonment had been an unfortunate compromise of principles."[1] In 1955, that compromise again reared its head.

The previous chapter traced the growth of private medical insurance schemes in Saskatchewan. While HSPC planners were preparing proposals for full public medical provision in the proposed regions, private insurers Medical Services Incorporated (MSI) and General Medical Services (GMS) combined efforts and put an alternative proposal before the two regional boards. The private group plan would provide broad coverage, but would not be controlled by a pubic board. In addition, the insurers argued that the provincial government had to increase the legal $50 premium limit in order for the insurance plan to be viable. This private proposal, unsurprisingly since it did not include any cap or limit on physician payments, received considerable organized public support from doctors. And so the Regina Rural and Assiniboia-Gravelbourg plans for public medical care coverage became a hotly contested political issue. In many ways, it was a precursor of the later campaign against province-wide medical coverage, which ultimately led to the 1962 physicians' strike. The SCPS engaged public relations experts, sent out speakers, and encouraged doctors in the regions to sign a pledge promising to refuse to work in a regional health board medical plan without SCPS approval.

The CCF government lost the Regina Rural and Assiniboia-Gravelbourg plebiscites by a significant margin. This led to some soul searching in the Department of Public Health. Milton Roemer, who had come to Saskatchewan in 1953 to become the director of the Medical and Hospital Services Branch, wrote a report analyzing the defeats. Roemer's report is fundamentally a political analysis, not a technical one. It begins with criticism of the unprecedented decision taken in June 1955 by the Council of the Regina Rural Health Region to "hold a vote of the electors," on the medical care scheme. Carefully tracing the history of the medical care plan in the model Swift Current Health Region No. 1—which had been established a decade earlier—Roemer pointed out there had not been a plebiscite on the introduction of medical services in Swift

Current and, furthermore, the public vote on the establishment of the Swift Current health region (as per the legislation) did not even mention medical care. It was only after the November 1945 vote on the establishment of the region, at a meeting of the regional council at Gull Lake in January 1946, that the decision was taken to inaugurate a prepaid medical plan. Roemer also pointed out that there was no public vote on the establishment of the SHSP "or any other of the various public medical plans in Saskatchewan which have since proved so successful." Roemer did not intend to criticize the lack of a plebiscite in Swift Current Health Region No. 1—quite the opposite. As he argued, "there are some 45 to 50 countries throughout the world with systems of governmentally required medical care insurance. In none of these has there been a public plebiscite on the issue."[2] Roemer further questioned "the entire wisdom of holding a plebiscite."

Roemer did a detailed analysis of voting patterns in the plebiscite according to two variables: first, prior experience with some form of medical care coverage (from municipal doctor plans to private insurance); second, rural or urban setting. Tellingly, the availability of private prepaid medical insurance schemes, especially MSI, increased support for a public scheme. Areas with the least support for the health region's plan were those rural municipalities that already had municipal doctor plans. In Roemer's view this was because of the success of the municipal doctor plans, which provided "extremely low-cost schemes of medical care," that were successful with the rural public.

This analysis is fascinating for a number of reasons. First, and perhaps surprisingly, it posits the plebiscites did not fail because the public preferred private plans. In other words, despite the loss of the plebiscite, Roemer believed the campaign by organized medicine and the private insurance counter-proposal were not decisive. Nor did Roemer believe that the outcome was a reflection of physician opposition at the local level. As Roemer put it:

if the opposition of the doctors were the predominant force affecting the vote, the opposite outcome would have been expected. Thus, the opposition of doctors would be expected to be greatest in communities under MSI contracts, yet the vote for the regional plan was strongest in these communities. Likewise, the opposition of doctors would be expected to be least in communities under municipal doctor schemes yet the opposition to the regional scheme was greatest in these communities.[3]

Roemer's report thus cautioned against giving medical opposition too much credit for the defeat of the schemes. There were other factors at work. Roemer was most convinced by the impact of the economic context, especially for rural farm voters. The price of wheat had fallen precipitously, making it difficult for voters to support the additional personal tax necessary to fund the medical care program:

> It must be kept in mind that serious illness and, therefore, high medical expenses in any given year affect only about 15 to 20 percent of the population. It is obvious that the remaining 80 to 85 percent of the population would spend less for medical care without a health insurance scheme than with one. In time of economic stress, therefore, 85 percent of the people might well prefer to "take a chance" and save money.

The main lessons to be learned from the failed votes, from Roemer's perspective, were, first, that the expansion of medical services could not be funded solely through personal levies as had been proposed. And, second, that medical insurance should be introduced at the provincial level as a next step, without local plebiscites. However, public medical insurance was not introduced in Saskatchewan until 1962.

In the years surrounding the CCF's election in 1944, health centres were considered a backbone of health care reform, and rural health care in particular. This model had a long transnational history into which Saskatchewan's experience fits comfortably. Their mention in planning discussions was frequent, inside and outside of government. The health centre model was embraced by Saskatchewan's grassroots health activists, such as the State Hospital and Medical League. And yet by the early 1950s, the health centre model was disappearing from view. It seems remarkable that this centrality faded so quickly. Indeed, historically, it has been all but forgotten. The 1951 Saskatchewan health survey barely mentioned health centres, instead referring to small community hospitals as the building blocks of rural health. This was partly the result of hospitalization insurance having already been established, and the absence of funding for publicly funded physician care. What use was a health centre with no physicians working in it? Medical treatment in hospitals was insured; medical treatment outside of the hospital was not. However, the retreat of the health centre was not a phenomenon unique to Saskatchewan. The most obvious point of comparison is the United Kingdom, where the Labour Party had endorsed health centres for over 30 years and yet, when in power, failed to implement them.

Models for socialized medicine in the late 1940s were not helped by the explicit endorsement of Soviet medicine and the close identification of the health centre model with Soviet health provision. It left the concept especially exposed to the Cold War ideological struggle that engulfed the debate over health care in the North Atlantic world. State Hospital and Medical League activist and trade unionist Joseph Thain recalled in a 1975 memoir about the League that responses to their eight-point plan were often framed by anti-communist rhetoric:

> When this document was released the Medical Profession, Boards of Trades, Nurses (under the influence of the doctors), Hospital Boards in larger centres, and many Councillors, and businessmen, commenced a very strong attack against the League and its supporters. Many were subjected to threats of

their jobs in hospitals, called "Reds," Communists and being that
there was a war on called "fifth columnists." This group was supported by the press and many Service Clubs, Lawyers and there
was little sympathy anywhere. Politicians started to condemn
the plan when they had not even given it any study ... several
of them were talking "revolution" and several of us that were
involved were subject to investigation by the RCMP and other
undercover organizations.[4]

Several elements of the health centre model were criticized by
organized medicine and other commentators as "socialistic" or "communistic." The issue was partly how doctors would be paid (salaried
or not), but that was not the only barrier from medicine's point of
view. For organized medicine, control over health organization and
delivery was paramount. Some elements of the model, such as health
education, were less politically threatening and easier to embrace.
But competition with the increasingly powerful private medical
marketplace was an open call to confrontation in the 1950s. The
eventual withdrawal of services by Saskatchewan doctors in 1962,
when the CCF took measures to insure physician care, revealed the
profession's fundamental antipathy to socialized health care. But
that confrontation was only one battle in a much longer conflict.

The shift away from the health centre model was not popular
in all quarters. Certainly, some grassroots activists believed that
by abandoning the health centre model, the CCF had chosen to
retreat from its commitment to socialized medicine. In retrospect,
some were bitter about the lost opportunity. Joseph Thain had been
appointed by the CCF to the HSPC advisory board, but his memoir recalls almost immediate frustration at the HSPC's direction.
Some of this may have been sour grapes, as Mindel Cherniack Sheps
had observed about some members of the League in her letters to
Sigerist. According to Thain, the League believed the HSPC's 1944
plan "was definitely not strong enough to withstand the onslaught

of the medical profession and business dominated Commission. The decisions to adopt and cut the plan into sections instead of tackling the main problems first created many anxious times for many ·Leaguers." For Thain, a major sticking point was the HSPC's failure to "put the medical and other professionals on salary." Thain resigned from the HSPC Advisory Board "after two years of continuous erosion of the plan. ... The people had been left out in the cold. It was no longer a State Hospital and Medical League Plan but a piece meal [sic] plan for political expediency."[5] Thain was perhaps more direct in his criticisms than most. But his memoir captures the political tensions on the left of the CCF, the movement for socialized medicine, and the feeling that the CCF had moved away from a model around which considerable political consensus had emerged by 1944.

Historians write to understand the past, on its own terms, not in relation to the present day. We try to resist the appeal of easy lessons. One of the compelling aspects of the health centre model's history, however, is the fact that many of the debates at its core—debates about physician power, the role of laypeople in determining their own health care, and the importance of equity and accessibility— have resurfaced again and again since the 1940s. The problem of health inequality has hardly resolved itself. Despite the many technological and societal differences between past and present, somehow these themes remain the same.

Progressive doctors still struggle to find a broad social relevance and a way to serve within a conservative profession. This is certainly what motivates projects such as "Upstream," a Saskatchewan "movement to create a healthy society through evidence-based, people-centred ideas. Upstream seeks to reframe public discourse around addressing the social determinants of health in order to build a healthier society."[6] In 2017, "Upstream" and the Canadian Federation of Medical Students published a collection of interviews with prominent Canadian physicians who share their perspective on health inequality. One of the book's editors is Dr. Ryan Meili, author of *A Healthy Society: How a Focus on Health Can Revive Canadian Democracy*, member of the Saskatchewan Legislature, and as of this writing, leader of the Saskatchewan New Democratic Party, and leader of the Official Opposition. *A Healthy Society's* preface speaks passionately about the social and political mission of physicians, with emotional echoes of physician commitment in the 1930s and 1940s. It speaks of working with patients and communities.[7] Much like the people whose lives are the subject of my book, Upstream practitioners are both inside and outside of their own profession.

Radical physicians were at the intellectual heart of movements for socialized medicine from the 1930s on. They were not the only knowledgeable people in the room, but they gained access to high-level health policy debates and, more importantly, existing health programs in a way that lay advocates could not. They had recognized expertise, social status, and university training. They could call upon scientific advancement as a tool for social equality and argue that medical knowledge belonged to "the people." They cared deeply about the health centre model, not only because they believed in its capacity to improve access and provide quality care regardless of financial status or where one resided, but also because it provided them with a way to live out their political principles and beliefs in a professional world that was largely hostile to their political instincts.

These "careniks," almost all men, formed an intimate network. Relationships ran deep and many lasted lifetimes. By the late 1940s, the Cold War had turned history against their health politics. Advocates like Milton Roemer were repeatedly investigated by security forces in the US for their alleged communism, and sometimes they lost their jobs. But they were also highly accomplished professionals and, like their mentor Sigerist, they looked out for each other. Occasionally women like Mindel Cherniack Sheps, who were feminist in their political orientation, entered this network, but their involvement was much less visible. Mindel's brief time in

Saskatchewan has left evidence of how gender and Jewish identity also shaped the health politics of the medical left.

It is interesting that a movement so focused on organization and service provision should thrive during the economic crisis of the 1930s. Although the health centre model had earlier transnational origins, the late 1930s through the early 1950s were its moment, when the concept seemed to take centre stage everywhere at the same time. Health centre advocates certainly understood the impact of poverty and wealth inequality upon health. Fred Mott spent a decade administering health co-operatives and programs for the poorest agricultural workers in the US—families in which illness and disability were constant threats. And yet he, with Milton Roemer and Mindel and Cecil Sheps, and like Norman Bethune before them, wanted to reform medicine itself. They saw health inequality as a dialectical problem: poverty and inadequate care were both important factors, and unequal access to modern medicine made people poor because it made them sick. For this generation of radical physicians, and for lay activists like the State Hospital and Medical League, the social relations of medicine were the social relations of capitalism. They chose sides in the struggle against health inequality by criticizing the unfairness, discrimination, and oppression that characterized health services in their day, and posing solutions that would make health care more accessible.

In Canada, we might take for granted that, whatever its flaws, medicare has mostly solved the problem of access. The claim of equal access to health care today is, of course, a myth. Indigenous health inequality is the most significant, although not the sole proof of that. But, prepared to ignore the gaps, Canadians have woven a sense of national identity around our embrace of medicare. Reflective of alleged shared communal values, medicare's history is framed as inevitable, as a fundamental symbol of what distinguishes us from Americans. This narrative is presentist. It ignores history.

Historians of Canadian Medicare have commonly argued

against any sense of historical inevitability. The introduction of publicly insured health care, they have shown, was the result of human effort and political struggle, dead ends and failures, as well as accomplisments. In recent years, a largely celebratory or descriptive literature written by firsthand participants or contemporary observers has moved into a deeper analysis of what went wrong, not just what went right. But this book is not meant as an indictment of the CCF's health program. It is more an attempt to understand how a powerful idea rose and then fell in the historical contingencies of place and time.

World historical forces such as the Depression and the Cold War played roles. Another significant factor over which Saskatchewan had little control was the policy direction of the federal Liberal governments. As Heather MacDougall has argued, the federal sponsorship of a public health insurance program, which seemed possible at the close of World War II, vanished "into thin air."[8] The CCF was in power in Saskatchewan for over a decade before funding from the federal government would provide meaningful support for the expansion of health programs in the province. Between 1947 and 1956, the province funded rapidly expanding hospital services largely from its own tax base, with municipal cost sharing. The 1946 hospital services legislation proved extremely popular. Better hospital access was needed across the rural parts of the province, which were underserviced, and local political leaders were anxious to get capital support for new buildings. But the greater the investments in hospitalization became, the further away receded the possibility of moving swiftly on other elements of the Sigerist plan. The consequent inability to afford medical care coverage province-wide was immediately a problem for the implementation of a health centre model. Health centres needed publicly funded practitioners. There was no feasible way to compel physicians to run group private practices from them. A medical care plan would have been a significant carrot for physicians, especially in rural areas, and it would have facilitated the growth of health regions with models similar to Swift Current. But Swift Current also told health planners how expensive it all would be. Having agreed to fee-for-service payment, Swift Current Health Region No. 1 had a very difficult time controlling costs. Had the fiscal capacity of the province been different, health planners and the provincial Cabinet would perhaps have made different choices.

It is difficult to say for certain, however. In the lead up to the 1944 election, Douglas had at times signaled hospital services would be prioritized as a first step towards socialized medicine.[9] The 1944 election platform, "Program for Saskatchewan," was fundamentally vague on how socialized medicine would be achieved, although it referred to a complete "network of health services," which intimated the sort of blueprint proposed by Henry Sigerist. Its main political message on health was to put the province's doctors on notice:

> In the working out of its health plans the CCF will seek the support and co-operation of the members of the medical, dental, and nursing professions; and will hope to get this. But it may, of course, have to rely mainly on the younger doctors and nurses with a more progressive viewpoint than that of some of the older members of the professions; and for the full success of its plan it may have to wait upon the training of those young men and women who would like a chance to become doctors, nurses, etc., but who have hitherto been prevented by a lack of money from getting the training which would enable them to make their more effective contribution to society.[10]

The platform discussed health and social provision in the same section, but did not make any explicit connection between poverty and ill health. It described old-age pensions as "a scandal and an insult," and promised income support for the physically disabled. There were only modest reforms to income support during the first two CCF mandates. The CCF established the province's first Department of Social Welfare in November 1944. Until that point, "relief" in Saskatchewan was funded partly by the province and partly by municipalities, but it was administered by municipal governments. The CCF called its new programs "social aid." The first major policy initiative was to provide free medical, hospital, dental, and nursing services for old-age pensioners and those on mothers' allowances and their dependents. This program was a national first. As Jim Pitsula has argued, "fewer people now had to turn to social aid to pay for medical care."[11] The Minister of Social Welfare, Oak Valleau, also established a schedule for minimum social aid to which the Department of Social Welfare hoped municipalities would adhere. Old-age pensions were to increase by $3 per month; mothers' allowances by $10 per month. Mothers' allowance benefits were extended to unmarried and divorced women.[12] Pitsula argues that these changes had limited impact because municipalities retained control over social-aid implementation, and many were punitive and discriminatory in their approach.

The major barrier to reforming social aid was, again, money. Social services (health, education, social aid, and labour) were consuming nearly half of the provincial budget by 1947–48, at a cost of $22.5 million annually. Only $800,000 of this was spent on social-aid programs. In 1947, the Economic Advisory Planning Board argued that the Province lacked the resources for significant wealth redistribution, and pinned responsibility on the federal failure to implement provincial equalization grants, which had been suggested by the Rowell-Sirois Commission. By 1952, the government's own Budget Bureau acknowledged that social-aid programs were failing to ensure that those in need were receiving adequate government assistance. In 1956–57, when the federal government starting contributing to the cost of social aid, the Province increased total expenditures on social aid by $450,000 a year, nearly 25 percent. Spending continued to increase through the 1950s.[13]

The health centre model demanded transformative measures difficult to reconcile with the realities of health politics and finance in Saskatchewan. This was not only about "regionalization." Yes, the model promoted a spatial organization that guaranteed equitable access to rural and urban working-class families and governance that gave them control over those services. But it also required taking health care out of the private marketplace, reining in the power of organized medicine and the hospital sector, the melding of prevention and cure, and the availability of multidisciplinary care, all in one site. In its architectural modernist iteration, the health centre represented elegant, affordable public solutions that offered dignity to patients and providers. From the buildings of Berthold Lubetkin in London to Vernon DeMars's Farm Security Administration clinics and rural hospitals (though unfortunately not in Saskatchewan), the health centre model employed the talents of creative and radical architects. The health centre ideal was partly utopian and served as a form of inspiration. But it has also been extremely resilient and flexible over time. It resurfaced in the community health centre movement of the 1960s and 1970s and the ideology of the New Left and other social movements, including feminism and anti-colonialism, when questions of gender and race reanimated the debate about the meaning of health equity.

The more recent history of the health centre has been, for me, a more personal one. Throughout my adult life, I have only on rare occasions been treated by a private-practice physician, usually a specialist. Leaving my rural community in Saskatchewan, I attended the student health centre at the University of Saskatchewan, and then McGill's student clinic. When I arrived in Winnipeg in the late 1980s, I became a patient at Klinic Community Health Centre, incorporated in 1973. The birth of my first son was attended by their physicians; now an adult, he is still a Klinic patient. When pregnant with my second child, I was cared for by a midwife who practiced out of a community health centre. Today, our family attends a health centre where we are often cared for by a nurse practitioner in a shared-care practice. I am in many ways grateful to be aware of the health politics and history this model of care embodies.

Historical continuities between the 1930s and 1940s and move-ments that emerged years later are a subject for another book.[14] Again, the story will have to be taken up across borders, through interconnecting networks of people and ideas. It will in all likelihood be a history of close relationships between passionate advocates, a story of ideas echoing across space, and a cautionary tale of the lim-its of electoral politics and the challenges of health reform. In the meantime, I hope this book has made a contribution to the longer history of the struggle for a more equitable health care system, of which we are still a part.

ENDNOTES

1   Joan Feather, "Impact of the Swift Current Health Region: Experiment or Model?," *Prairie Forum* 16, 2 (1991): 228.

2   Yale University Library Manuscripts and Archives (hereafter YULMA), MS 1786, Milton Irwin Roemer Papers, Box 38, "Analysis of the Public Vote on a Prepaid Medical Care Plan in the Regina Rural Region," December 28, 1955.

3   YULMA, MS 1786, Milton Irwin Roemer Papers, Box 38, "Analysis of the Public Vote on a Prepaid Medical Care Plan in the Regina Rural Region," December 28, 1955.

4   Saskatchewan Archives Board (hereafter SAB), R-690.1, State Hospital and Medical League, File 8, "My Memories of the State Hospital and Medical League by Joseph A. Thain," 3–4.

5   SAB, R-690.1, State Hospital and Medical League, File 8, "My Memories of the State Hospital and Medical League by Joseph A. Thain," 5–6.

6   http://www.thinkupstream.net/ Accessed February 4, 2018.

7   Andrew Bresnahan et al., eds., *Upstream Medicine: Doctors for a Healthy Society* (Vancouver: University of British Columbia press, 2017), xiii–xv, https://www.ubcpress.ca/upstream-medicine.

8   Heather Macdougall, "Into Thin Air: Making National Health Policy, 1939-1945," in *Making Medicare: New Perspectives on the History of Medicare in Canada*, ed. Gregory P. Marchildon (Toronto: University of Toronto Press, 2012), 41–70.

9   A.W. Johnson, *Dream No Little Dreams: A Biography of the Douglas Government of Saskatchewan, 1944-1961* (Toronto: University of Toronto Press, 2004), 50–51.

10 University of Saskatchewan Archives, Sophia Dixon Fonds, "CCF Program for Saskatchewan," 1944, 7-8.

11 James M. Pitsula, "The CCF Government in Saskatchewan and Social Aid, 1944-1964," in *Building the Cooperative Commonwealth": Essays on the Democratic Socialist Tradition in Canada*, ed. J. William Brennan (Regina: Canadian Plains Research Centre, University of Regina, 1984), 207.

12 Johnson, *Dream No Little Dreams*, 89.

13 Pitsula, "The CCF Government in Saskatchewan and Social Aid," 210–12.

14 See *Comrades in Health: U.S. Health Internationalists, Abroad and at Home*, ed. Anne-Emanuelle Birn and Theodore M. Brown (New Brunswick, NJ and London: Rutgers University Press, 2013).

INDEX

BIBLIOGRAPHY

Abbott, Philip. "Titans/Planners, Bohemians/Revolutionaries: Male
Empowerment in the 1930s." *Journal of American Studies* 40, 3 (2006):
463–85.

Allan, John. *Berthold Lubetkin, Architecture and the Tradition of Progress.*
London: RIBA Publications, 1992.

Arnup, Katherine. *Education for Motherhood: Advice for Mothers in Twentieth
Century Canada.* Toronto: University of Toronto Press, 1993.

Baillargeon, Denyse. *Babies for the Nation: The Medicalization of Motherhood in
Quebec, 1910-1970.* Waterloo: Wilfred Laurier University Press, 2009.

Balin, Carole B. "The Call to Serve: Jewish Women Medical Students in
Russia, 1872-1887." In *Jewish Women in Eastern Europe,* edited by Chaeran
Freeze, Paula Hyman, and Antony Polonsky, 133-152. Oxford: The
Littman Library of Jewish Civilization, 2005.

Barnhart, Gordon Leslie, ed. *Saskatchewan Premiers of the Twentieth Century.*
Regina: University of Regina, Canadian Plains Research Center, 2004.

Beach, Abigail. "Potential for Participation: Health Centres and the Idea of
Citizenship 1920-1940." In *Regenerating England: Science, Medicine and
Culture in Interwar Britain,* edited by C. Lawrence and A.K. Mayer,
203–30. Amsterdam: Rodopi, 2000.

Berridge, Virginia. "Health and Medicine." In *The Cambridge Social History of
Britain, 1750-1950,* edited by F.M. L. Thompson, 171–242. Cambridge, UK:
Cambridge University Press, 1990.

——. "Polyclinics: Haven't We Been There Before?" *British Medical Journal*
336 (2008): 1161–62.

Birn, Anne-Emanuelle and Theodore M. Brown, eds. *Comrades in Health:
U.S. Health Internationalists, Abroad and at Home.* New Brunswick, NJ:
Rutgers University Press, 2013.

Bliss, Michael. *Banting: A Biography.* Toronto: McClelland and Stewart, 1984.

Bresnahan, Andrew, Mahli Brindamour, Christopher Charles, and Ryan
Meili, eds. *Upstream Medicine: Doctors for a Healthy Society.* Vancouver:
University of British Columbia press, 2017.

Brinkley, Alan. "The New Deal and the Idea of the State." In *The Rise and Fall
of the New Deal Order 1930-1980,* edited by Steve Fraser and Gary Gerstle,
85–121. Princeton NJ: Princeton University Press, 1989.

Brockway, Fenner. *Bermondsey Story: The Life of Alfred Salter.* London:
Independent Labour Publications, 1995.

Brooke, Stephen. *Labour's War: The Labour Party During the Second World
War.* Oxford: Clarendon, 1992.

Bryder, Linda, and John Stewart. "'Some Abstract Socialistic Ideal or Principle': British Reactions to New Zealand's 1938 Social Security Act." *Britain and the World* 8, 1 (March 2015): 51–75.

Bullock, Neil. "Fragments of a Post-War Utopia: Housing in Finsbury, 1945-51." *Urban Studies* 26 (1989): 46–58.

Cherry, Steven. "Medicine and Public Health, 1900-1939." In *A Companion to Early Twentieth-Century Britain*, edited by C. Wrigley, 405-23. Oxford: Blackwell Publishing, 2003.

Christie, Nancy. *Engendering the State: Family, Work and Welfare in Canada.* Toronto: University of Toronto Press, 2000.

Coe, P., and M. Reading. *Lubetkin and Tecton: Architecture and Social Commitment.* Bristol: Arts Council of Great Britain, 1981.

Collins, Sheila D., and Gertrude Schaffner Goldberg, eds. *When Government Helped: Learning from the Successes and Failures of the New Deal.* New York: Oxford University Press, 2014.

Comacchio, Cynthia R. *Nations Are Built of Babies: Saving Ontario's Mothers and Children, 1900-1940.* Montreal and Kingston: McGill-Queen's University Press, 1998.

Connor, J.T.H. "'One Simply Doesn't Arbitrate Authorship of Thoughts': Socialized Medicine, Medical McCarthyism, and the Publishing of *Rural Health and Medical Care*," *Journal of the History of Medicine and Allied Sciences*, 72, 3 (2017): 245-71.

Couto, Robert. "Heroic Bureaucracies." *Administration and Society* 23, 1 (1991): 123–47.

David-Fox, Michael. *Showcasing the Great Experiment: Cultural Diplomacy and Western Visitors to the Soviet Union, 1921-1941.* New York: Oxford, 2012.

Derickson, Alan. *Health Security for All: Dreams of Universal Health Care in America.* Baltimore: Johns Hopkins University Press, 2005.

———. "The House of Falk: The Paranoid Style in American Health Politics." *American Journal of Public Health* 87, 11 (November 1997): 1836–43.

Diani, Mario. "Network Analysis." In *Methods of Social Movement Research*, edited by Bert Klandermans and Suzanne Staggenborg, 173–200. Minneapolis: University of Minnesota Press, 2002.

Dickinson, Harley D, and Renée Torgerson. "Medicare: Saskatchewan's Gift to the Nation?" In *Perspectives of Saskatchewan*, edited by Jene M. Porter, 175-96. Winnipeg: University of Manitoba Press, 2009.

Dubinsky, Karen, Adele Perry, and Henry Yu, eds. *Within and Without the Nation: Canadian History as Transnational History.* Toronto: University of Toronto Press, 2015.

Duffin, Jacalyn, and Lesley Falk. "Sigerist in Saskatchewan: The Quest for Balance in Social and Technical Medicine." *Bulletin of the History of Medicine* 70, 4 (1996): 658–83.

Duffin, Jacalyn. "The Guru and the Godfather: Henry Sigerist, Hugh
MacLean, and the Politics of Health Care Reform in 1940s Canada."
Canadian Bulletin of Medical History 9 (1992): 191–218.

Dyck, Erika. *Facing Eugenics: Reproduction, Sterilization, and the Politics of
Choice.* Toronto: University of Toronto Press, 2013.

———. "Prairie Psychedelics: Mental Health Research in Saskatchewan, 1951-
1967." In *Mental Health and Canadian Society,* edited by James E. Moran
and David Wright, 221–44. Montreal and Kingston: McGill-Queen's
University Press, 2006.

Efron, Noah J. *A Chosen Calling: Jews in Science in the Twentieth Century.*
Baltimore: Johns Hopkins University Press, 2014.

Ewing, Sally. "The Science and Politics of Soviet Insurance Medicine." In
Health and Society in Revolutionary Russia, edited by Susan Gross
Solomon and John F. Hutchinson, 69–96. Bloomington and Indianapolis:
Indiana University Press, 1990.

Eyler, John M. *Sir Arthur Newsholme and State Medicine, 1885-1935.* Cambridge;
New York: Cambridge University Press, 1997.

Falk, I. S. "The Present and Future Organization of Medicine." *Milbank
Memoral Fund Quarterly* 12, 2 (1934): 115–25.

Falk, L. A. "E. Richard Weinerman, M.D., M.P.H. (July 17, 1917--February 21,
1970)." *The Yale Journal of Biology and Medicine* 44, 1 (August 1971): 3–23.

Feather, Joan. "From Concept to Reality: Formation of the Swift Current
Health Region." *Prairie Forum* 16, 1 (1991): 59–80.

———. "Impact of the Swift Current Health Region: Experiment or Model?"
Prairie Forum 16, 2 (1991): 225–48.

Fee, Elizabeth. "The Pleasures and Perils of Prophetic Advocacy: Socialized
Medicine and the Politics of American Medical Reform." In *Making
Medical History: The Life and Times of Henry E. Sigerist,* edited by
Elizabeth Fee and Theodore M. Brown, 197–228. Baltimore and London:
Johns Hopkins University Press, 1997.

Field, Mark G. *Soviet Socialized Medicine: An Introduction.* New York: The Free
Press, 1967.

Fitzpatrick, Sheila, and Carolyn Rasmussen, eds. *Political Tourists: Travellers
From Australia to the Soviet Union in the 1920s-1940s.* Carlton, VIC:
Melbourne University Publishing, 2008.

Frager, Ruth. *Sweatshop Strife: Class, Ethnicity, and Gender in the Jewish Labour
Movement of Toronto, 1900-1939.* Toronto: University of Toronto Press, 1992.

Freidenreich, Harriet Pass. *Female, Jewish and Educated: The Lives of Central
European University Women.* Bloomington: University of Indiana Press,
2002.

Giesbrecht, Jodi. "Accommodating Resistance: Unionization, Gender, and Ethnicity in Winnipeg's Garment Industry, 1929-1945." *Urban History Review* 39, 1 (2010): 5–19.

Glancey, Jonathan. "A Vision Still Worth Fighting For." *The Independent.* March 29, 1995.

Gleason, Mona. *Small Matters: Canadian Children in Sickness and Health.* Montreal and Kingston: McGill-Queen's University Press, 2013.

Goodwin, Jeff, James M. Jasper, and Francesca Polletta. *Passionate Politics: Emotions and Social Movements.* 1st edition. Chicago: University of Chicago Press, 2001.

Gordon, Linda. *Woman's Body, Woman's Right: A Social History of Birth Control in America.* New York: Penguin Books, 1977.

Goss, Sue. *Local Labour and Local Government.* Edinburgh: Edinburgh University Press, 1988.

Graves, Pamela. *Labour Women: Women in British Working-Class Politics 1918-1939.* Cambridge: Cambridge University Press, 1994.

Grey, Michael R. *New Deal Medicine: The Rural Health Programs of the Farm Security Administration.* Baltimore and London: Johns Hopkins University Press, 1999.

Gutkin, Harry. *Journey Into Our Heritage: The Story of the Jewish People in the Canadian West.* Toronto: Lester and Orphen Dennys, 1980.

Hannant, Larry. *The Politics of Passion: Norman Bethune's Writing and Art.* Toronto: University of Toronto Press, 1998.

Hendricks, Rickey. *A Model for National Health Care: The History of Kaiser Permanente.* Health and Medicine in American Society. Piscataway, NJ: Rutgers University Press, 1994.

Hendricks, Rickey L. "Liberal Default, Labor Support, and Conservative Neutrality: The Kaiser Permanente Medical Care Program After World War II." *Journal of Policy History* 1, 2 (1989): 156–80.

Hoffmann, Beatrix. *Health Care for Some.* Chicago: University of Chicago Press, 2012.

Hollander, Paul. *Political Pilgrims: Travels of Western Intellectuals to the Soviet Union, China and Cuba, 1928-1978.* New York: Oxford University Press, 1981.

Hollis, Patricia. *Ladies Elect: Women in English Local Government 1865-1914.* Oxford: Clarendon, 1987.

Honigsbaum, Frank. *Health, Happiness, and Security: The Creation of the National Health Service.* London and New York: Routledge, 1989.

———. *The Division in British Medicine: A History of the Separation of General Practice From Hospital Care, 1911-1968.* London: Kogan Page, 1979.

Hopkins, Charles Howard. *John R. Mott, 1865-1955: A Biography.* Grand Rapids, MI: Eerdmans, 1979.

Horlick, Louis. J. *Wendell Macleod: Saskatchewan's Red Dean.* Montreal and
Kingston: McGill-Queen's University Press, 2007.

Houston, C. Stuart. *36 Steps on the Road to Medicare: How Saskatchewan Led
the Way.* Montreal and Kingston: McGill-Queen's University Press, 2013.

Hyman, Paula. *Gender and Assimilation in Modern Jewish History: The Roles and
Representation of Women.* Seattle: University of Washington Press, 1995.

Jasper, James M. *The Art of Moral Protest: Culture, Biography, and Creativity in
Social Movements.* Chicago: University of Chicago Press, 1999.

Johannisson, K. "The People's Health: Public Health Policies in Sweden." In
The History of Public Health and the Modern State, edited by Dorothy
Porter, 165–82. Amsterdam: Rodopi, 1994.

Johnson, A.W. *Dream No Little Dreams: A Biography of the Douglas Government
of Saskatchewan, 1944-1961.* Toronto: University of Toronto Press, 2004.

Jones, Esyllt W. *Influenza 1918: Disease, Death and Struggle in Winnipeg.*
Toronto: University of Toronto Press, 2007.

———. "Nothing Too Good for the People: Local Labour and London's
Interwar Health Centre Movement." *Social History of Medicine* 25, 1 (2011):
84–102.

Kelm, Mary-Ellen. *Colonizing Bodies: Aboriginal Health and Healing in British
Columbia, 1900-1950.* UBC Press, 1999.

Kinnear, Mary. *In Subordination: Professional Women 1870-1970.* Montreal and
Kingston: McGill-Queen's University Press, 1995.

Klein, Jennifer. "A New Deal Restoration: Individuals, Communities, and the
Long Struggle for the Collective Good." *International Labor and Working-
Class History* 74, 1 (2008): 42–48.

———. *For All These Rights: Business, Labor, and the Shaping of America's Public-
Private Welfare State.* Princeton, NJ: Princeton University Press, 2004.

Kline, Wendy. *Building a Better Race: Gender, Sexuality and Eugenics from the
Turn of the Century to the Baby Boom.* Berkeley: University of California
Press, 2001.

Kuznick, Peter. *Beyond the Laboratory: Scientists as Political Activists in 1930s
America.* Chicago: University of Chicago Press, 1987.

Lawson, Gordon S. "The Road Not Taken: The 1945 Health Services Planning
Commission Proposals and Physician Remuneration in Saskatchewan."
In *Making Medicare: New Perspectives on the History of Medicare in
Canada,* edited by Gregory P. Marchildon, 151–82. Toronto: University of
Toronto Press, 2012.

Lebas, Elizabeth. "The Making of a Socialist Arcadia: Arboriculture and
Horticulture in the London Borough of Bermondsey after the Great War."
Garden History 27 (1999): 219–37.

———. "'When Every Street Became a Cinema': The Film Work of Bermondsey Borough Council's Public Health Department, 1923-1953." *History Workshop Journal* 39, 1 (1995): 42–66.

Lepore, Jill. "Historians Who Love Too Much: Reflections on Microhistory and Biography," *The Journal of American History* 88, 1 (June 2001): 129-44.

Levene, Alysa, Martin Powell, and John Stewart. "Patterns of Municipal Health Expenditure in Interwar England and Wales." *Bulletin of the History of Medicine* 78 (2004): 635–39.

———. "The Development of Municipal General Hospitals in English County Boroughs in the 1930s." *Medical History* 50 (2006): 3–28.

Lipset, Seymour Martin. *Agrarian Socialism: The Cooperative Commonwealth in Saskatchewan.* Berkeley: University of Chicago Press, 1950.

Lux, Maureen K. "Perfect Subjects: Race, Tuberculosis and the Qu'Appelle BCG Vaccine Trial." *Canadian Bulletin of Medical History* 15, 2 (1998): 277–95.

———. *Separate Beds: A History of Indian Hospitals in Canada, 1920s-1980s.* Toronto: University of Toronto Press, 2016.

MacDougall, Heather. "Into Thin Air: Making National Health Policy, 1939-1945." In *Making Medicare: New Perspectives on the History of Medicare in Canada,* edited by Gregory P. Marchildon, 41–70. Toronto: University of Toronto Press, 2012.

MacLeod, Wendell, Libbie Park, and Stanley B. Ryerson. *Bethune: The Montreal Years.* Toronto: James Lorimer & Company, 1978.

Madison, Donald L. "Remembering Cecil." In *Cecil G. Sheps Memoral Volume,* edited by Donald L. Madison. Chapel Hill: Cecil G. Sheps Center for Health Services Research, 2005.

Maioni, Antonia. *Parting at the Crossroads: The Development of Health Insurance in Canada and the United States.* Princeton, NJ: Princeton University Press, 1998.

McBain, Lesley. "Caring, Curing and Socialization: The Ambiguities of Nursing in Northern Saskatchewan, 1944-57." In *Caregiving on the Periphery: Historical Perspectives on Nursing and Midwifery in Canada,* edited by Myra Rutherdale, 278-308. Montreal and Kingston: McGill-Queen's University Press, 2010.

McCallum, Mary Jane Logan. *Indigenous Women, Work, and History: 1940-1980.* Winnipeg: University of Manitoba Press, 2000.

McGrane, David. "A Mixed Record: Gender and Saskatchewan Social Democracy." *Journal of Canadian Studies/Revue d'études Canadiennes* 42, 1 (2008): 179–203.

McKay, Ian. "For A New Kind of History: A Reconnaissance of 100 Years of Canadian Socialism." *Labour / Le Travail* 46 (Fall 2000): 69-125.

McKay, Marion. "Region, Faith, and Health: The Development of Winnipeg's
Visiting Nursing Agencies, 1897-1926." In *Place and Practice in Canadian
Nursing History*, edited by Jane Elliott, Meryn Stuart, and Cynthia
Toman, 70-90. Vancouver: University of British Columbia Press, 2008.

McLeod, Thomas H., and Ian McLeod. *Tommy Douglas: The Road to Jerusalem.*
2nd ed. Regina: Fifth House Publishers, 2004.

McWilliams, Roland Fairburn, and Margaret McWilliams. *Russia in 1926.*
London and Toronto: J.M. Dent, 1927.

Medovy, Harry. "The Early Jewish Physicians in Manitoba." In *Jewish Life and
Times: A Collection of Essays*, 23–39. Winnipeg: Jewish Historical Society
of Western Canada, 1983.

Millar, W.P.J. "'We Wanted Our Children Should Have It Better': Jewish
Medical Students at the University of Toronto, 1910-1951." *Journal of the
Canadian Historical Association* 11, 1 (2000): 109–24.

Mombourquette, Duane. "An Inalienable Right: The CCF and Rapid Health
Care Reform, 1944-1948." *Saskatchewan History* 43, 3 (1991): 101–16.

Mott, Frederick Dodge, and Roemer, Milton I. *Rural Health and Medical Care.*
New York: McGraw-Hill, 1948.

Nadeau, Gabriel. "A T.B.'s Progress, the Story of Norman Bethune." *Bulletin of
the History of Medicine*, 8 (1940): 1135–72.

Naylor, David. *Private Practice, Public Payment: Canadian Medicine and the
Politics of Health Insurance, 1911-1966.* McGill-Queen's Press - MQUP, 1986.

Nelson, Alondra. *Body and Soul: The Black Panther Party and the Fight Against
Medical Discrimination.* Minneapolis: University of Minnesota Press, 2013.

Newsholme, Arthur, and John Adams Kingsbury. *Red Medicine: Socialized
Health in Soviet Russia.* Garden City, New York: Doubleday, 1933.

Ostry, Aleck. "Prelude to Medicare: Institutional Change and Continuity in
Saskatchewan, 1944-1962." *Prairie Forum* 20, 1 (1995): 87–105.

Panitch, Leo. "Back to the Future: Contextualizing the Legacy." In *Jewish
Radicalism in Winnipeg, 1905-1960*, edited by Daniel Stone, 10-28.
Winnipeg: Jewish Heritage Centre of Western Canada, 2002.

Patrias, Carmella. "Socialists, Jews and the 1947 Saskatchewan Bill of Rights."
Canadian Historical Review 87, 2 (2006): 1-16.

Pitsula, James M. "The CCF Government in Saskatchewan and Social Aid,
1944-1964." In *"Building the Cooperative Commonwealth": Essays on the
Democratic Socialist Tradition in Canada*, edited by J. William Brennan,
205–25. Regina: Canadian Plains Research Centre, University of Regina,
1984.

Porter, Dorothy. *Health Citizenship: Essays in Social Medicine and Biomedical
Politics.* Berkeley: University of California Medical Humanities Press, 2011.

Powell, Martin. "Socialism and the British National Health Service." *Health
Care Analysis* 5, 3 (1997): 187–94.

Quiring, David M. *CCF Colonialism in Northern Saskatchewan: Battling Parish Priests, Bootleggers, and Fur Sharks*. Vancouver: University of British Columbia Press, 2004.

Reiter, Ester. *A Future Without Hate or Need: The Promise of the Jewish Left in Canada*. Toronto: Between the Lines, 2016.

Revie, Linda. ""More Than Just Boots!": The Eugenic and Commercial Concerns behind A. R. Kaufman's Birth Controlling Activities." *Canadian Bulletin of Medical History* 23, 1 (2006): 119–43.

Rogers, Naomi. "Feminists Fight the Culture of Exclusion in Medical Education, 1970-1990." In *Women Physicians and the Cultures of Medicine*, edited by Ellen S. More, Elizabeth Fee, and Manon Parry, 205-241. Baltimore: Johns Hopkins University Press, 2008.

Ryan, Michael. "Health Centre Policy in England and Wales." *The British Journal of Sociology* 19, 1 (1968): 34–46.

Sangster, Joan. *Dreams of Equality: Women on the Canadian Left, 1920-1950*. Toronto: McClelland and Stewart, 1989.

Sigerist, Henry E. *Socialised Medicine in the Soviet Union*. London: Victor Gollancz, 1937.

Smith, Doug. *Joe Zuken: Citizen and Socialist*. Toronto: James Lorimer & Company, 1990.

Smith, Susan Lynn. *Sick and Tired of Being Sick and Tired: Black Women's Health Activism in America, 1890-1950*. Philadelphia: University of Pennsylvania Press, 1995.

Solomon, Susan Gross. "The Expert and the State in Russian Public Health: Continuities and Changes Across the Revolutionary Divide." In *The History of Public Health and the Modern State*, edited by Dorothy Porter, 183–223. Amsterdam: Rodopi, 1994.

———. "Foreign Expertise on Russian Terrain: Max Kuczynski on the Kirghiz Steppe, 1923-24." In *Soviet Medicine: Culture, Practice, and Science*, edited by Frances L. Bernstein, Christopher Burton, and Dan Healey, 71–91. DeKalb, IL: Northern Illinois University Press, 2010.

———. "Social Hygiene and Soviet Public Health, 1921-1930." In *Health and Society in Revolutionary Russia*, edited by Susan Gross Solomon and John F. Hutchinson, 175-99. Bloomington and Indianapolis: Indiana University Press, 1990.

Srebrnik, Henry. "Birobidzhan on the Prairies: Two Decades of Pro-Soviet Jewish Movements in Winnipeg." In *Jewish Radicalism in Winnipeg, 1905-1960*, edited by Daniel Stone. Winnipeg: Jewish Heritage Centre of Western Canada, 2002.

Starks, Tricia. *The Body Soviet: Propaganda, Hygiene, and the Revolutionary State*. Madison, WI: University of Wisconsin Press, 2008.

Stern, Alexandra Minna. *Eugenic Nation: Faults and Frontiers of Better Breeding in Modern America*. Berkeley: University of California Press, 2005.

Stern, Ludmila. *Western Intellectuals and the Soviet Union, 1920-40: From Red Square to the Left Bank*. London: Routledge, 2007.

Stewart, John. "'For a Healthy London': The Socialist Medical Association and the London County Council in the 1930s." *Medical History* 42 (1997): 417–36.

———. "Socialist Proposals for Health Reform in Inter-War Britain: The Case of Somerville Hastings." *Medical History* 39, 3 (1995): 338–57.

———. *The Battle for Health: A Political History of the Socialist Medical Association, 1930-51*. Aldershot: Ashgate, 1999.

———. "'The Finest Hospital Service in the World?': Contemporary Perceptions of the London County Council's Hospital Provision, 1929-39." *Urban History* 32 (2005): 327–44.

Stewart, Roderick, and Sharon Stewart. *Phoenix: The Life of Norman Bethune*. Montreal and Kingston: McGill-Queen's University Press, 2011.

Stone, Daniel. *Jewish Radicalism in Winnipeg, 1905-1960*. Winnipeg: Jewish Heritage Centre of Western Canada, 2002.

———. "Moving South: The Other Jewish Winnipeg Before the Second World War." *Manitoba History* 76 (2014): 2-9.

Super, Ava Block. "Preserving Winnipeg's Jewish History." *Canadian Jewish Studies* 23 (2015): 138-43.

Tanner, Duncan. "The Politics of the Labour Movement, 1900-1939." In *A Companion to Early Twentieth-Century Britain*, edited by C. Wrigley. Oxford: Blackwell Publishing, 2003.

Taylor, Graham. *Ada Salter: Pioneer of Ethical Socialism*. London: Lawrence and Wishart, 2016.

Taylor, Malcolm. *Health Insurance and Canadian Public Policy: The Seven Decisions That Created the Health Insurance System and Their Outcomes*. McGill-Queen's Press, 1987.

Thane, Pat. "Visions of Gender in the Making of the British Welfare State: The Case of Women in the British Labour Party and Social Policy." In *Maternity and Gender Policies: Women and the Rise of the European Welfare States 1880s-1950s*, edited by Gisela Bock and Thane, 93–118. London: Routledge, 1991.

———. "Women in the British Labour Party and the Construction of State Welfare, 1906-1939." In *Mothers of a New World: Maternalist Politics and the Origins of Welfare States*, edited by Seth Koven and Sonya Michel, 343–77. London: Routledge, 1993.

Thomas, Lewis H., ed. *The Making of a Socialist : The Recollections of T.C. Douglas*. Edmonton: University of Alberta Press, 1984.

Towers, Graham. *Shelter Is Not Enough: Transforming Multi-Storey Housing.* Bristol: The Policy Press, 2000.

Trachtenberg, Henry. "The Winnipeg Jewish Community and Politics: The Inter-War Years, 1919-1939." *Manitoba Historical Society Transactions* Series 3, no. 35 (1978).

Usiskin, Roz. "Winnipeg's Jewish Women of the Left: Traditional and Radical." In *Jewish Radicalism in Winnipeg, 1905-1960*, edited by Daniel Stone, 106-21. Winnipeg: Jewish Heritage Centre of Western Canada, 2002.

Viseltear, Arthur J. "The California Medical-Economic Survey: Paul A. Dodd Versus the California Medical Association." *Bulletin of the History of Medicine* 44, 2 (1970): 141–53.

Waiser, Bill. *Saskatchewan: A New History.* Calgary: Fifth House Publishers, 2005.

Waiser, Bill, and Stuart Houston. *Tommy's Team: The People Behind the Douglas Years.* 1st edition. Markham, ON: Fifth House Publishers, 2010.

Webb, Sydney, and Beatrice Webb. *Soviet Communism: A New Civilization?* New York: C. Scribner's Sons, 1935.

Webster, Charles. "Beveridge after 50 Years." *British Medical Journal* 305, 6859 (October 17, 1992): 901–2.

———. *The Health Services Since the War, Vol. 1.* London: Her Majesty's Stationery Office, 1988.

Weinbren, Dan. "Sociable Capital: London's Labour Parties, 1918-45." In *Labour's Grass Roots: Essays on the Activities of Local Labour Parties and Members, 1918-45*, edited by Matthew Worley, 194–215. Aldershot: Ashgate, 2005.

Weindling, Paul. "Public Health in Germany." In *The History of Public Health and the Modern State*, edited by Dorothy Porter, 119–31. Amsterdam: Rodopi, 1994.

Weissman, Neil B. "Origins of Soviet Health Administration: Narkomzdrav, 1918-1928." In *Health and Society in Revolutionary Russia*, edited by Susan Gross Solomon and John F. Hutchinson, 97–120. Bloomington and Indianapolis: Indiana University Press, 1990.

Williams, Christopher. "The Revolution from above in Soviet Medicine, Leningrad 1928-1932." *Journal of Urban History* 20, 4 (August 1994): 512.

Young, Ken, and Patricia Garside. *Metropolitan London: Politics and Urban Change 1837-1981.* New York: Holmes and Meier Publishers, 1982.

Esyllt W. Jones is the award-winning author or editor of six books, including *Influenza 1918: Disease, Death and Struggle in Winnipeg* (University of Toronto Press, 2007).

Dr. Jones is currently Professor of History at the University of Manitoba and Dean of Studies at St. John's College in Winnipeg. She is a member of the College of Artists, Scholars and Scientists of the Royal Society of Canada.